# LIFESPAN
# PERSPECTIVES
## *on the* FAMILY
## *and* DISABILITY

**JUDY O. BERRY**

*University of Tulsa*

**MICHAEL L. HARDMAN**

*University of Utah*

*Foreword by*

**Eunice Kennedy Shriver**

**Allyn and Bacon**

Boston • London • Toronto • Sydney • Tokyo • Singapore

Series Editor: Ray Short
Editorial Assistant: Christine Svitila
Marketing Manager: Kris Farnsworth
Sr. Editorial Production Administrator: Susan McIntyre
Editorial Production Service: Ruttle, Shaw & Wetherill, Inc.
Composition Buyer: Linda Cox
Manufacturing Buyer: Megan Cochran
Cover Administrator: Suzanne Harbison
Text Design and Electronic Composition: Publishers' Design and Production Service, Inc.

Library of Congress Cataloging-in-Publication Data
Berry, Judy O.
   Lifespan perspectives on the family and disability / Judy O.
Berry, Michael L. Hardman.
     p. cm.
   Includes bibliographical references and index.
   ISBN 0-205-19395-1
   1. Handicapped children—Family relationships. 2. Handicapped children—Care. I. Hardman, Michael L. II. Title.
HQ773.6B477 1997
306.87—dc21
                                       97-16309
                                          CIP

**Photo Credits:** p. 1 © Mary Ellen Leponika, p. 25 © Will Hart, p. 47 © Robert Harbison, p. 71 © Robert Harbison, p. 99 © Robert Harbison, p. 123 © Brian Smith, p. 151 © Robert Harbison, p. 183 © Will Faller, p. 213 © Will Faller, and p. 245 © Will Faller.

Printed in the United States of America

10 9 8 7 6 5 4 3      RRD     04 03 02 01 00

*With love and appreciation for John, Doug, and Ryan, my husband and sons. You guys are the best. (Berry)*

*With love for my mom, Betty, who has always been there for each of her four sons in the best and worst of times. (Hardman)*

# CONTENTS

CHAPTER 10
*Families and the Adult Years*     *245*

Wᴛᴛʜ ᴛʜɪꜱ ʙᴏᴏᴋ, ᴡᴇ ʙʀɪɴɢ ᴏᴜʀ ʀᴇᴀᴅᴇʀꜱ scholarship with a heart. Profession-ally, we teach, consult, publish, and conduct research on issues concerning disability and family. Personally, we receive continuing education from cherished teachers within our own families. As the mother (Berry) and brother (Hardman) of men with developmental disabilities, our personal lifespan journeys enable us to bring to our readers a message that combines scholarly pursuit with personal experience.

Our book is about people with disabilities, their families, and the profession-als who provide the services and support that enhance their lives. We examine how families cope, adapt, and grow through the challenge of living with a child with a disability and how family members nurture and support the child's devel-opmental journey to adulthood. A nested focus of the child within the family and the family within the community is presented in a lifespan framework. When a child has a disability, it affects the parents and other family members as individ-uals, the family as a system, and the parental role. Parents have to move broadly and deeply beyond the family into the community in order to meet the needs of their sons and daughters. In order to do this, parents need information, support from a variety of professional and community resources, and skills that facilitate both coping and empowerment. This book is based on the premise that family members are the most important people in the lives of individuals with disabili-ties, and their only constant.

We represent two different professional backgrounds, psychology (Berry) and special education (Hardman) and appreciate the value and the challenge of interdisciplinary effort. We have designed this book for a variety of professionals, including educators, psychologists, social workers, therapists, and medical per-sonnel. Our intent is to help professionals, both individually and as members of a team, to better understand and support families.

## ORGANIZATION

The first half of the book addresses topics important to understanding families from a historical perspective, supporting them in the present, and preparing them for future challenges. In Chapter 1, the depiction of discrimination and isolation is brightened by the recent impact of family-driven advocacy efforts and the far-reaching results in the development of home/professional partnerships. Chapters 2 and 3 consider the family as an interactive unit in which disability influences all members and the lives they lead. Chapter 4 examines family stress, how family members cope, and ways to support each individual. Chapter 5 addresses the needs of each family member from an ecological perspective that looks broadly at the community and at social policy. Finally, in Chapter 6, effective communication and collaboration with families is addressed for the individual professional and the interdisciplinary team.

Chapters 7–10 address the particular needs and experiences of families at four lifespan phases: infancy and early childhood, the school years, transition from school to adult life, and the adult years. The focus is understanding the particular issues faced by individuals with disabilities and their families at each of these life stages and how to provide effective and appropriate support.

## FEATURES TO ENHANCE LEARNING

Throughout the book, windows provide a forum for individuals with disabilities, parents, siblings, and professionals to provide illustration and meaning to the concepts presented with their "voices from the heart." In addition, we provide focus questions and statements in each chapter to guide understanding and integration of the material. At the end of each chapter, we highlight and summarize these focus areas, providing an in-depth chapter review.

OUR FAMILIES, OUR STUDENTS, and our fellow professionals provided the inspiration for this book and deserve our gratitude. We are thankful as well for our excellent support system at Allyn and Bacon. Special thanks to Ray Short, our editor, and Christine Svitila, editorial assistant, for their knowledgeable guidance throughout this project. We thank our reviewers, Rebecca R. Fewell, University of Miami; Donna E. Dugger Wadsworth, University of Southwestern Louisiana; and Vicki Stayton, Western Kentucky University, whose careful attention to our manuscript allowed us to revise, fine-tune, and improve the quality of our book. We also thank doctoral student Melissa Berry (who provided astute and conscientious attention to detail that helped keep us on track) and Chris Clark, who assisted throughout with editing and permissions. Finally, we are grateful we had the opportunity to work together. We come from different backgrounds, but share a professional philosophy and personal commitment of caring and optimism toward people with disabilities and their families.

I AM PLEASED TO HAVE A PART in introducing to you this new book, *Lifespan Perspectives on the Family and Disability*. Through my thirty years in the Special Olympics movement and as the executive vice president of the Joseph P. Kennedy, Jr. Foundation, I have had the opportunity to meet thousands of people with mental retardation, and their family members. I have often listened to parents talk of their struggles in finding needed services for their child, the challenges of communicating their hopes and dreams to professionals, and the triumphs of having their child succeed—whether it be successfully completing a school assignment or as a Special Olympics athlete on the field of competition. Through it all, I have gained a genuine love and respect for each and every one of these exceptional families.

This book is about the lives of exceptional families—parents, grandparents, and siblings of children and adults with disabilities. It is about families that have emerged through years of discrimination and isolation into a new era of social reform and community participation. Institutions are closing all over this country while family support, community and school programs continue to grow. As a society, we now provide more family assistance than ever before in our history. People with disabilities now have opportunities that only a few years ago seemed out of reach, such as access to schooling, employment, and community living. One example of these expanding opportunities has been in education. Our public schools now serve more than 5 million children with disabilities from ages 3 through 21 years. Access to special education has opened new life experiences for these children, better preparing them to live as more independent adults.

Today, parents of children with disabilities have the right to participate with professionals in planning and implementing services for their child in areas such as education and social services. Research suggests that the professional and parent partnership is a critical factor not only in helping the child with a disability grow and learn, but also as a means to solidify the family's ability to function as a unit.

Yet, although much has been accomplished in supporting families who have a child with a disability, more remains to be done. That is why this book is so important. It addresses many of the complex issues that affect the family on a continual basis and throughout the life of the individual with a disability. The intended audience for this book is you, the *prospective professional*, who will someday have the responsibility of working directly with parents in their never-ending endeavors to help build a quality life for their child.

It is also important for you to know that the authors of *Lifespan Perspectives on the Family and Disability* bring both a professional and personal perspective to their writing. Dr. Judy Berry is a psychologist and a mother of a young man with multiple disabilities. Dr. Michael Hardman is an educator and a brother of a man with mental retardation and epilepsy. Both Dr. Berry and Dr. Hardman have experienced life on both sides of the curtain, seeing professionals from the standpoint of the family and seeing the family from the eyes of professionals.

Professionals charged with the responsibility of providing services for individuals with disabilities, whether they be special educators, nurses, psychologists, physicians, or social workers, are faced with some difficult challenges. They must first and foremost respond to the individual needs of each child or adult with a disability. Second, they must always view the individual as a part of a diverse family unit. Finally, they must find ways to go beyond individual needs and support family members as they attempt to be a part of the neighborhood and community in which they live. This book helps to make the challenges facing the newly prepared professional just a little easier. The voices of real people, heard throughout this book, bring meaning to the often impersonal research that supports the importance of building partnerships between families and professionals. It is my hope that you find this book a helpful resource in your quest to better the lives of people with disabilities and the family members who love and support them.

Eunice Kennedy Shriver
April 1997

# CHAPTER ONE

# Disability and the Family through Time

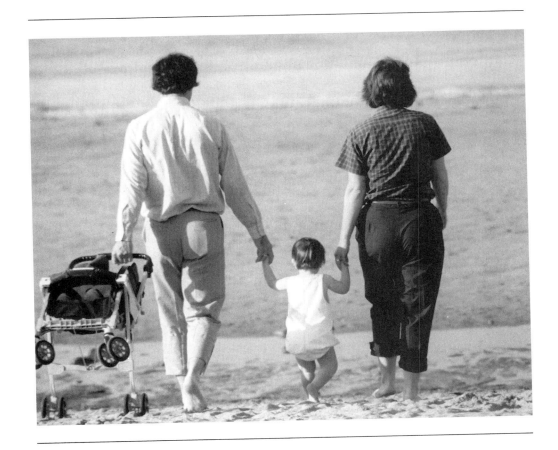

---

★ **WINDOW 1.1**

---

## *But I Wanted to Go to Italy!*

Whenever you're going to have a baby, it's like you're planning a vacation to Italy. You are all excited. Seeing the Coliseum . . . the Michelangelo . . . the gondolas of Venice. You get a whole bunch of guidebooks. You learn a few phrases in Italian so you can order in restaurants and get around. When it comes time, you excitedly pack your bags, head for the airport, and take off for Italy . . . only when you land, the stewardess announces "Welcome to Holland."

You look at one another in disbelief and shock saying, "Holland? What are you talking about—Holland? I signed up for Italy!" But they explain that there's been a change of plans and the plane has landed in Holland—and there you must stay.

"But I don't know anything about Holland! I don't want to stay here," you say. "I never wanted to come to Holland!" "I don't know what to do in Holland and I don't want to learn!" But you do stay. You go out and buy some new guidebooks. You learn some new phrases in a whole new language and you meet people you never knew existed.

But the important thing is that you are not in a filthy, plague-infested slum full of pestilence and famine. You are simply in another place, a different place than you had planned. It's slower paced than Italy; less flashy than Italy; but after you've been there a little while and have had a chance to catch your breath, you begin to discover that Holland has windmills . . . Holland has tulips . . . Holland even has Rembrandts.

But everyone else you know is busy coming and going from Italy. And they're all bragging about what a great time they had there. And for the rest of your life you will say, "Yes, that's where I was going, that's where I was supposed to go, that's what I had planned." And the pain of that will never ever go away.

**And you have to accept that pain because the loss of that dream, the loss of that plan is a very significant loss. But if you spend your life mourning the fact that you didn't get to Italy, you will never be free to enjoy the very special, the very lovely things about Holland.**

*Source:* Copyright © 1990 by the American Association on Mental Retardation.

---

This book is about people—individuals with disabilities, their families, the professionals who provide care, education, and support, as well as the communities that guide their lives. Each child brings a unique set of mental, physical, and behavioral characteristics into the world. Far from the isolation of the womb, the newborn child is immediately thrust into a system that is the oldest and most enduring of all human institutions: the family. From the very beginning of life, child and family interact continually as they attempt to create a balance between individual needs and the dynamics of the group. The family becomes the reference point through which children gain a sense of who they are and how they will learn and cope with the expanded life space of community and society. At the same time, the child becomes one lens through which family members see the world, a lens through which relationships both within and external to its members are shaped. Parental perceptions of their children may range from sheer joy, in which they see their offspring as an extension of themselves, to the view that a child is an expensive, emotionally draining inconvenience dramatically hampering their lifestyle. Siblings may see each other as mirror images, competitors for attention, or sources of pride or embarrassment.

The family system is extremely complex and demanding, oftentimes rewarding, sometimes dysfunctional, and constantly in flux. It becomes even more complicated with the advent of a child with a disability. As the metaphor in Window 1.1 so aptly describes, family members may find themselves feeling like the misguided traveler, saying "What are you talking about—Holland? I signed up for Italy!" Well, in this book, we are going to Holland. The purpose of our journey is to gain a better understanding of people with disabilities and their families as they live, love, and learn from birth through the adult years. We examine how families cope, adapt, and grow through the challenges of living with a child with a disability. These challenges include working directly with professionals from many fields as well as the supports and services intended to help the person with a disability gain access to the opportunities needed for a more independent and fulfilling life.

We begin with an examination of people with disabilities and their families through time. Our discussion focuses on how families have struggled, survived, sometimes even thrived, and at the very least significantly changed through three periods of civilization: early history, the industrial age, and today's information age.

## THREE WAVES OF SOCIAL CHANGE

⊞ **FOCUS 1**

*Identify three waves of change that have redefined the meaning of civilization over time.*

One constant for the human race is that we change, undergo social upheaval, and continually redefine the meaning of civilization. Toffler and Toffler (1995) describe three great waves of social change, "each one largely obliterating earlier cultures or civilizations and replacing them with a way of life inconceivable to those who came before" (p. 19). These authors describe the first wave as the agricultural revolution, beginning in about 8000 B.C., when people cultivated and lived off the land. The second wave was the rise of industrialization that began in the mid-seventeenth century and was characterized by the building of factories, mills, and plants; the manufacturing of products; and blue-collar assembly line workers. Toffler and Toffler suggest that industrialization still plays a major role in today's society as we move toward the twenty-first century. Industrialization peaked in

Three Waves of Social Change

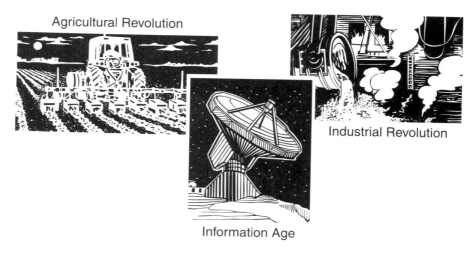

Agricultural Revolution

Industrial Revolution

Information Age

the years following World War II, and a third wave of change, "the information-age society," took root in the 1950s and is cresting as the year 2000 nears. We must cope with the impact of high technology on the way we do our jobs and how we structure our economy, political philosophy, and family lifestyle.

In the next two sections, we take a brief look at the societal roles for people with disabilities and their families during early history (the agricultural revolution) and during the industrial age. In the final section, we examine how the information age is affecting families and what its impact may be on the lives of people with disabilities in the twenty-first century.

## EARLY HISTORY: SURVIVAL OF THE FITTEST

*As to the exposure and rearing of children, let there be a law that no deformed child shall live . . .*

*Aristotle*

### ⊕ FOCUS 2

*Why is early history often described in terms of "survival of the fittest"?*

Although Aristotle's stark statement on the killing of deformed children in the fourth century B.C. is inconceivable in today's world, it describes the views once held by many civilizations. From the beginning of recorded history until well into the eighteenth and nineteenth centuries, children, many of whom had disabilities, were vulnerable to such practices as infanticide, slavery, physical abuse, and abandonment (Hewett & Forness, 1984). Early civilizations were patriarchies in which fathers had the absolute right to make life-and-death decisions regarding their children. Mentally and physically capable male children were highly prized, whereas the birth of a daughter or a deformed male child could bring shame upon the family. Weir (1984) suggested that infanticide was common practice for centuries in many early civilizations. The killing of firstborn children was widely viewed by ancient Hebrews as a sacrifice that signified religious obedience. Other civilizations accepted infanticide as a necessary means of controlling population growth and ensuring that only the strongest would survive in societies highly dependent on agriculture.

Early Greek and Roman patriarchies also openly practiced selected eugenics. Eugenics is the science of improving the human race through the careful selection of parents and the improvement of offspring. History records widespread practices in which fathers of deformed children would throw their offspring off mountain cliffs, sell them into slavery, or abandon them to professional beggars who would maim their bodies and then use them to "solicit alms from a charitable passerby" (Barclay, cited in Hewett and Forness, 1984, p. 4).

There were some notable exceptions to the barbarism that marked this early period. The ancient Egyptians viewed infanticide as a crime (Durant, 1966). Ancient China was concerned with the plight of persons with mental illness and revered those who were blind and exhibited unique talents as storytellers, musicians, and scholars (Kirtley, 1975). But for many early civilizations, deformed children represented weakness, shame, and an unnecessary burden on the family and society.

Threats to a deformed child's very survival continued into the Middle Ages, although this period was characterized by some humanitarian reform that resulted in better care for people with physical afflictions, retardation, sensory loss, or emotional disturbance. However, in many societies, superstitious beliefs still flourished, and the prevailing belief was that "mental afflictions" were the direct result of divine intervention. The question was whether it was a good or an evil spirit that had invaded the person's body. People possessed by so-called good spirits were admired and respected as soothsayers, magicians, and prophets. However, if a person's diminished cognitive capacity or psychological disturbance was considered a possession by an evil spirit, the individual was thought to have made a pact with the devil. Feeblemindedness (retardation) or "deranged behavior" was then viewed as a result of divine punishment. Demons were believed to be residing in these deformed creatures and therefore needed to be exorcized or the person destroyed. Early treatment techniques included "trephining" (drilling holes in the skull to force out the evil spirits).

As the industrial age approached and knowledge of medicine expanded, these superstitious beliefs were challenged by some professionals who saw mental and psychological abnormalities as physical diseases. A person with diminished mental capacity or exhibiting abnormal behavior was considered ill, thus the origin of the term *mental illness*. A person with mental illness became a patient in need of medical treatment.

## THE INDUSTRIAL REVOLUTION AND HUMANITARIAN REFORM

### *The Early Reformers*

⊕ **FOCUS 3**

*Identify the contributions of the eighteenth- and nineteenth-century reformers to our understanding of people with disabilities and their families.*

As many civilizations were making the transition from an agrarian- to an industry-based economy, two contrasting beliefs about people with disabilities emerged. From one perspective, people with disabilities were seen as potential contributors to the economic growth of a community. Others, however, saw people with disabilities as useless burdens on society. Those who were deaf or blind had the potential to make contributions to society because their intellect and physical abilities were essentially intact. However, deafness could also be associated with inferior intelligence because some people with hearing loss were not able to express themselves through speech. This belief resulted in the emergence of the term *deaf and dumb*. Although many people with physical disabilities ("cripples" as they were often referred to during this time) were of less value because they could not labor in the fields, others with physical limitations were recognized for their intellectual contributions. However, people described as idiots or insane were deemed hopeless, and any attempt at education or rehabilitation was viewed as fruitless. Using terminology from the emerging medical model, most physicians of the eighteenth century described idiots and the mentally ill as "incurable."

The nineteenth century ushered in the first sustained efforts at humanitarian reform. Among the early reformers were Philippe Pinel (1742–1826) and John Locke (1632–1704), both of whom revolutionized society's perception of deviance from the demonological and superstitious beliefs of the Middle Ages to an understanding of the person as physically and mentally sick. Locke attempted to distinguish idiocy from insanity; Pinel advocated that people who were insane or idiots should be treated humanely. However, Pinel emphasized that such individuals were essentially incurable, and Locke described the mind as a blank slate with potential for new learning. The polar positions of Pinel and Locke represent the classic nature versus nurture controversy that continues today: What roles do heredity and environment play in determining the abilities of an individual?

Jean-Marc Itard (1775–1838), a protégé of Pinel and a young physician specializing in diseases of the ear and education of the deaf, became very interested in the contrasting views of Locke and Pinel. As a product of the French Revolution, Itard espoused the belief that every human being has value and dignity and deserves a chance to rise above the squalor of family poverty and the lack of opportunity to learn and grow. In 1801, Itard had the chance to test his theory that every child can learn when he encountered Victor, the so-called wild boy of Aveyron.

> Victor was 12 years old when found in the woods by hunters. He had not developed any language, and his behavior was virtually uncontrollable, described as savage or animal like. Ignoring . . . the diagnosis that the child was an incurable idiot, Itard took responsibility for Victor and put him through a program of sensory stimulation that was intended to cure his condition. After five years, Victor developed some verbal language and became more socialized as he grew accustomed to his new environment. Itard's work with Victor documented for the first time that learning is possible even for individuals described as . . . totally helpless. (Hardman, Drew, & Egan, 1996, p. 19)

The work of Itard and others provided hope for families and professionals that treatment and education could make a difference. The first schools and specialized facilities were established in western Europe in the early 1800s. Itard mentored Edouard Séguin, who began the first French school for training the feebleminded. Séguin emigrated to the United States in 1850 and was instrumental in establishing early schools and residential facilities for people with mental retardation. Other reformers, such as Anne Sullivan, who worked with Helen Keller, and Benjamin Rush (the father of American psychiatry), focused attention on the potential of people with disabilities to learn and to become contributors to society.

Unfortunately, hope eventually turned to despair for many people with disabilities and their families. The success of the early reformers in demonstrating that people with disabilities had the potential to learn was tempered by the realities of the industrial age. People with disabilities were not being cured of their afflictions, and the public began to wonder whether they would forever be hopelessly dependent on society.

## Families and Industrialization

### ⊞   FOCUS 4

*What was the impact of the industrial age on people with disabilities and their families?*

> They [idiots] are unable in all cases to take care of themselves, though many are capable of performing some labor, often sufficient to pay the expenses of their maintenance. Nearly all who have the use of their limbs are capable of

learning something useful, or of establishing habits of cleanliness and order; many can learn to read, to write, to sing, to enjoy a limited knowledge and be taught to labor advantageously. . . . [However] many of this class are suffered to grow up mere animals, to be a burden and affliction to their friends, or a public charge. (State of New York Committee on Medical Societies and Colleges, 1846, cited in Blatt, 1973, p. 328)

Whereas early civilizations were characterized by their dependency on the land and survival of the fittest, the industrial age began to flourish in the late eighteenth century, ushering in an era of factories, mass production, and the use of "less valued" people as cheap, unskilled labor. Toffler and Toffler (1995) suggest that "masses of peasants were forced off the land to provide workers for the new . . . mills and factories that multiplied over the landscape" (p. 28). The need for unskilled laborers forced many children from impoverished homes into the factories where they worked for long hours with little pay and no protection from physical and mental abuse.

For people with disabilities and their families, the industrial age was an era in which wealthy industrialists determined the value of the less fortunate on the basis of their ability to work. Families changed from households in which many generations lived together in order to work the land to small nuclear units expected to labor in the factories and be self-sufficient. Knoblock (1987) suggested that during this period, "Disability became an economic category . . . that applied more to the whole family rather than to a specific child. . . . Disability was a subcategory of poverty" (p. 348). If families with children who were disabled could not work or take care of themselves without help from the outside, they were considered a social liability.

There was a concerted attempt to keep these families-in-need together. Relatives and friends were expected to pitch in and provide direct financial assistance. In some cases, families and their children with disabilities were either forced to leave the community or to live together in poorhouses with little provisions or other means of support from society. For many families, the hardships and discrimination they faced only strengthened their resolve, and they bonded together more than ever. For others, the burden of a child with a disability became too great, and they abused their children or abandoned them to the streets.

## Families and the Eugenics Scare

As the twentieth century began, people with disabilities and their families faced some marked contradictions in government support. On the one hand, treatment and education that had been denied for centuries were becoming more accessible. More and more schools were offering special classes for slow learners, children with physical disabilities, and those who were deaf and blind. On the other hand, the societal view of these families was becoming increasingly more negative and accusatory. Parents were blamed for the genetic inferiority of their children and held responsible for not being able to take care of their needs without additional government support. The fear grew that many disabilities were passed on from generation to generation and that eventually these so-called defectives would defile the human race.

> We must come to recognize feeblemindedness, idiocy, imbecility and insanity as largely communicable conditions or diseases, just as the physician recognizes smallpox, diphtheria, etc. as communicable. (Sprattling, 1912; cited in Wolfensberger, 1975)

In the United States, the initial response to the eugenics scare was the passage of laws in many states that prohibited "mental and moral defectives" from marrying. Eventually the legislation was expanded to include sterilization. Some state lawmakers were so concerned about genetic inferiority and social deviance that they extended sterilization beyond the feebleminded and insane to people with epilepsy, the sexually promiscuous, and convicted felons. In Nazi Germany, the eugenics scare came full circle from early Greek and Roman history to reach its pinnacle in 1939 with the planned extermination of the "mentally and physically disabled" under what was referred to as Operation T4. People with disabilities were openly targeted by Adolf Hitler for the "final solution." The German government actively terminated the lives of people with disabilities as a means to "purify" the human race and put these "wretched" individuals out of their misery.

But in most other countries, the eugenics scare of the early twentieth century evolved from marriage and sterilization laws to planned social isolation rather than to extermination. The earlier emphasis in the United States on keeping families together at all costs changed to a perspective that advocated removing the child with disabilities from the family into a controlled, large congregate living facility, which was believed to be in the best interests of society, the family, and the child. Such isolation would prevent the further spread of genetic and social deviance as well as protect society from the defective person.

Large congregate living facilities for deviant populations were subsumed under many different labels, such as institution, hospital, colony, prison, school, or asylum. In some cases, the initial purpose for segregated facilities was to rehabilitate the person so he or she could return to society; however, most focused on custodial care in an isolated environment. The move away from therapy to custodial care increased over a period of fifty years as these congregate care facilities grew in size and financial resources did not keep pace. U.S. institutions continued to grow, and by the 1920s every state had a mental hospital, and the numbers of large, isolated institutions for persons with mental retardation were multiplying rapidly. Families faced the dilemma of either keeping the child at home, often with no medical, educational, or social supports, or giving the child over to professionals for 24-hour care where he or she could be with others of "their own kind." This situation remained virtually unchanged for nearly five decades and declined even further during the depression years of the 1930s and 1940s, when funds and human resources were in short supply. By the 1950s, more than 500,000 persons had been committed to mental hospitals in the United States. Comparable numbers were placed in institutions for persons with mental retardation.

### Education as a Privilege, Not a Right

⊞     **FOCUS 5**

*Why were many children with disabilities excluded from public education throughout most of the twentieth century?*

In spite of the growth of hospitals and segregated institutions well into the 1950s, most people with disabilities remained at home within their families. For the most part, families that made the choice to keep the child at home were on their own with little or no outside support. As suggested by Bradley, Knoll, and Agosta (1992), government resources were directed at support that was outside of the family, often even beyond the community in which they resided. Many families that had a child with a disability were unable to get help for basic needs such as medical and dental care, social services, or education.

Throughout most of the twentieth century, public education for children with disabilities in the United States was considered a privilege, not a right. The public schools of the early 1900s were ill prepared for any nontraditional learners. Fewer than 10 percent of all children graduated from high school. The emphasis in education was on learning the basics and then leaving school to work in the expanding number of factories, to return to labor the land, or to go on for further education at a college or university. Educating children with disabilities was not a priority. In fact, educators were seeking ways to determine who would benefit from an education and who should be excluded on the basis of ability. This resulted in the use of an intelligence test first developed in 1905 by Alfred Binet and Theodore Simon in France. The test was translated into English in 1908 and became known as the Stanford-Binet Intelligence test. It provided a way to identify children who deviated significantly from the average in intellectual capability and thus were not good candidates for a public education (Hardman et al., 1996).

From the 1920s into the 1960s, public school programs for children with disabilities were *allowed* in some states, but not required. Local schools could choose who would and would not be served. Decisions were based on whether the child fit the existing program, not whether the program could be adapted to the child.

When special education programs were available in a local area, most often they were held in separate classes for children with mild learning problems and those with hearing and vision loss. Special classes for children with physical disabilities gained momentum in the 1930s with separate schools becoming a primary service model in the 1950s. Most professionals believed that these schools were best for children with physical disabilities because they could be specially equipped with elevators, ramps, and modified doors, toilets, and desks.

The 1950s saw an increase in the number of public school special classes for children with mild mental retardation and emotional disturbance. However, these classes were offered at the discretion of the local school district, and children could be excluded if they did not fit the existing program. This practice continued throughout the United States until the 1970s.

## Parents as Reformers and Advocates for Their Children

### ⊞   FOCUS 6

*Identify the roles parents played in the reform of social and educational programs for people with disabilities in the mid-twentieth century.*

Throughout the twentieth century, people with disabilities and their families have struggled with a society that in the best of times was apathetic to their needs and in the worst of times was clearly discriminatory (see Window 1.2 on page 12). Parents were often identified as the source of their child's problems. The eugenics movement characterized parents as the cause of their child's disability because of genetic inferiority that was passed on from one generation to the next. Other societal perspectives focused on the fact that many children with disabilities came from an impoverished environment. The problems of these children were thought to have resulted directly from parents subjecting them to destitution and squalor. Some professional views held that the child's disability was the result of poor parenting. Parents of children with disabilities were described as totally inadequate in the practice of child rearing. Bettelheim (1950) described mothers of children with autism as the source of their child's condition because they were cold and unresponsive to the child's needs. He characterized these parents as "refrigerator mothers."

Another factor contributing to apathy and discrimination in both social and educational services for people with disabilities was that, in spite of the efforts of the reformers of the eighteenth and nineteenth centuries, these individuals could not be cured in the traditional sense. As such, why should society invest limited funds into a population that would never be able to contribute but would always consume resources? At best, all that could be done was to care for and manage people with disabilities, not teach or treat them.

---

✯ **WINDOW 1.2**

---

## *Advocating for Chris*

ACCORDING TO THE DICTIONARY, an advocate is one who pleads the cause of another. Without realizing exactly what had taken place through the years, I had become Chris's advocate, a role I will need to fill for the rest of my life.

As a parent, I was prepared for certain duties and obligations inherent in caring for children: speaking for them when they're too young to do so for themselves; intervening in situations that they can't handle; supporting them until they're ready to leave home. But the advocacy role I had grown into was almost a public function. I would have to interact across a broad spectrum of organizations and individuals for Chris. Parenting had a new slant. It was as if I didn't have a choice; Chris's situation required it of me. Advocating for Chris was very different from advocating for our other children, whose basic human rights were rarely, if ever, in question. With Chris's situation, I had to be vigilant to see that his rights were not overlooked, that he would receive services to which he was entitled, and that he was treated fairly and with equity.

I found definite disparities between how special-needs students and regular students were treated. For instance, I never had to advocate for the right of the other children to be taught to read, but I had to press to make sure Chris had that same opportunity. Students without disabilities are given a choice about which vocational areas to study; students with disabilities may be tested, but the courses they are offered are not so much a reflection of what they need but of what the school offers. The criteria are not always fair to the student. In one situation, Chris was said to be not suitable for a vocational program because he hadn't learned the skill of getting his lunch alone and reporting to another building on time. However, no one even considered teaching him those skills so that he could get to the training program on time. As a result, he was eliminated from the program.

Advocacy for children with special needs doesn't end when children are no longer in school. It will continue throughout their lifetimes as they need housing, jobs, recreation, medical and dental care, and other services. When the parents are no longer alive or able to be advocates, others, whether family members or agency workers, will have to take up the role.

*Source:* Taken from *Parenting a Child With Special Needs* by Rosemary S. Cook. Copyright © 1992 by Rosemary S. Cook. Used by permission of Zondervan Publishing House.

---

Although many organizations for persons with disabilities had been in existence since the early twentieth century (such as the National Association for the Deaf, the American Association on Mental Deficiency,[1] and the American Federation for the Blind), there was a major surge in parent associations in the 1950s and 1960s. In response to the apathy and discrimination that permeated their lives, new parent groups advocating for the rights of children with disabilities began to organize on a national level around 1950. The United Cerebral Palsy

---

[1]Now the American Association on Mental Retardation.

Organization (UCP) was founded in 1949, and the National Association for Retarded Children[2] (NARC) began in 1950. These organizations had similar goals. Both were concerned about educating the public regarding the people they represented; both wanted to ensure the rights of full citizenship for people with disabilities through access to medical treatment, social services, and education. Other parent groups followed the lead of these two landmark organizations, including the National Society for Autistic Children (1961) and the Association for Children with Learning Disabilities[3] (1964).

The advent of parent organizations as advocates for people with disabilities coincided with the civil rights movement in the 1950s. As courts throughout the country reaffirmed the civil rights of ethnic minorities, parent organizations seized the opportunity to lay a foundation for a stronger federal and state role in meeting the needs of individuals with disabilities. In 1956, only two years after the landmark U.S. Supreme Court decision in *Brown* v. *Board of Education of Topeka* declared that separate education for people of color was inherently unequal, NARC presented a call to action for the federal government to expand teaching and research in the education of children with mental retardation. Other parent and professional organizations followed suit. By 1960 the Congress and state legislatures were actively engaged with both parents and professionals concerned with improving the lives of people with disabilities.

These organizations received a major boost in 1961 with the election of John F. Kennedy. President Kennedy, through the strong encouragement of his sister Eunice Kennedy Shriver and out of a strong family commitment to his sister Rosemary (who was mentally retarded), elevated the needs of people with disabilities to a major national concern. The President's Committee on Mental Retardation and legislation that eventually resulted in the establishment of the Bureau of Education for the Handicapped in the U.S. Office of Education were among his many federal initiatives for people with disabilities. Kennedy was also a strong advocate for institutional reform.

> We as a Nation have long neglected the mentally ill and mentally retarded. This neglect must end. . . . We must act . . . to stimulate improvements in the level of care given the mentally disabled in our State and private institutions, and to reorient those programs to a community centered approach. (President John F. Kennedy, October 31, 1963)

Spurred on by an emerging federal role in services for people with disabilities and the expanding U.S. civil rights movement, parents moved to the courts as a

---

[2]The National Association for Retarded Children became the Association for Retarded Citizens in 1974. It is now known as ARC—A National Organization on Mental Retardation.

[3]The Association for Children with Learning Disabilities is now known as the Learning Disabilities Association (LDA).

means to fight discrimination in social and educational services. In a 1972 case *Wyatt* v. *Stickney*, parents of institutionalized persons in the state of Alabama filed suit, claiming that people with mental retardation who were institutionalized in Bryce Hospital were being deprived of their right to individual treatment that would give them a realistic opportunity for habilitation. The court described the institution as a human warehouse steeped in an atmosphere of psychological and physical deprivation. The state was ordered to ensure that people residing in the institution had a therapeutic environment. The *Wyatt* case led to the development of federal standards for institutions across the country that mandated specific rights for persons with disabilities, including privacy, management of their own affairs, freedom from physical restraint and isolation, and an adequate medical program. The *Wyatt* case was followed by other landmark decisions on institutional reform, such as *Halderman* v. *Pennhurst State School and Hospital, Youngberg* v. *Romeo*, and *Homeward Bound* v. *Hissom Memorial Center*. In the case of *Homeward Bound* v. *Hissom Memorial Center* (1988), a U.S. district judge ruled that people with mental retardation residing at an Oklahoma institution had been denied opportunities for a quality life. The state of Oklahoma was directed to close the institution and create community alternatives for supported living, employment, education, medical needs, and social services. Hissom closed its doors in 1994.

Parents were equally active in their efforts to reform the education system. In 1971, parents from the Pennsylvania Association for Retarded Citizens (PARC) filed a class-action suit (*PARC* v. *The Commonwealth of Pennsylvania*) claiming their children were being denied the right to a free and appropriate public education on the basis of mental retardation. The court ordered Pennsylvania schools to provide a free public education to all children with mental retardation between the ages of 6 and 21. Later that same year, the Pennsylvania decision was expanded to include all children with disabilities in the case of *Mills* v. *District of Columbia Board of Education*. *PARC* and *Mills* were catalysts for several court cases and legislation in the years that followed, culminating in the passage of federal legislation in 1975 mandating a free and appropriate public education for all students with disabilities. The passage of Public Law 94-142[4] brought together all of the various pieces of state and federal legislation into a national law requiring parent involvement in the education of their children, multidisciplinary and non-discriminatory testing, education in the least restrictive environment, and the development of an individualized education plan for every student (see Chapter 8).

The culmination of parent and professional advocacy on behalf of 43 million persons with disabilities in the United States was the passage of the Americans with Disabilities Act (ADA). ADA was initiated and developed by the National Council on Disability in 1988. This fifteen-person council, many of whom were parents of children with disabilities, proposed the law as a means to combat dis-

---

[4]Public Law 94-142, the Education for All Handicapped Children's Act, was renamed the Individuals with Disabilities Education Act (IDEA) in 1990.

crimination against people with disabilities in all sectors of society and every aspect of daily living (West, 1991).

Hailed as the most sweeping civil rights legislation since the passage of the Civil Rights Act of 1964, ADA provided a national mandate to end discrimination against individuals with disabilities in private sector employment, all public services, and public accommodations, transportation, and telecommunications. As suggested by Hardman et al. (1996), "much as the Civil Rights Act of 1964 gave clout to the African American struggle for equality, the ADA has promised to do the same for those with disabilities. Its success in eliminating the fear and prejudices of the . . . community remains to be seen" (p. 14) (see Chapter 10).

## INTO THE TWENTY-FIRST CENTURY: FAMILY SUPPORT AND THE INFORMATION AGE

### ⊞   FOCUS 7

*How have families changed over the past one hundred years? What has been the impact of this change on families who are raising a child with a disability?*

> [The information age] . . . brings with it a genuinely new way of life based on diversified, renewable energy sources; on methods of production that make most factory assembly lines obsolete; *new non-nuclear families*; on a novel institution that might be called the "electronic cottage," and on radically changed schools and corporations for the future. (Toffler & Toffler, 1995, p. 20)

As we move headlong into the information age of the twenty-first century, the dramatic changes in society over the past one hundred years and their impact on people with disabilities and their families become clear.

- Six times as many people now graduate from high school.
- Agricultural jobs have declined by about 300 percent; jobs in wholesale, retail, finance, and service industries have increased tenfold.
- Expectations for postsecondary education have increased dramatically; ten times as many people complete four or more years of college.
- The mortality rate for children ages 1 through 4 is one hundred times lower; today two out of every three children born with a severe disability will be alive at age 21.
- Overall life expectancy has increased from 47 to 76 years of age (see Point of Interest 1.1 on page 16).

Only forty years ago, the majority of families consisted of a working father, a mother who stayed at home, and about two school-age children. The family

◆ **POINT OF INTEREST 1.1**

*A U.S. Profile: Then and Now*

| *THEN (The Industrial Age)* | *NOW (The Information Age)* |
|---|---|
| Population in 1900: 76 million | Population in 1995: 262.6 million |
| Average household size in 1900: 4.76 persons | Average household size in 1995: 2.67 persons |
| Infant mortality rate in 1915: 99.9 babies died per 1,000 births | Infant mortality rates in 1993: 8.3 babies died per 1,000 births |
| Leading causes of death in 1900 (in order): pneumonia and influenza, tuberculosis, intestinal ulcers, heart disease, strokes, kidney disease, all accidents, cancer, senility, diphtheria | Leading causes of death in 1993 (in order): heart disease, cancer, stroke, lung disease, accidents, pneumonia and influenza, diabetes, HIV, suicide, homicide |
| Mortality rate for children ages 1–4 who died in 1900: 4.350 per 100,000 | Mortality rate for children ages 1–4 who died in 1992: 43.6 per 100,000 |
| Number of agricultural workers in 1900: 9.7 million | Number of agricultural workers in 1993: 3.1 million |
| Number of manufacturing workers in 1900: 6.1 million | Number of manufacturing workers in 1993: 19.6 million |
| Number in wholesale, retail, and finance industries in 1900: 3.2 million | Number in wholesale, retail, and finance industries in 1993: 32.7 million |
| Number in service industries in 1900: 3.9 million | Number in service industries in 1993: 41.8 million |
| Americans who could not read or write a simple message in any language in 1900: 10.7% | Americans who could not read or write a simple message in any language in 1993: 21% |
| Those 25 years of age or older who had four years of high school in 1910: 13.5% | Those 25 years of age or older who had four years of high school in 1993: 81.5% |
| Those 25 or older with four or more years of college in 1910: 2.7% | Those 25 or older with four or more years of college in 1993: 21.9% |

*Source:* Copyright © 1995 by *U.S. News and World Report.*

was traditionally defined as a group of individuals, all of whom were bonded biologically, living under one roof with a father and a mother. This model is no longer the case in the 1990s. The family has become a diverse organizational unit with many different constellations. Jaynes and Williams (1989) delineated demographic changes occurring over the past three decades for American families.

These changes include lower rates of marriage, later ages at first marriage, higher divorce rates, lower birthrates, a higher proportion of births to unmarried mothers, an increase in mothers who are employed outside the home, a higher percentage of children living in poverty, and an increase in female-headed households. For example, about 25 percent of all children are living in single-parent families with the mother as the head of the household in 90 percent of the cases. More than half of all children will experience living in a single-parent household at some time before the age of 18. Almost 50 percent of all American children living in a family whose head is a person 25 years of age or younger are poor. One-third of all children living in a family whose head is a person 30 years of age or younger are poor. About 25 percent of all homeless persons in the United States are children. Families with children are the fastest growing segment of the homeless population (National Association of State Directors, 1991).

The family, now more divergent and under considerable stress in the 1990s, faces even greater challenges raising a child with a disability. These challenges may result in two very different outcomes. As suggested by Shelton, Jeppson, and Johnson (1987), the birth of a child with a disability may throw the family into further crisis, weakening emotional bonds and imposing serious financial problems. However, in spite of the considerable pressure on today's families, many are resilient in the face of adversity. The effect of raising a child with a disability can actually unify some family units by strengthening bonds and building stronger relationships (Hardman et al., 1996). Whether the challenges of raising a child with a disability in the twenty-first century result in a unification or further dissolution of the family will depend on internal factors as well as the societal supports available to its members (McDonnell et al., 1995).

## *Reforms of the Twentieth Century and Their Impact on Families*

### ⊞ FOCUS 8

*How have the reforms of the past three decades changed the lives of people with disabilities and their families?*

The evolution of family support has come full circle from the early history of infanticide, the emphasis on keeping families-in-need together at all costs during the industrial revolution, a return to selective eugenics and social isolation in the first half of the twentieth century, and finally an era of rights and family support as we move toward the twenty-first century. The legal and humanitarian reforms of the past three decades have made significant changes in the lives of people with disabilities and their families.

In community services, federal and state support for residential living is being redirected from isolated large, congregate care settings to small, community-based residences located within local neighborhoods. The large institutions (such as the Hissom Memorial Center in Oklahoma, the Mansfield Training Center in Connecticut, and Willowbrook School in New York) are closing down to make way for semi-independent homes and apartments, as well as small group homes.

Although the unemployment rate of people with disabilities is the highest of any population in the world, legislative reforms are expanding the traditional sheltered workshop model for people with more severe disabilities to a supported employment model with an emphasis on real jobs, earning wages, and working side by side with nondisabled people. With the passage of the Americans with Disabilities Act, employers are now required to make "reasonable efforts" to hire people with disabilities. Employers are prohibited from discriminating against a worker or applicant who has a disability.

For families in which the person with a disability remains in the home, there has been an expansion in services, such as respite care and in-home assistance, to provide help in coping with everyday stress. Nisbet, Clark, and Covert (1991) suggest that respite care services "enable family members to become more socially active and in return reduce their feelings of social isolation" (p. 135). Family counseling and skills training programs assist families in dealing with relationships and interactions within the immediate family, with the extended family, and with friends and the community at large. As described by Bronicki and Turnbull (1987), "all parts of the family are interrelated; furthermore, each family has unique properties, understood only through careful observations of the relationships and interactions among all members" (p. 22).

People with disabilities and their families are also experiencing a stronger emphasis on individualization through coordinated planning and service delivery across agencies. Through individualized program planning, myriad agencies (such as social services, vocational rehabilitation, health care, social security) can be brought together with adults with disabilities and their families to plan, develop, and implement the supports necessary for an individual to participate in the life of the community (Point of Interest 1.2).

Individualization is at the core of educational reform for children with disabilities. Legal reforms, as mandated in the Individuals with Disabilities Education Act (formerly known as Public Law 94-142), now require that parents have the opportunity to participate actively in the development of an appropriate education for their son or daughter based on an individualized education program (IEP). It was only a few years ago that parents were being prosecuted as public nuisances for demanding educational services for their child with disabilities. Today, parents must be members of a parent–professional team responsible for making critical decisions about the specially designed instruction necessary for each student with a disability to receive an appropriate education.

The reforms of the last half of the twentieth century have had a dramatic impact on the lives of people with disabilities and their families. However, as we

## Statement in Support of Families and Their Children

THESE PRINCIPLES SHOULD GUIDE PUBLIC POLICY TOWARD FAMILIES OF CHILDREN WITH DEVELOPMENTAL DISABILITIES . . . AND THE ACTIONS OF STATES AND AGENCIES WHEN THEY BECOME INVOLVED WITH FAMILIES:

All children, regardless of disability, belong with families and need enduring relationships with adults. When states or agencies become involved with families, permanency planning should be a guideline philosophy. As a philosophy, permanency planning endorses children's rights to a nurturing home and consistent relationships with adults. As a guide to state and agency practice, permanency planning requires family support, encouragement of a family's relationship with the child, family reunification for children placed out of home, and the pursuit of adoption for children when family reunification is not possible. Families should receive the supports necessary to maintain their children at home.

Family support services must be based on the principle "whatever it takes." In short, family support services should be flexible, individualized, and designed to meet the diverse needs of families.

Family supports should build on existing social networks and natural sources of support. As a guiding principle, natural sources of support, including neighbors, extended families, friends, and community associations, should be preferred over agency programs and professional services. When states or agencies become involved with families, they should support existing social networks, strengthen natural sources, and help build connections to existing community resources. When natural sources of support cannot meet the needs of families, professional or agency-operated support services should be available.

Family supports should maximize the family's control over the services and supports they receive. Family support services must be based on the assumption that families, rather than states and agencies, are in the best position to determine their needs.

Family supports should support the entire family. Family support services should be defined broadly in terms of the needs of the entire family, including children with disabilities, parents, and siblings.

Family support services should encourage the integration of children with disabilities into the community. Family support services should be designed to maximize integration and participation in community life for children with disabilities.

When children cannot remain with their families for whatever reason, out-of-home placement should be viewed initially as a temporary arrangement and efforts should be directed toward reuniting the family. Consistent with the philosophy of permanency planning, children should live with their families whenever possible. When, due to family crisis or other circumstances, children must leave their families, efforts should be directed at encouraging and enabling families to be reunited.

When families cannot be reunited and when active parental involvement is absent, adoption should be aggressively pursued. In fulfillment of each child's right to a stable family and an enduring relationship with one or more adults, adoption should be pur-

*continued*

---

♦ **POINT OF INTEREST 1.2** *(continued)*

sued for children whose ties with their families have been broken. Whenever possible, families should be involved in adoption planning and, in all cases, should be treated with sensitivity and respect. When adoption is pursued, the possibility of "open adoption," whereby families maintain involvement with a child, should be seriously considered.

While a preferred alternative to any group setting or out-of-home placement, foster care should only be pursued when children cannot live with their families or with adoptive families. After families and adoptive families, children should have the opportunity to live with foster families. Foster family care can provide children with a home atmosphere and warm relationships and is preferable to group settings and other placements. As a state or agency-sponsored program, however, foster care seldom provides children the continuity and stability they need in their lives. While foster families may be called upon to assist, support, and occasionally fill in for families, foster care is not likely to be an acceptable alternative to fulfilling each child's right to a stable home and enduring relationships.

*Source:* Reprinted with permission of the Center on Human Policy.

---

move toward the twenty-first century and the expanding information age, it will be important to remain diligent about how people with disabilities can be included more effectively in the life of the family, school, and community.

## REVIEW

*FOCUS 1: Identify three waves of change that have redefined the meaning of civilization over time.*

- The first wave was the agricultural revolution, beginning in about 8000 B.C., when people cultivated and lived off the land.

- The second wave was the rise of industrialization that began in about the mid-seventeenth century and was characterized by the building of factories, mills, and plants, the manufacturing of products, and blue-collar assembly line workers.

- The third wave is the information age that began in the 1950s and is cresting as the year 2000 nears. We must cope with the impact of high technology on the way we do our jobs and how we structure our economy, political philosophy, and family lifestyle.

*FOCUS 2: Why is early history often described in terms of "survival of the fittest"?*

- People with disabilities were considered the weakest link in society and were vulnerable to practices of infanticide, slavery, physical abuse, and abandonment.
- Early Greek and Romans openly practiced selected eugenics.
- In some societies, people with disabilities were thought to be possessed by the devil. Demons residing in the individual had to be exorcized or the person destroyed.

*FOCUS 3: Identify the contributions of the eighteenth- and nineteenth-century reformers to our understanding of people with disabilities and their families.*

- Early reformers such as John Locke distinguished mental retardation from mental illness; Philippe Pinel advocated that people with disabilities be treated humanely.
- Jean-Marc Itard demonstrated that treatment and education of a person with a disability could make a difference. His work documented that it is possible for persons with severe disabilities to learn.
- Others, including Edouard Séguin, Anne Sullivan, and Benjamin Rush, focused attention on the potential of people with disabilities to learn and become contributors to society.

*FOCUS 4: What was the impact of the industrial age on people with disabilities and their families?*

- Many families changed from households where multiple generations lived together as a means to work the land to small, nuclear units expected to labor in factories and be self-sufficient.
- Families faced contradictions in government support. Although treatment and education were becoming more accessible for their children with disabilities, more and more parents were seen as the genetic cause of their child's problems and were held responsible for their care.
- The eugenics scare of the industrial age resulted in the passage of discriminatory marriage and sterilization laws as well as the eventual social isolation into large institutions of people with disabilities, who were viewed as a public threat.

*FOCUS 5: Why were many children with disabilities excluded from public education throughout most of the twentieth century?*

- It was the prevailing view that these children would not benefit from an education because they lacked the ability to learn basic academic skills. Public schools were not prepared to meet the needs of the nontraditional learner.

*FOCUS 6: Identify the roles parents played in the reform of social and educational programs for people with disabilities in the mid-twentieth century.*

- New national parent organizations evolved for the purpose of educating the public and advocating for the rights of their children.

- As the U.S. civil rights movement gathered momentum, parents moved to the courts as a means to fight discrimination in social and educational services (e.g., *Wyatt* v. *Stickney*; *Halderman* v. *Pennhurst, PARC* v. *Pennsylvania*).

- Parents played a key role in the development and passage of the Americans with Disabilities Act of 1990.

*FOCUS 7: How have families changed over the past one hundred years? What has been the impact of this change on families who are raising a child with a disability?*

- The family, traditionally defined as a group of individuals all of whom were bonded biologically, has become a diverse organizational unit with many different constellations. The traditional family in which the father works and the mother stays home is now only one of several definitions of family. Today, more children are living in single-parent families with the mother as the head of the household; families with children are the fastest growing segment of the homeless population.

- The family, now more divergent and under considerable stress in the 1990s, faces even greater challenges raising a child with a disability. A child with a disability may throw a family into further crisis. Or, raising a child with a disability may unify family members, strengthening bonds and building stronger relationships.

*FOCUS 8: How have the reforms of the past three decades changed the lives of people with disabilities and their families?*

- In community services, support for residential living is being redirected from large, congregate care settings to small, community-based residences located within local neighborhoods.

- Employment programs are expanding from traditional sheltered workshops to supported employment with an emphasis on real jobs, earning wages, and working side by side with nondisabled people.

- There has been an expansion of family support services in the areas of respite care and in-home assistance.

- People with disabilities and their families are experiencing more of an emphasis on individualization through coordinated planning and service delivery across agencies.

# REFERENCES

Aristotle. (1941). Politics. In R. McKeon (Ed.), *The basic works of Aristotle (Book 7)* (p. 1302). New York: Random House.

Bettelheim, B. (1950). *Love is not enough.* New York: Macmillan.

Blatt, B. (1973). *Souls in extremis: An anthology on victims and victimizers.* Boston: Allyn & Bacon.

Bradley, V. J., Knoll, J., & Agosta, J. M. (1992). *Emerging issues in family support.* Washington, DC: American Association on Mental Retardation.

Bronicki, G. J., & Turnbull, A. P. (1987). Family-professional interactions. In M. E. Snell (Ed.), *Systematic instruction of persons with severe handicaps* (pp. 9–35). Columbus, OH: Merrill.

Center on Human Policy. (1987). *Statement in support of families and their children.* Syracuse, NY: Author.

Cooke, R. S. (1992). *Parenting a child with special needs.* Grand Rapids, MI: Zondervan.

Crutcher, D. M. (1990). Quality of life versus quality of life judgments: A parent's perspective. In R. L. Schalock (Ed.), *Quality of life: Perspectives and issues* (pp. 17–22). Washington, DC: American Association on Mental Retardation.

Durant, W. (1966). *The life of Greece.* New York: Simon & Schuster.

Hardman, M. L., Drew, C. J., & Egan, M. W. (1996). *Human exceptionality* (5th ed.). Boston: Allyn & Bacon.

Innovative approaches to family support: Chicago pilot program for home care. (1990, Fall). *Family Support Bulletin*, p. 9.

Hewett, F. M., & Forness, S. (1984). *Education of exceptional learners* (3rd ed.). Boston: Allyn & Bacon.

Jaynes, G. D., and Williams, R. M. (Eds.). (1989). *A common destiny: Blacks and American society.* Washington, DC: National Academy Press.

Kennedy, J. F. (1963, October 31). *Remarks upon signing Bill for the construction of the Mental Retardation Facilities and Community Mental Health Centers.* Washington, DC: The White House.

Kirtley, D. D. (1975). *The psychology of blindness.* Chicago: Nelson-Hall.

Knoblock, P. (1987). *Understanding exceptional children and youth.* Boston: Little, Brown.

McDonnell, J., Hardman, M. L., McDonnell, A. P., & Kiefer-O'Donnell, R. (1995). *Introduction to persons with severe disabilities.* Boston: Allyn & Bacon.

National Association of State Directors of Special Education. (1991, March). *Reference notes for speechmaking or understanding the forces at work which are driving social policy.* Washington, DC: Author.

Nisbet, J., Clark, M., & Covert, S. (1991). Living it up! An analysis of research on community living. In L. H. Meyer, C. A. Peck, & L. Brown (Eds.), *Critical issues in the lives of people with severe disabilities* (pp. 115–144). Baltimore: Brookes.

Rosellini, L. (1995, August 28/September 4). Our century. *U.S. News and World Report*, pp. 58–83.

Shelton, T. L., Jeppson, E. S., & Johnson, B. H. (1987). *Family-centered care for children with special health-care needs.* Washington, DC: Association for the Care of Children's Health.

Toffler, A., & Toffler, H. (1995). *Creating a new civilization: The politics of the third wave.* Atlanta: Turner.

Weir, R. (1984). *Selective nontreatment of handicapped newborns.* New York: Oxford University Press.

West, J. (1991). Implementing the act: Where we begin. In J. West (Ed.), *The Americans with Disabilities Act: From policy to practice* (pp. xi–xxxi). New York: Milbank Memorial Fund.

Wolfensberger, W. (1975). *The origin and nature of our institutional models.* Syracuse, NY: Human Policy Press.

# CHAPTER TWO

# The Family as an Interactive Unit

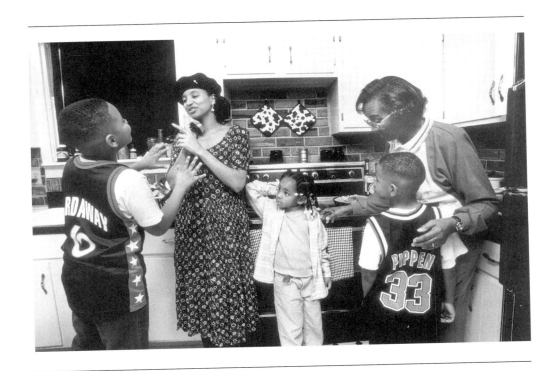

---

✴ **WINDOW 2.1**

---

## *Caring for Frankie*

WE WERE LOOKING FORWARD TO A CHILD and thought we'd have a big family. I still remember the look on the obstetrician's face when he came to see me. He told me that Dr. Ellison was going to see Frank Jr. and would tell us what the score was. Dr. Ellison told us there was a lot of brain damage. He wasn't sure first whether Frank would live and, if he were to live, how well he would do. He was going to get a specialist in babies to look at Frankie. And it seemed that life, a part of my life, ended right then and there.

We were both upset. I guess I showed it more than Jean. I tend to get very agitated when I can't settle something. No matter how hard we try, neither of us can remember that first week. Jean really took care of Frankie and I guess, me, for a while.

From that time on, we've been surrounded by Jean's family. She has two older sisters who live not too far from us. It seems they're around all the time. It's unfair to look at it that way, I guess, because they have been very helpful and try to do what they can to help Jean. At this time Frankie can do so little for himself. He requires constant attention. But I haven't had any privacy—we haven't had any privacy—since then. I began to wonder whether I really will ever have a wife again, or what kind of a wife and husband we are going to be.

*Source:* Reprinted with the expressed consent and approval of *Exceptional Parent*, a monthly magazine for parents and families of children with disabilities and special health care needs. Subscription cost is $32 per year for 12 issues; Call 1-800-247-8080. Offices at 555 Kinderkamack Rd. Oradell, N.J. 07649.

---

JUST DEFINING WHAT IS MEANT BY *FAMILY* can be challenging. The word tends to evoke a traditional image of a provider husband, homemaker wife, and children. As we noted in Chapter 1, however, that image is not reality for most American families today. Indeed, Berger (1994) reported the following:

> If current trends continue, only a minority—about 40 percent—of American children born in the 1990's will live with both biological parents from birth to age 18. Another 30 percent will begin life with married parents who will later divorce, while the remaining 30 percent will be born to an unmarried woman. . . . In addition, many children in the latter two groups will experience several changes in household composition—spending part of childhood living with a grandparent, or with a stepparent, or with a parent's live-in lover—and several marital transitions, from divorce to remarriage to divorce again. (p. 345)

Furthermore, over two-thirds of American mothers are currently employed outside the home, including over half of mothers with children under 3 (Voydanoff, 1993).

Families vary in size, age, and relationship patterns as well as cultural heritage, beliefs, and values. Thomas (1992) defined family as "any group of people

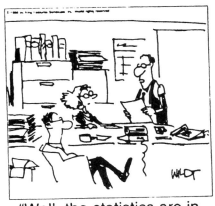

"Well, the statistics are in.
There is no typical
American family."

*Source:* Copyright © Chris Wildt.

who are related legally or by blood, or who are perceived to be family by an individual" (p. 36). Typical risk factors for families include greater numbers of children, children spaced close together, families adjusting to parental divorce and remarriage, single-parent families, very young parents, geographical isolation, and health problems.

These situations, however, may not be problematic if the family has a strong support system through extended family and friends and/or support agencies, or the financial resources to acquire outside help. Also, cultural diversity need not be a risk factor but will become so if professionals providing services to families do not recognize and accept ethnic, cultural, and value differences between themselves and the families they serve. Situations that are likely to be problematic and are unfortunately on the rise include child poverty, family violence, and substance abuse (Bennett, 1994; Emery, 1989). These situations require a variety of professional interventions ranging from crisis intervention to preventive approaches.

The impact of family size, family composition, and particular family problems on various family members is best understood when the family is viewed as an interactive system. Okun and Rappaport (1980) characterize this system as an organizational structure with specific goals and strategies for meeting those goals. They also perceive the family to be "an ongoing process of changing relationships among its members" (p. 6). Social science has borrowed from the fields of biology, engineering, economics, and general systems theory to address the organization and operation of families (Bertalanffy, 1968). Family systems theory views the family as an open, interactive system guided by family rules or norms that organize interactions. This theory has been translated into therapeutic approaches to family intervention (e.g., Kerr & Bowen, 1988; Minuchin, 1981).

According to McCubbin et al. (1993), each family has a schema or unique character that results from the fundamental convictions and values as well as the cultural and ethnic beliefs of the family system. In addition, families have paradigms that provide a framework for family behaviors and patterns of functioning. McCubbin et al. (1993) provided this metaphor of the family system, applicable to all families, but particularly salient for families that include a member with disabilities:

> The meaningful relationship between family schema and paradigms may be described by using the metaphor of a simple umbrella intended to provide protection, in this case to help a family unit cope with stress. At the top, the

center of the umbrella is the hub, the family schema consisting of its shared and fundamental values and convictions.

Emanating from the hub are a series of ribs, or spokes, each with a specific purpose designed to define and bring breadth, balance, and stability to the umbrella. These spokes may be viewed as family paradigms designed to guide different aspects of family life—the marital relationship, parenting, work and family, intergenerational relationships, and health care. Each is linked to the hub, but each has a unique purpose in guiding and supporting family coping and functioning. To complete the metaphor, the umbrella, characterized as the family's appraisal process, is designed to provide protection to the family system, particularly during periods of adversity and inclement conditions. (p. 1065)

This chapter presents the family as an interactive system. We discuss the impact of disability on this system as well as how disability affects each of the family subsystems: parental, marital, sibling, and extended family.

## THE FAMILY AS A SYSTEM CHARACTERIZED BY CHANGE

⊕    **FOCUS 1**

*How does disability affect the family as an interactive system?*

In this section, we address the issues of change within the family system, family rules and roles, and family goals, first from the perspective of any family and then from the perspective of families that include a member with a disability.

### Family Change

The family is a dynamic system of interdependent parts that is virtually *characterized* by change. Members are added by birth, adoption, and marriage. Members depart through death and divorce. Some family members may live far away but stay very involved; others are physically close, but psychologically distant. Other changes within families include aging, developmental change, and changes in roles and interests outside the family. Changes for individual family members affect other family members as well as the family as a whole. This is particularly true of change that involves stress.

The relationship between the system and its components is called wholeness. The system as a whole is more than its component elements. However, a change in any part of the system can cause a change for other parts and for the system as a whole. Homeostasis means a tendency toward a stable state. So the dynamic and changing family seeks homeostasis, or stability. Disequilibrium in the family is inevitable as well as necessary for growth to occur, but homeostasis restores equilibrium in this dynamic system. As Sieburg (1985) stated, "Homeostasis does not imply sameness or reversibility to a prior state; it simply means the capacity of the family to adjust to changing conditions by finding a new balance that still falls within an acceptable range" (p. 29). For example, easy, open communication between a mother and her young son may change when the son reaches adolescence. A mother facing this situation arranged to take her son out to dinner alone once a week. She commented, "He loves to eat and when he eats he talks." This mother accomplished homeostasis and facilitated family communication.

According to Papero (1983), the family system perspective attempts to understand the behavior of individual family members as "the product of a balance of forces in the family" (p. 139). The first force is the togetherness force that directs families to maintain closeness, preserve harmony, and assume responsibility for one another. The second force is the force toward individualization, whereby the individual develops personal goals and assumes personal responsibility. These forces operate continuously in families, with the system seeking to maintain balance or homeostasis that supports both togetherness and individuality. When these forces are out of balance, anxiety may occur, which can be transferred from one family member to another.

The caregiving and educational needs of a child with disabilities result in changes for the family as a whole and for individual family members and can upset the balance between togetherness and individuality. For example, the child's needs may affect the financial stability of the family as a whole and the career paths of both parents. A mother may have to go on welfare long enough to finish her high school degree because she needs a better-paying job to meet the increased expenses. This change may be motivated by a togetherness force or family need, but it can contribute to individual achievement as well. A father may have to seek a job that involves less travel so he can be available to help his wife with their twins with developmental disabilities, thereby sacrificing individuality for togetherness, at least temporarily. These changes and choices are complicated for all families and particularly for families that include a son or daughter with a disability. Families may need help in decision making that can lead to achieving homeostasis and maintaining the balance between togetherness and individuality (Falik, 1995).

## Family Rules and Roles

Families are characterized by rules and roles. Rules are expectations for behavior that guide how families operate. They can be spoken (or even written) or unspoken, and they can be negotiated. Sieburg (1985) stated that rules "permit the system to remain open to new environmental inputs, to regulate itself, and to adjust collectively to the stress it encounters" (pp. 14–15). Rules may be reflected in family routines, such as having dinner together. The role a person plays is determined by the needs of the family and may be influenced by roles within a person's family of origin. For example, a mother may assume primary responsibility for child care because she is not employed and is more available for this role or because her mother played this role and she therefore assumes it will be her role, even if she is employed outside the home.

Disability can bring about change in rules and roles. The organizational structure of the family may change. A child with feeding problems may necessitate a new routine at the dinner hour, for example. Role changes can also occur, for example, when the oldest daughter's role changes from being a child to being a co-parent to the child with a disability. Victoria Hayden (1993) wrote about her responsibilities for her younger sister Mindy who was hearing impaired. She described a scary time when Mindy wandered away while under her supervision. "After a thorough but fruitless search of the neighborhood, my mother hysterically told me that if anything happened to Mindy I would be to blame. I felt terrified and guilty. I was seven" (p. 93).

### Family Goals

Families set goals and revise them as change occurs within the family system. Some goals are influenced by the togetherness force, such as buying a home with a family room for family activities. Others reflect goals of an individual family member but may require financial and schedule accommodations by other family members, such as a daughter's goal to play on the basketball team or a father's goal to seek a graduate degree. Some goals are set by one or more family members on behalf of another family member, for example when parents set up college education funds for their children.

The presence of a child with a disability may change current family goals, and the ongoing needs of this child will affect future planning and goal setting. For example, the goal to have additional children may be threatened as the family attempts to discover a cause of the child's condition and whether it is likely to occur again. The parents must also determine if there are sufficient family resources—particularly time, energy, and money—to support an additional child while meeting the needs of the child with disabilities. This situation is reflected in the story of Marina and Katya (Carlyle, 1993) (Window 2.2).

Individual goals may also be affected and may have to be modified or postponed. For example, a mother may have to put aside for a while her goal of returning to work in order to have more time to carry out her child's home therapy program. Or a family may postpone a move to a rural community because they cannot leave the medical care needed by their child that is available only in a large city. Some goals, however, may not change. Margaret Hansen (1993) wrote about her daughter Martha and expressed a single goal for all her children: "We worked toward giving them the guidance and encouragement that would produce independent, responsible adults. As Martha's challenge arose in our lives, we decided that we would keep that goal in place for all four children" (p. 2). Furthermore, new goals can be created. After successfully advocating for their own child, advocating and performing volunteer services for others with disabilities may become a family goal.

---

✶ **WINDOW 2.2**
_____

## *Marina and Katya*

A FEW YEARS AFTER KATYA'S BIRTH, my husband and I decided to try to have another child. To state that more truthfully, my husband Peter wanted to have another child and I agreed to try while inwardly rejecting the idea with every fiber of my being. Aside from the fact that we were dealing with a couple of medical problems that continued to physically and financially exhaust us in regard to Katya's care, I had come to know more than anyone should ever be forced to know about the things that can go wrong from the moment that sperm meets ovum. Anyone who has ever spent much time in newborn and pediatric intensive care units tends to learn those things. It's not a matter of choice—it "just happens."

For more than three years, Peter tried to conceive and my body refused. . . .

[Then] I was definitely pregnant.

I sat down and cried in the bathroom. . . .

And so began my pregnancy with Marina. At the very beginning of Peter's attempt to conceive, I had told my gynecologist that if I got pregnant I wanted to undergo chorion villi sampling (CVS). I didn't want to wait the extra time for amniocentesis. . . . [She ended up having both of these prenatal tests.]

Eventually the results came back. All was well—at least all that could be tested for was well—and we settled into a holding pattern. Peter happily, me blocking out the entire idea as much as possible. . . .

[When it was time for the birth] I suddenly realized that if Marina wanted to stay in the womb until it was time for college, maybe that wasn't such a bad idea. I could put off facing the outcome of this pregnancy for 18 more years. I was happy with our family just the way it was. I was used to Katya and we functioned well the way we were. I didn't like surprises. Katya had provided us with enough surprises for a lifetime, for several lifetimes. Why were we doing this? . . .

Now Marina is four. She sings, she dances, she runs like the wind. She draws rainbows. . . .

So, we won the lottery with both Marina and Katya. I love each of them fiercely. And you couldn't pay me 47 million dollars to go through it again.

*Source:* Copyright © 1993 by Brookline Books.

## FAMILY RELATIONS

Within the family are units called subsystems or combinations. Many combinations are possible, but particular combinations include the parental subsystem, the marital subsystem, the sibling subsystem, and the extended family subsystem. Families can also be assessed on continuums of cohesion, adaptability, and openness. In terms of cohesion, families may be enmeshed—overprotective and overinvolved with one another without appropriate boundaries. The other end of the cohesion continuum is disengaged, or not adequately interested in or concerned about one another. Adaptability is assessed on a continuum ranging from rigid to chaotic, which essentially means too many rules and expectations or too few. Families that are overly rigid and/or enmeshed tend to be closed or isolated physically or psychologically from the community beyond the family. Disability increases the risk for relationship problems within and outside the family. For example, the needs of an infant with medical problems may result in a family that is overprotective, rigid, and closed or isolated from others. This family is attempting to meet the needs of the infant, but at a cost to all family members. Professionals can assist families in forming and maintaining relationships that are growth promoting for all family members (Duck & Wood, 1995). To do this, professionals need an understanding of relationship dynamics within the various family subsystems.

## Parental Subsystem

### ⊞   FOCUS 2

*What is the impact of a family member with a disability on the parental subsystem?*

The impact of a child with a disability on the parental subsystem includes both the satisfaction and stress involved in the day-to-day caregiving of the child with disabilities and the other children in the family for parents and, in some families, for stepparents as well. Both parent reports and studies involving control groups support the idea that parents of children with disabilities have increased stress. However, these parents also acknowledge the good times, including developmental gains, sibling relationships, and family fun, as well as enjoying a sense of humor—their children's and their own (Klein & Schleifer, 1993; Moss, 1995).

Studies addressing stress in the parent–child relationship have typically focused on mothers. Fathers, however, are beginning to receive more attention, and studies that compare mothers and fathers of children with disabilities (Beckman, 1991; Krauss, 1993) point to some differences. Specifically, mothers reported more stress stemming from demands of the parental role and relationship with spouse, whereas fathers reported more stress as a result of the child's temperament and problems with attachment to the child. In addition, mothers reported external social support to be more important in mediating stress than fathers did (Goldberg et al., 1986). Historically, the literature on parenting a child with a disability has been for and about mothers. This is beginning to change. Hornby (1992) reviewed personal accounts of fathers of children with disabilities and delineated seven common themes:

- the high intensity of their feelings at the time of their child's diagnosis
- existential conflicts experienced in the process of adaptation to the disability

- negative feelings toward professionals and resentment toward attitudes and lack of help from neighbors and workmates
- the stress of caring for the child and the consequent negative effects on fathers' lives, their wives, and their marriages
- concern about finding suitable care, especially in the longer term
- high intensity of positive and negative feelings toward their children with disabilities
- acknowledgment of personal growth from parenting a child with disabilities.

The growing literature on fathers attests to the importance of addressing the needs and feelings of fathers and mothers as individuals. Accounts of parent–child relationships, such as David's relationship with his father, attest to particular strengths of both male and female parents over the lifespan (Window 2.3 on page 34).

Clearly, professionals can help children with disabilities by helping their parents. Parents can be so involved in their parental role that they stop seeing themselves as individuals. Professionals can help parents realize that taking care of themselves is one of the most important ways they can help their child. As Buscaglia (1983) commented:

> To raise an exceptional child in our culture will demand the best parents have to give. In fact, it will perhaps become their life's second greatest challenge. The main challenge to any person will always be *personal* growth, development, and self-actualization. Parents can only give to their children, or anyone else, what they themselves have and know. For parents the main responsibility will always be to themselves. This may sound selfish but it becomes less so when one considers that ignorance only creates more ignorance, while only wisdom can create wisdom. No dead person has ever taught life, as no loveless person has ever been able to teach love. One must have these qualities first, before sharing them with others. (p. 85)

Parents also need safety zones for expressing their feelings. For some this may mean referral for individual counseling. Others may profit from the sharing that takes place in parent support groups. Parents need a break from their responsibilities to pursue personal interests, so referrals for babysitting and respite care are important as well.

## Marital Subsystem

**⊞  FOCUS 3**

*What is the impact of a family member with a disability on the marital subsystem?*

The responsibility of parenting a child with a disability can strain the marital relationship. However, it is important to remember that the presence of any child

---

★ **WINDOW 2.3**
_____

## A Father's Gift

DAVID RACED INTO THE HOUSE AND ANNOUNCED to everyone who would listen, "We caught 19 sunnies and on the way home, I saw three deer!" A couple weeks later, David rushed into the kitchen and shouted, "My team won by one touchdown. I gotta go call Dad—he owes me a quarter!"

These may sound like typical scenes in the lives of children who spend time participating in recreational activities with their parents. But David is our 26-year-old son who has mental retardation and attention-deficit/hyperactivity disorder. When he was younger and living at home, we privately called him the "white tornado," because he moved so fast. Today, he lives in a group home with three other young men.

Even though David has a developmental delay and some challenging behaviors, his father included him, whenever possible, in his own favorite activities—watching sporting events, fishing, and hunting. . . .

David's outings with Dad have resulted in many unanticipated benefits. At our house, David feels like he is one of us. While he is aware of his limitations, he feels accepted because we have emphasized what he _can_ do. By including him in recreational activities, David's father helped him develop interests that are appropriate for a man; more importantly, these activities have given David lots to talk about!

When David meets someone, he might ask, "Did you see the game—who won?" or "Did you know they traded the catcher?" This small talk is socially appropriate and has helped other people accept David. Sometimes, people don't know what to say to a person with a disability. But all of our family members and friends have lots to talk about with David because of his interests and involvement in these leisure-time activities. . . .

Through many outings, David's father gave him the priceless gift of time—time to be together, to share and to learn. Because of this gift, David has learned to talk about and enjoy a number of leisure activities. This happened because David's father was willing to share an even greater gift—the gift of love.

_Source:_ Reprinted with the expressed consent and approval of _Exceptional Parent_, a monthly magazine for parents and families of children with disabilities and special health care needs. Subscription cost is $32 per year for 12 issues; Call 1-800-247-8080. Offices at 555 Kinderkamack Rd. Oradell, N.J. 07649.

---

influences the marital relationship. Belsky (1990) summarized multiple research findings this way: "We discover repeatedly that children's presence and marital quality tend to be inversely related" (p. 172). In light of the research evidence on the potential detrimental effect of marital tension and divorce on all children (Hetherington, Hagan, & Anderson, 1989), marital stress experienced by these families should be taken quite seriously.

Marital stress can result from difficulties in communicating feelings about the child (Lichtenstein, 1993). For example, Fern Kupfer was feeling pessimistic and depressed about Zach (their baby son with severe disabilities) at a point when her husband, Joe, was feeling more optimistic, and this led to marital tension. Joe stated, "I have to believe things will get better with Zach. I lash out at Fern because I feel her trying to bring me down with her. Sometimes she is more of a burden to me than Zach is" (Kupfer, 1982, p. 105).

Marital stress is also related to the pressures of the parental role. Research documents high demands on the time and energy of mothers of children with disabilities (Breslau, 1983; Traustadottir, 1991). For married mothers, help with child care from their spouse has been identified as a valued source of support and as a predictor of marital satisfaction for both parents (Willoughby & Glidden, 1995).

Young and Roopnarine (1994) were interested in fathers' child-care involvement with preschool children with disabilities. They suggested that visibility of the disability and care demands at this age might mean less participation for fathers of children with disabilities than for fathers of children with typical development. However, they found no differences. Although it was encouraging that fathers of these young children were not less involved, they may need to be more involved, especially if the child is severely disabled. Helping married parents communicate feelings and accomplish role sharing can be important to the marital satisfaction of both parents.

An understanding of marital stress and adjustment in these families is necessary for professionals working with children with disabilities and their parents. Benson and Gross (1989) reviewed studies that addressed marital adjustment in families with a child with congenital disabilities, and Sabbeth and Leventhal (1984) reviewed research on marital satisfaction in relation to chronic childhood illness. Benson and Gross found that in the bulk of the studies, separation and divorce rates were not elevated for these families. Studies of marital satisfaction and adjustment, however, yielded mixed findings. Most of the studies reviewed indicated that the marriages were affected by the presence of a child with disabilities, but the influence was found to be negative in some cases (increased stress) and positive in others (increased cohesiveness). These authors criticized the reviewed studies for problems in methodology and for failure to address factors that contribute to marital adjustment.

Studies reviewed by Sabbeth and Leventhal (1984) that utilized a control group (of parents of children without disabilities) revealed that parents of children with disabilities were not more likely to divorce but were more likely to experience marital dissatisfaction and stress. They also expressed concern for what is not included in current research findings—specifically, studies that address communication, decision making, problem solving, and role flexibility.

When viewed as a whole, these studies imply that having a child with a disability does not automatically mean the marriage is in trouble. Although some families find this situation stressful in ways that affect relationships, other families seem to grow stronger. However, it is appropriate to consider these families at risk for marital tension and stress and to provide appropriate supports when needed.

When parents of a child with a disability do divorce, professional support in negotiating roles for shared custody may be needed. In circumstances in which one parent has sole or primary custody, external sources of support are particularly important ("He didn't take responsibility," 1991). This support may come from extended family, friends, or an agency. Often, what a single parent needs most is help in assessing needs and options for both short- and long-term support.

Professionals can support married parents through preventive approaches such as referral for services that provide appropriate child care so parents can spend time alone. Professional referral for marriage counseling is appropriate in some cases, and families that include a son or daughter with a disability may particularly need counseling and other support services for circumstances involving divorce, custody, stepparenting, and blended families.

## Sibling Subsystem

**FOCUS 4**

*What is the impact of a family member with a disability on the sibling subsystem?*

Being a sibling is both an introductory peer relationship and often the longest relationship of a person's life. This relationship provides early lessons in loving and being loved, cooperation, competition, and conflict resolution. Learning social skills through play, observation, teaching, and advising also occurs, as well as nurturance and caregiving. The societal movement away from institutional care for children with disabilities has meant that siblings without disabilities are more likely to be involved in day-to-day family interactions that are influenced by disability. Similarly, inclusion within the school setting means these siblings are likely to share a school experience. So, what does it mean to be the brother or sister of someone with a disability? Is it a positive or negative experience? Research findings support both positive and negative outcomes but, more importantly, suggest ways to influence positive outcomes.

Common perceptions of outcomes for siblings present a highly negative or, occasionally, overly positive picture. However, recent studies do not support these extreme perceptions. Lobato (1990) reviewed carefully controlled studies comparing siblings of children with and without disabilities and did not find a higher rate of major personality or behavior disorders among children with a brother or sister with a disability as compared to control samples. An overly positive perception, supported by older studies not involving control samples (e.g., Cleveland & Miller, 1977), is that these siblings are more likely to choose careers in the helping professions. However, a study that included a control group (Konstam et al., 1993) found no significant differences in occupation and career choices between the two groups.

Instead, children with a brother or sister with a disability or chronic illness can be considered at risk for problems with adjustment and self-esteem, including aggressive behavior, poor peer relations, anxiety, somatization, and depression (Lobato, Faust, & Spirito, 1988). Factors influencing this risk have been addressed by researchers. Early studies (Grossman, 1972) found increased risk with more severe disability, but a later, carefully controlled study by Breslau, Weitzman, and Messenger (1981) found no differences in sibling or parental adjustment related to the severity of the disability.

Two publications (Lobato, 1990; Powell & Gallagher, 1993) combine research findings with self-report information from siblings to give a rich picture of what life is like for these brothers and sisters. Although research findings from carefully controlled studies provide an encouraging picture of sibling adjustment, negative feelings reported by siblings should not be denied or underestimated. These siblings report feeling angry, guilty, embarrassed, resentful, and jealous. They also express anxiety about future caregiving responsibilities and their own future parenthood. However, siblings also provide evidence of social and psychological strength as they describe being empathic, altruistic, mature, and patient. They also convey a sense that their family is different in positive and negative terms, describing both activity limitations and increased closeness. And they cringe from expressions of pity or inappropriate praise. Sibling David Hansen (1993) expressed it this way: "I learned to despise the sickening smiles of people who talked about how strong we were, or how noble, or how courageous. I felt that they understood us the least" (p. 7).

Powell and Gallagher (1993) have stressed the importance of studying sibling interactions. Of particular interest are findings indicating that brothers and sisters of children with disabilities assumed greater responsibility for teaching, helping, and directing (Stoneman et al., 1987) and assumed dominant leadership roles even if they were younger siblings (Abramovitch et al., 1987). This teaching role, helping role, and the role asymmetry of these relationships may play a part in the advocacy role often assumed by these siblings as they reach adulthood (Stoneman et al., 1987).

Stress and coping is another area of potential vulnerability for siblings. However, Gamble and McHale (1989) found no significant differences in frequency of stressful events or of anger felt and no gender differences between a group with siblings with disabilities and a control group without a sibling with disabilities. These siblings of persons with disabilities did report being teased or provoked more often, and they had significantly higher affect ratings in response to their sibling being hurt or sick. This ties in with the findings of sadness and anxiety reported by Wilson, Blacher, and Baker (1989).

Parents going through the struggle of adjusting to the child with a disability may be less available physically and emotionally to the sibling. A mother wrote the following about her two young sons, Nathan, who has Down syndrome, and his younger brother, Wess. "I was expending all my time and energies on Nathan, figuring that Wess would do all right. After all, he was normal. But was he? Would he be?" (Therrien, 1993, p. 47). From a sibling's perspective, Hayden (1993) wrote of her life with her sister Mindy, who is deaf. "Mother and Daddy 'expected more' from me, but it seems to me that they gave me less" (p. 93).

Gender, birth order, and age spacing are also predictive, to some extent, of sibling adjustment. In terms of gender and birth order, older sisters and younger brothers of siblings with disabilities have higher rates of behavior problems, probably due to increased caregiving responsibility by the older sister and role tension for the younger brother (Lobato, Faust, & Spirito, 1988). The likelihood of adjustment problems decreases as the age differences between siblings with and without disabilities increases (Breslau, 1982). Age proximity means more overlap in school and other activities that can increase caregiving responsibilities and complicate peer relationships. An adolescent sibling wrote about his life with a brother, 16 months older, with severe disabilities. He conveyed the pressure he felt when asked a simple question about what grade his brother was in. "I either had to lie or divulge something about myself that I was unprepared to reveal. At a time when blending in was the most important thing in my life, I stood out" (Siegel & Silverstein, 1994, p. 7).

A potential source of stress for everyone in the family occurs when the younger sibling's development surpasses that of the older sibling with disabilities. A mother of children with and without disabilities wrote about this situation in her family:

> Without realizing it the process of parenting this normal child becomes a double-edged sword. We are thrilled and delighted with each accomplishment. It brings us great joy to see this child developing and progressing so well. However, at the same time, the experience can be one of pain—a spark that ignites the flames of chronic sorrow. This is especially true when the normal child surpasses the sibling with a disability. It is a very happy time that can produce, without warning, sadness. (Michalegko, 1993, p. 52)

Several studies provide insight into factors that predict more positive adjustment for these siblings. Dyson, Edgar, and Crnic (1989) found that family factors, including parental stress and resources, perceived family social support, family relationship, family's emphasis on personal growth, and maintenance of family system contributed to all measured aspects of adjustment for children with a sibling with a disability. They found a strong relationship between self-concept of the siblings studied and parental stress and resources. These findings suggest that the best way to help and support siblings is to help and support their parents. Parental acceptance of the child with disabilities has also been linked to more positive outcomes for siblings (Konstam et al., 1993) and is supported by a sibling's comments concerning lessons learned from his parents. Concerning his brother with disabilities, this sibling learned "to meet his [disabled sibling's] needs, . . . enjoy his engaging personality, and accept what seemed impossible to change. The model of caring consistently displayed by our parents made it easier for my brother and me to assume this kind of acceptance" (Bodenheimer, 1979, p. 292).

Both the research literature and interviews with siblings provide guidelines for supporting siblings. From their families, these brothers and sisters need to know that they are loved and valued. They do not need to be overburdened with responsibilities. They need a safe place to share feelings. Ideally, this will occur within the family, but may need to be supplemented through counseling, sibling support groups, or programs such as Sibshops (Meyer & Vadasy, 1994), workshops designed especially for siblings of children with special needs.

Siblings need information. They need to be able to ask questions and to receive answers from their parents and from professionals providing services for their family. Participation in programs such as Sibshops allows for the sharing of information among siblings in addition to the, probably more important, sharing of feelings. They also need to be taught ways to become more involved in their siblings' lives, for example, learning sign language (Berry, 1987). Meyer (1994) discusses information needs of siblings from a lifespan perspective and encourages professionals to include siblings as part of the team (see Point of Interest 2.1 on page 40).

These siblings also need coping strategies, including how to explain their brother or sister to their friends and how to handle the situation if their brother or sister is teased. They need to be taught strategies for managing their siblings' behavior when it is annoying or embarrassing—and especially if it is rough or destructive.

Although there has been increased interest and research in this area, many unanswered questions about sibling adjustment and support remain. Lobato, Faust, and Spirito (1988) stated,

> Parents' and siblings' ability to communicate expectations and feelings openly, to flexibly adjust routines to meet individual members' needs, and to problem-solve effectively have been alluded to the most in clinical interviews with siblings but examined the least in empirical research. (p. 403)

The literature does, however, attest to both problems and benefits for siblings and can perhaps be summed up by the statement of David Hansen (1993) about his life with his sister Martha. "Growing up with a sibling who had disabilities was painful but rich. It continues to enrich me" (p. 8).

♦ **POINT OF INTEREST 2.1**

## Information Needs of Siblings

THROUGHOUT THEIR LIVES, the types of information siblings need—as well as how it is optimally presented—will vary with the siblings' age. . . .

### Preschoolers

Preschoolers need to know that they cannot catch their siblings' disability, nor did they cause the condition. These concepts—while obvious to adults—may not be clear to a young child who has caught her sister's cold and has a preschooler's sense of causality.

Explanations of disabilities or illness to children at this age should be as clear as possible. . . . One way to explain a disability is to describe it in terms of differences in behavior or routine. A 4-year-old who accompanies his 2-year-old sister to an early intervention program may understand his sister's disability this way: "Down syndrome means you have to go to school to learn how to talk. . . ." While clearly incomplete, a definition like this can be the foundation for more involved explanations at later ages.

### School-Aged Children

During their grade-school years, siblings need information to answer their own questions about the disability or illness as well as questions posed by classmates, friends or even strangers. . . .

School-age children may have more specific questions than preschoolers. They may ask: "Why can some people with cerebral palsy walk and some can't?" "What does amniocentesis mean?" "What's physical therapy? Does it hurt?" . . .

### Teenagers

Because they can envision a life beyond their parents, teenagers and young adults require additional information about their siblings' future and what role they will play in that future. If parents have not made plans by this time, it is critical that they begin and encourage brothers and sisters to be a part of this planning. . . .

### Into the Loop

Inviting—but not requiring—siblings to attend meetings with service providers can benefit all parties. When included, siblings can obtain helpful, reassuring information about a sibling's condition, and can contribute by providing information, and unique, informed (and frequently unsentimental) perspectives on issues such as barriers to inclusion with neighborhood peers, or a sibling's ability to accomplish household and self-care responsibilities. . . .

When invited to meet with service providers, siblings are brought "into the loop." A message is sent to family members and service providers alike that brothers and sisters are valued members of the child's "team." Including them acknowledges the important roles they play in their siblings' lives and, for many, roles they will have as adults. . . .

*Source:* Reprinted with the expressed consent and approval of *Exceptional Parent*, a monthly magazine for parents and families of children with disabilities and special health care needs. Subscription cost is $32 per year for 12 issues; Call 1-800-247-8080. Offices at 555 Kinderkamack Rd. Oradell, N.J. 07649.

## Extended Family Subsystem

**⊞ FOCUS 5**

*What is the impact of a family member with a disability on the extended family subsystem?*

Grandparents, aunts, uncles, cousins, and other family members can be sources of support or sources of additional stress for parents of children with disabilities. Although the research literature on this topic is sparse, it does endorse the positive influence of intergenerational support on mothers and fathers of children with disabilities (Hornby & Ashworth, 1994; Vadasy, Fewell, & Meyer, 1986; Weisbren, 1980). However, this support may not be forthcoming because grandparents may be grieving both for their grandchild and for their son or daughter (Gabel & Kotsch, 1981; McPhee, 1982). Other feelings may get in the way of supportive interactions. Seligman (1991) suggested that "the birth of a disabled grandchild introduces uncertainty about the future, anger at the resumption of a parental role in the face of their child's crisis, and a sense of powerlessness" (p. 149). Most distressing of all can be blame, which may be directed by the grandparents toward the daughter-in-law or son-in-law. Elizabeth Pieper (1976) wrote of experiencing blame from her mother-in-law upon the birth of her son with multiple disabilities, but also of learning to understand her mother-in-law's feelings. "Her harsh words to me in the hospital were a way of expressing the same protectiveness towards her son [the baby's father] that I was now feeling towards mine" (p. 6). And sometimes the support itself can be stressful, as it was for Frankie's parents (Window 2.1).

As the baby with disabilities becomes a child with disabilities, reality dawns within the entire family system that problems and challenges are here to stay. Some families rally to meet these changing but continuing demands, and some do not. Carly McClure, the mother of Josh, a preschool child with severe developmental disabilities, commented on her extended family:

> I'm struggling with my brothers. As Josh has gotten bigger, less babylike, and obviously disabled, they have withdrawn from him to the point of not even saying "hello" or "goodbye" to the child. Now that Rachel [her baby daughter] is here, I can see that it is clearly Joshua's being disabled that causes this reaction, and not an inability to relate to kids. I'm angry with them. They say "cop out" things like "I just can't handle it." I want to say back to them "Tough, I've *had* to handle it. This is how it is." I haven't communicated with them in over a month. I'm regrouping and planning to write to them in a while. It never ends, does it? I feel OK about Josh, but have to prod the family to do the same. I expect strangers to have difficulty, I suppose I expected more from kin. (McClure, 1993, p. 173)

Professionals can help parents by offering to share information with extended family members, by addressing ways to involve family members in the child's program, and by sharing positive ideas developed by other families. One such idea is "project cousins." The parents of Kevin, who has cerebral palsy, invited near-age cousins for visits and outings that resulted in friendship bonds between their son and his cousins that have strengthened over time (Darby, 1995). In addition, professionals can refer family members to services such as grandparent support groups, where grandparents can talk about their feelings with others who will understand (Bell & Smith, 1996; Johnson, 1995). One grandmother provided the following example of both peer support and positive intergenerational communication:

> Our daughter was kind enough to give us a few pamphlets that helped us learn about our new grandson's condition. We also talked with some other friends of ours who have a granddaughter with Down syndrome. They didn't know a whole lot more than we did, but the talking did us both some good. (Hardman et al., 1993, p. 429)

Finally, professionals can help families find sources of support beyond the extended family so that relationships between parents and extended family members are not dominated by caregiving needs.

Clearly, disability does not just affect the family member who has received the diagnosis. It has profound consequences for parents as individuals, for the marital relationship, for siblings, for extended family members, and for the family system. Chapter 3 considers these consequences in the daily lives of family members and on the family life cycle.

## REVIEW

*FOCUS 1: How does disability affect the family as an interactive system?*

- A change in any part of the family system, such as the diagnosis of disability, can cause change for all members of the family and the family as a whole. Disability will impose disequilibrium, but the family system will seek to adjust and achieve homeostasis.

- Disability can bring about change in rules and roles and the organizational structure of the family.

- The presence of a child with disabilities may change current family goals, and the ongoing needs of this child will affect future planning and goal setting.

*FOCUS 2: What is the impact of a family member with a disability on the parental subsystem?*

- The impact of a child with a disability on the parental subsystem includes the grief response and both the pleasure and stress involved in day-to-day caregiving of the child with disabilities and the other children in the family.
- The needs and feelings of both the mother and father must be considered by professionals providing services to families.

*FOCUS 3: What is the impact of a family member with a disability on the marital subsystem?*

- The responsibility of parenting a child with disabilities can stress the marital subsystem, placing the marital relationship at risk.
- The marriage itself may be at risk, but stress within the marital relationship is a more likely occurrence.

*FOCUS 4: What is the impact of a family member with a disability on the sibling subsystem?*

- The sibling subsystem also involves risk. Both positive and negative consequences are reported by the research literature and by siblings themselves.
- Support for siblings is a critical component of family support.

*FOCUS 5: What is the impact of a family member with a disability on the extended family subsystem?*

- The extended family subsystem can be a source of support for parents of a child with disabilities or a source of additional stress.
- Extended family members need information about disability and support for their own feelings in order to form positive, supportive relationships with the child with a disability and to be of help to his or her parents.

# REFERENCES

Abramovitch, R., Stanhope, L., Pepler, D. J., & Corter, C. (1987). Patterns of sibling interaction among preschool-age children. In M. E. Lamb & B. Sutton-Smith (Eds.), *Sibling Relationships* (pp. 61–68). Hillsdale, NJ: Erlbaum.

Beckman, P. J. (1991). Comparison of mothers' and fathers' perception of the effect of young children with and without disabilities. *American Journal on Mental Retardation, 95,* 585–595.

Bell, M. L., & Smith, B. R. (1996). Grandparents as primary caregivers: Lessons in love. *Teaching Exceptional Children, 28,* 18–19.

Belsky, J. (1990). Children and marriage. In F. D. Fincham & T. N. Bradbury (Eds.), *The psychology of marriage* (pp. 172–200). New York: Guilford.

Bennett, W. J. (1994). *The index of leading cultural indicators.* New York: Simon & Schuster.

Benson, B. A., & Gross, A. M. (1989). The effect of a congenitally handicapped child upon the marital dyad: A review of the literature. *Clinical Psychology Review, 9,* 747–758.

Berger, K. S. (1994). *The developing person through the lifespan* (3rd ed.). New York: Worth.

Berry, J. O. (1987). Involving siblings in sign language. *Communication Outlook, 8,* 8–9.

Bertalanffy, L. (1968). *General systems theory: Foundations, development, applications.* New York: Braziller.

Blaska, J. K. (1994, May). A father's gift. *Exceptional Parent,* pp. 19–20.

Bodenheimer, C. (1979). For the sake of others. *Journal of Autism and Developmental Disorders, 9,* 291–293.

Breslau, N. (1982). Siblings of disabled children: Birth order and age spacing effects. *Journal of Abnormal Child Psychology, 10,* 85–96.

Breslau, N. (1983). Care of disabled children and women's time use. *Medical Care, 21,* 620–629.

Breslau, N., Weitzman, M., & Messenger, K. (1981). Psychologic functioning of siblings of disabled children. *Pediatrics, 67,* 344–353.

Buscaglia, L. (1983). *The disabled and their parents: A counseling challenge* (2nd ed.). Thorofare, NJ: Slack.

Carlyle, K. (1993). And the winner of the rainbow lottery is . . . In J. A. Spiegle & R. A. van den Pol (Eds.), *Making changes: Family voices on living with disabilities* (pp. 153–158). Cambridge: Brookline.

Cleveland, D., & Miller, N. (1977). Attitudes and life commitments of older siblings of mentally retarded adults: An exploratory study. *Mental Retardation, 15,* 38–41.

Darby A. (1995, December). "Project cousins": Discovering the joys of family. *Exceptional Parent,* pp. 39–40.

Duck, S., & Wood, J. T. (1995). *Confronting relationship challenges.* Thousand Oaks: Sage.

Dyson, L., Edgar, E., & Crnic, K. (1989). Psychological predictors of adjustment by siblings of developmentally disabled children. *American Journal on Mental Retardation, 94,* 292–302.

Emery, R. E. (1989). Family violence. *American Psychologist, 44,* 321–328.

Falik, L. H. (1995). Family patterns of reaction to a child with a learning disability: A mediational perspective. *Journal of Learning Disabilities, 28,* 335–341.

Gabel, H., & Kotsch, L. S. (1981). Extended families and young handicapped children. *Topics in Early Childhood Special Education, 1,* 29–35.

Gamble, W. G., & McHale, S. M. (1989). Coping with stress in sibling relationships: A comparison of children with disabled and nondisabled siblings. *Journal of Applied Developmental Psychology, 10,* 353–373.

Goldberg, S., Marcovitch, S., MacGregor, D., & Lojkasek, M. (1986). Family responses to developmentally delayed preschoolers: Etiology and the father's role. *American Journal of Mental Deficiency, 90,* 610–617.

Grossman, F. K. (1972). *Brothers and sisters of retarded children: An exploratory study.* Syracuse, NY: Syracuse University Press.

Hansen, D. (1993). Let her do it. In J. A. Spiegle and R. A. van den Pol (Eds.), *Making changes: Family voices on living with disabilities* (pp. 5–8). Cambridge: Brookline.

Hansen, M. (1993). Insisting on the positive possibility. In J. A. Spiegle and R. A. van der Pol (Eds.), *Making changes: Family voices on living with disabilities,* (pp. 1–4). Cambridge: Brookline.

Hardman, M. L., Drew, C. J., Egan, M. W., & Wolf, B. (1993). *Human exceptionality: Society, school, and family* (4th ed.). Boston: Allyn & Bacon.

Hayden, V. (1993). The other children. In S. D. Klein and M. J. Schleifer (Eds.), *It isn't fair!* (pp. 91–96). Westport, CT: Bergin & Garvey.

"He didn't take responsibility when they were younger." Divorce and children. (1991, January/February). *Exceptional Parent*, pp. 40–42.

Hetherington, E. M., Hagan, M. S., & Anderson, E. R. (1989). Marital transitions: A child's perspective. *American Psychologist, 44,* 303–312.

Hornby, G. (1992). A review of fathers' accounts of their experiences of parenting children with disabilities. *Disability, Handicap & Society, 7,* 363–374.

Hornby, G., & Ashworth, T. (1994). Grandparents' support for families who have children with disabilities. *Journal of Child and Family Studies, 3,* 403–412.

"I don't know where we're going." Marital problems and the young family. (1991, June). *Exceptional Parent*, pp. 50–52.

Johnson, J. (1995, December). Grandparents have special needs, too. *Exceptional Parent*, pp. 30–31.

Kerr, M., & Bowen, M. (1988). *Family evaluation: An approach based on Bowen theory.* New York: Norton.

Klein, S. D., & Schleifer, M. J. (1993). *It isn't fair!* Westport, CT: Bergin & Garvey.

Konstam, K., Drainoni, M., Mitchell, G., Houser, R., Reddington, D., & Eaton, D. (1993). Career choices and values of siblings of individuals with developmental disabilities. *The School Counselor, 40,* 287–292.

Krauss, M. W. (1993). Child-related and parenting stress: Similarities and differences between mothers and fathers of children with disabilities. *American Journal on Mental Retardation, 97,* 393–404.

Kupfer, F. (1982). *Before and after Zachariah.* New York: Delacorte.

Lichtenstein, J. (1993). Help for troubled marriages. In G. H. S. Singer & L. E. Powers (Eds.), *Families, disability and empowerment* (pp. 259–277). Baltimore: Brookes.

Lobato, D. J. (1990). *Brothers, sisters and special needs: Information and activities for helping young siblings of children with chronic illness and developmental disabilities.* Baltimore: Brookes.

Lobato, D., Faust, D., & Spirito, A. (1988). Examining the effects of chronic disease and disability on children's sibling relationships. *Journal of Pediatric Psychology, 13,* 389–407.

McClure, C. (1993). Happily ever after? In J. A. Spiegle & R. A. van den Pol (Eds.), *Making changes: Family voices on living with disabilities* (pp. 161–193). Cambridge: Brookline.

McCubbin, H. I., Thompson, E. A., Thompson, A. I., McCubbin, M. A., & Kaston, A. J. (1993). Culture, ethnicity, and the family: Critical factors in childhood chronic illness and disabilities. *Pediatrics, 91,* 1063–1070.

McPhee, N. (1982, June). A very special magic: A grandparent's delight. *The Exceptional Parent*, pp. 13–16.

Meyer, D. J. (1994, December). Information needs of siblings. *Exceptional Parent*, p. 49.

Meyer, D. J., & Vadasy, P. F. (1994). *Sibshops: Workshops for siblings of children with special needs.* Baltimore: Brookes.

Michalegko, P. M. (1993). A sibling born without disabilities: A special kind of challenge. In S. D. Klein and M. J. Schleifer (Eds.), *It isn't fair!* (pp. 51–54). Westport, CT: Bergin & Garvey.

Minuchin, S. (1981). *Families and family therapy.* Cambridge, MA: Harvard University Press.

Moss, J. (1995, June). Learning the "ability words." *Exceptional Parent*, p. 96.

Okun, B. F., & Rappaport, L. J. (1980). *Working with families: An introduction to family therapy.* Belmont, CA: Wadsworth.

Papero, D. V. (1983). Family systems theory and therapy. In B. B. Wolman & G. Striker (Eds.), *Handbook of family and marital therapy* (pp. 137–158). New York: Plenum.

Pieper, E. (1976, April). Grandparents can help. *The Exceptional Parent*, pp. 6, 7–10.

Powell, T. H., & Gallagher, P. A. (1993). *Brothers and sisters: A special part of exceptional families*. Baltimore: Brookes.

Sabbeth, B. F., & Leventhal, J. M. (1984). Marital adjustment to chronic childhood illness: A critique of the literature. *Pediatrics, 73*, 762–768.

Seligman, M. (1991). Grandparents of disabled grandchildren: Hopes, fears, and adaptation. *Families in Society, 72*, 147–152.

Sieburg, E. (1985). *Family communication: An integrated systems approach*. New York: Gardner.

Siegel, B., & Silverstein, S. (1994). *What about me? Growing up with a developmentally disabled sibling*. New York: Plenum.

Stoneman, Z., Brody, G. H., Davis, C. H., & Crapps, J. M. (1987). Mentally retarded children and their older same-sex siblings: Naturalistic in-home observations. *American Journal on Mental Retardation, 92*, 290–298.

Therrien, V. L. (1993). For the love of Wess. In S. D. Klein and M. J. Schlerfer (Eds.), *It isn't fair!* (pp. 45–49). Westport, CT: Bergin & Garvey.

Thomas, M. B. (1992). *An introduction to marital and family therapy*. New York: Merrill.

Traustadottir, R. (1991). Mothers who care: Gender, disability and family life. *Journal of Family Issues, 12*, 211–228.

Vadasy, P. F., Fewell, R. R., & Meyer, D. J. (1986). Grandparents of children with special needs: Insights into their experiences and concerns. *Journal of the Division for Early Childhood, 10*, 36–44.

Voydanoff, P. (1993). Work and family relationships. In T. H. Brubaker (Ed.), *Family relations: Challenges for the future* (pp. 98–111). Newbury Park, CA: Sage.

Weisbren, S. E. (1980). Parents' reactions after the birth of a developmentally disabled child. *American Journal of Mental Deficiency, 84*, 345–351.

Willoughby, J. C., & Glidden, L. M. (1995). Fathers helping out: Shared child care and marital satisfaction of parents of children with disabilities. *American Journal on Mental Retardation, 99*, 399–406.

Wilson, J., Blacher, J., & Baker, B. L. (1989). Siblings of children with severe handicaps. *Mental Retardation, 27*, 167–173.

Young, D. M., & Roopnarine, J. L. (1994). Father's childcare involvement with children with and without disabilities. *Topics in Early Childhood Special Education, 14*, 488–502.

# CHAPTER THREE

# Families: Day to Day and across the Lifespan

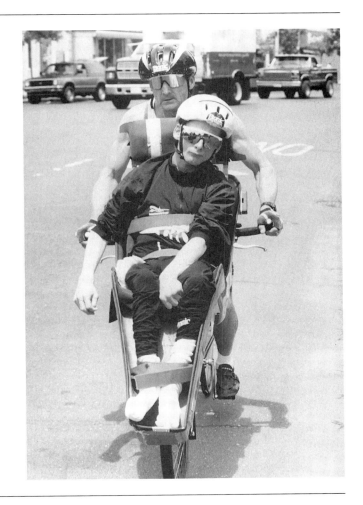

★ **WINDOW 3.1**

## Welcome to Our Family, Casey Patrick

"*WELCOME TO OUR FAMILY, CASEY PATRICK. WE LOVE YOU.*" The brightly colored banner greeted us as Roger and I drove up to the house on April 13, 1981, with our newborn son. Our older boys, Sean, 8, and Ryan, 4, had printed the message in huge letters and stretched the banner across the garage.

The next morning, Roger came home from work to drive me to the doctor's office so Casey could have a quick, routine phenylketonuria (PKU) test. Since Casey had been born in a hospital 40 miles from our hometown, we were anxious for our regular doctor to see him. We figured we'd be in and out like a flash.

But our long-time pediatrician and friend gave Casey a very thorough exam, during which he asked a lot of questions. I became amused. "Boy," I thought, "Irwin really has changed his newborn visits in the last 4 years. He must have attended some seminars that emphasized the psychological aspects of parenting."

I remember his asking, "How do you plan to raise Casey? Do you plan to do anything differently than you did with Sean and Ryan?" That seemed to be a strange question, but since we'd known each other a long time and since he seemed to be in this psychological mode, I didn't give it much thought.

"Gosh, Irwin, he's the third one. I'm an old hand at this. I'm sure I'll be a lot easier on him. Besides, Sean and Ryan are 180 degrees apart in personality. Casey has to fit somewhere in between. So raising him will be a piece of cake."

A few minutes later, Irwin put Casey back in my arms. Then, with tears in his eyes, he said, "I strongly suspect Casey has Down syndrome."

CRASH! Our world fell apart. And with it crumbled all that confidence.

Over the years, our confidence has returned. Through trial and error, we've learned some principles that have helped us in parenting a child with a *difability*, a term I prefer to use because it reminds me to look at Casey's *different* abilities rather than his *dis*, or lack of, abilities.

As it turns out, raising Casey has not been a piece of cake. But in this day and age, raising any child conscientiously is no easy task.

*Source:* From *Cognitive Coping, Families, and Disability* by A. P. Turnbull et al. Copyright © 1993 Brookes Publishing Co., P.O. Box 10624, Baltimore, MD 21285-0624.

---

THE ARRIVAL OF ANY CHILD INTO A FAMILY represents change and the potential for stress as the family adapts to this change. Parental stress appears to be an inevitable and ongoing component of parenthood because it represents loss of resources such as time, energy, and money as well as the potential for daily hassles (Berry & Jones, 1995; Crnic & Greenberg, 1990). However, parenting is also a source of satisfaction, joy and renewal. The arrival and ongoing parenting of a child with a disability combines the predictable parental stress just described with a special circumstance involving loss. The loss of the healthy and developmentally normal child the parents expected to raise may be further complicated by greater than usual loss of resources such as energy, money, sleep, and control (Berry & Zimmerman, 1983; Davis, 1987). Resource and support needs, along with societal attitudes and availability or lack of services, influence how families operate on a day-to-day basis as well as how they adjust and readjust over time.

This chapter discusses feelings experienced by parents both when the child's disability is diagnosed and across the family lifespan. In addition, we consider family functions, or what families do, from the perspective of disability. Finally, we present an overview of the family lifespan as well as the developmental stages of the family member with a disability.

## FAMILIES AND FEELINGS

### FOCUS 1

*What are the feeling states typically experienced by parents?*

Much research has focused on the dynamic of loss, bereavement, and ensuing grief by drawing on stage models based on the work of Kubler-Ross (1969) with people who were terminally ill. These models presume that the birth or diagnosis of a child with a disability brings about an initial period of shock followed by a period of disorganization and disequilibrium which can include feelings of denial, anxiety, guilt, blame, depression, anger, and fear. Bargaining or shopping (for a cure or better diagnosis) may also occur. These negative feelings are eventually replaced by acceptance and reorganization.

This model has been criticized by parents of children with disabilities as being too simplistic (Searl, 1978) and by researchers as being too rigid and overly negative (Blacher, 1984). It is true that parents are not likely to experience these emotions in a orderly fashion, move on, and not look back. In fact, this is not possible considering that feelings about the loss of the expected child are superimposed on the day-to-day tasks of caring for the real child (Berry & Zimmerman, 1983). Furthermore, according to Davis (1987), "The relationship between disability and grief is complex, because it must take into account the variety of disabilities and individuals who live with them" (p. 352).

Yet there is evidence that these families are at risk for anxiety and depression (Breslau, Staruch, & Mortimer, 1982), parental stress (Beckman, 1991; Berry & Jones, 1995), and social isolation (Breslau, 1983). Furthermore, the writings of parents themselves attest to these feelings (Featherstone, 1980; Kupfer, 1982; Speigle & van den Pol, 1993; Turnbull & Turnbull, 1985).

Rather than a systematic stage process, Moses (1987) addresses feeling states that may occur with some order, but may vary according to the characteristics and needs of the child and of the parents themselves. He views the diagnosis of disability as loss because it ends the dreams and plans of the parents both for their child and for themselves as parents. He also believes that parents must be allowed to experience these feelings in order to "separate from the lost dream and generate new, more attainable dreams" (p. 8). Instead of a step-by-step process, he suggests a pattern of experiencing these feeling states (Figure 3.1).

Denial is the first feeling state likely to be experienced by parents when they learn of their child's disability. Denial is psychologically necessary and highly adaptive. It cushions the blow of bad news and softens the initial effects of the parents' shattered dreams. This allows parents time to gather resources—both internal and external—to deal with this crisis. Denial can become maladaptive if parents isolate themselves from others to avoid facing reality or if denial keeps their child away from needed services.

The next feeling state likely to be experienced is anxiety. Anxiety is an unpleasant feeling, but it can be useful. Anxiety can provide energy and mobilize parents to seek answers concerning their child and to seek support in meeting their child's needs and their own needs (Moses, 1987). Anxiety may turn to fear as the parental focus changes from the present situation to the predicted future needs of the child and to the parents' ability to meet these needs. Mothers and fathers may feel a sense of abandonment and vulnerability, but they may then be able to move on and begin to create new dreams (Moses, 1987).

Guilt is another emotion that parents are likely to experience. For example, in some situations the child's condition is a result of an action on the part of one or both parents such as physical or emotional abuse or prenatal substance abuse. Sometimes, negative thoughts or feelings about the child are unrealistically blamed. In other cases, there is genetic causation, which may cause guilt for parents and extended family even though the problem could not have been prevented. A grandmother commented on her family's experience when her grandson was born with multiple disabilities. The baby's diagnosis "was a multisyllabic disease, very rare and genetic. Grandparents and great-grandparents gasped! That diagnosis set both

**FIGURE 3.1**  *Grieving/Coping Model*

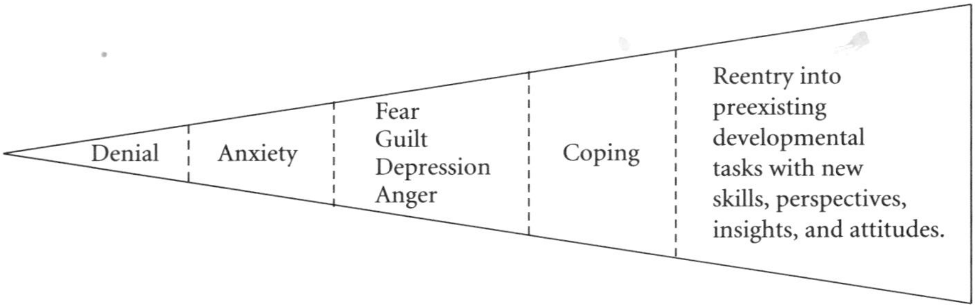

Source: Moses (1991).

sides of the family busy rattling skeletons trying to prove that each was pure and not responsible for the present suffering" (McPhee, 1982, p. 13). Another guilt-producing circumstance may occur when disability results from accident or injury. Adam, an 8-year-old, suffered brain damage as a result of an accident at day camp. His distressed mother said, "I kept thinking, if I hadn't insisted that Adam go to camp that morning, he wouldn't have gotten hurt" (Moore, 1990, p. 7).

Guilt allows parents to assess the reality of these concerns. If an action on the part of the parents was responsible for the child's disability, the parents can begin the hard work of change for the child's and their own benefit. If a genetic condition is present, the parent can seek information to aid in better understanding of the child's condition and for future family planning. In most cases, parents bear no responsibility for what has occurred and did not have the power to achieve a different outcome. Experiencing guilt can be important to gaining a sense of control and a sense of explaining the unexplainable (Moses, 1987).

Depression and anomie (which is a sense of meaninglessness and powerlessness) are also common feelings experienced by parents in response to their child's diagnosis. Parents use words like *devastated* when describing their reaction to their child's diagnosis. This feeling of great sadness as well as the accompanying tears is a necessary part of the work of grieving.

Anger, although natural and necessary, is one of the most disconcerting of the feeling states—both for the person expressing anger and for the people in the path of the anger. But there is reason for parents to feel angry. Their dreams have been shattered, and their sense of justice has been challenged (Moses, 1987). They are also angry about the struggles that lay ahead for their child. Some of this anger may take the form of blame—self-blame, blame of spouse or other family members, or blame of the service delivery system.

Again, these feelings are necessary for adjustment to loss, not reflections of pathology or maladjustment. However, the feelings of parents can frighten and dismay helping professionals. One of the most important lessons for professionals is that they must allow parents to grieve and to feel their feelings. This can be difficult. Parents must be allowed denial until they have the psychological resources to deal with the reality of their child's problems. They must be allowed to feel sad and angry and to express these feelings. However, there are many ways to help parents. Information and referral for services can help alleviate anxiety and fear. Discussion of guilt feelings can lead to reassurance. Also, anger is often justified because the service delivery system or other support system has let parents down. Professionals should try not to be put off by anger or by sadness, but instead be willing to listen and serve as a safety zone where these feelings can be expressed.

Professional support can be especially important because typical sources of support from friends and family may not be available. Friends may stay away because they do not know what to do or say or because they feel their own healthy children would be upsetting to these parents. Family members, especially grandparents, may be dealing with their own grief (Seligman, 1991). In a two-parent family, the marital pair grieves as individuals, perhaps limiting their ability to support one another.

## REOCCURRENCE OF FEELINGS

**✛   FOCUS 2**

*What is meant by the reoccurrence of feeling states and the impact of societal attitudes?*

Although the feelings of grief are likely to be most intense at the time of initial diagnosis, they do not go away. The phenomenon of reoccurrence of feeling states was labeled chronic sorrow by Olshansky (1962) and was later empirically demonstrated by Wikler, Wasow, and Hatfield (1981). Furthermore, grieving was found to be an ongoing feature of rearing a child with intellectual disabilities and more intense for mothers than for fathers in research by Bruce and colleagues (1994).

Comments by parents reinforce this point. A mother, Donna Lea Johnson (1993), expressed these feelings:

> The last really bad depression was Eric's third birthday. I remembered what one of Eric's therapists told me about the grieving process usually taking three years. I guess I thought I could wave a magic wand when Eric turned three and be finished with the grieving process. No such luck. When the realization hit me that I wasn't finished grieving in the allotted three years, I really got depressed. Grieving is the pits! (p. 153)

At a point further along the lifespan, the mother of a 21-year-old woman with severe disabilities commented, "Sometimes it is too painful to see my friend, who has a child the same age. Often I avoid contact with her. Her daughter has her driving license and is at university. This is very painful. It hurts" (Bruce et al., 1994, p. 45). Davis (1987) stressed the need for helping professionals to view chronic sorrow as a natural reaction (rather than expecting grief to be resolved and put aside) because she felt this would lead to offering a continuum of appropriate support services.

Chronic sorrow does not mean continual sorrow, but rather it means vulnerability to recurrent sorrow. Predictable points of reoccurrence are linked to developmental stages (Wikler, Wasow, & Hatfield, 1981), such as "the time he should have started to walk" or "the time she should be attending college," as suggested by the mother of the 21-year-old. Transition points may also be difficult.

For example, anxiety may return when a child leaves a home-based infant program for a center-based preschool program or when a young adult is employed for the first time. But parents also report being blindsided by feelings. Fern Kupfer wrote of her feelings about her son Zach who has severe disabilities (Window 3.2).

The impact of societal attitudes on parental feelings and adjustment should also not be underestimated. Although parents report fewer negative reactions as society becomes better informed about disability, they continue to document a sense of being on public view and of being judged. This was portrayed poignantly by Kathryn Morton (1985), who described grocery shopping with her daughter, Beckie:

> "I took her shopping with me only if I felt up to looking groomed, cheerful, competent, and in command of any situation . . . to look tired and preoccupied with surviving . . . would have turned both of us into objects of pity." (p. 144)

Both negative and overly positive reactions can be distressing to parents. Marilyn Trainer (1991) wrote about the "cringe factor" in describing her feelings when people would extol her and her husband for being "wonderful," "remarkable," and "inspiring" as they raised their daughter with Down syndrome. She felt that people who use these words are influenced by out-of-date attitudes. "They

---

★ **WINDOW 3.2**

### *Changing Seasons in Iowa*

ONLY LAST WEEK, AS SEASONS BEGAN TO SHIFT IN IOWA, and I was sorting out our summer clothes from where they are stored under the big window seat in the yellow bedroom, I came across something in a paper bag pressed down into the back corner of the big chest. I knew immediately what it was: a baseball glove my father had bought for Zach when he was only a few weeks old. I took out the glove, rubbed the soft palm, smelled the leather of that tiny glove. I felt such a rush come, the pain so engulfing that I could no longer stand upright, and I dropped on the bed and lay amid the halter tops and jean cutoffs and terry beach robes, bellowing and crying in rage and despair. Then lying spent in soggy grief, I watched the second hand on the clock radio go around for the third time and said aloud, "You either make it or you don't." I put the glove back in the bag among turtleneck sweaters and put it all back in the chest. . . . Then I went downstairs and started thinking about supper.

*Source:* From *Before and After Zacharian* by F. Kupfer. Copyright © 1982 by Dell Publishing Group, Inc.

want to say something—anything—to make us, and themselves, feel better, so they come up with effusive platitudes. I certainly can't fault people for trying to be kind, but I cringe just the same" (p. 136).

This discussion of feelings puts a somewhat negative spin on parental response to disability. Yet if parents are allowed to grieve, they can move on to coping very effectively and to finding happiness and satisfaction in the parenting experience, as expressed by Casey's mother (see Window 3.1 on page 48).

## FAMILY FUNCTIONS

### ⊞    FOCUS 3

*Identify seven family functions affected by a family member with a disability.*

Family feelings and family relationships are superimposed on the work the family has to do, or how the family functions. Turnbull, Summers, and Brotherson (1984, 1986) delineated seven family functions, or needs, that the family must meet: economic, daily care, recreation, socialization, affection, self-definition, and educational/vocational. These tasks are common to all families but are likely to be affected by the presence of a family member with a disability.

### Economic

Disability is expensive. Medical and therapy services, special equipment, and adapted toys and clothing are examples of the financial impact of disability. Poverty is a risk factor for birth problems and delayed development (Kopp & Kaler, 1989), and the financial demands of disability may drain already limited financial resources for some families, thereby placing them at increased risk.

In addition to bearing added expenses, earning a living may require the presence of both parents in the workplace. Meeting both workplace demands and family responsibilities and acquiring suitable child care are difficult tasks for many parents (Voydanoff, 1993). Families with a son or daughter with disabilities are likely to have more work–family conflict because of the child's medical needs, therapy appointments, and school conferences. These needs are not specific to children. Parents often attend team meetings and medical appointments with their adult sons and daughters, even if they are living away from the family. In addition, parents may have difficulty finding persons and agencies qualified and willing to care for their child, which may become more problematic and expensive as children get older. These family demands can place parents at risk for not receiving raises or promotions or even for losing their jobs. In some families the needs of the child are so high and the care options so limited that one parent must remain unemployed, even if the additional salary is greatly needed. Family members may also be less able to transfer to a new job in another city. An educational and family support system developed in one city may not be available elsewhere.

## Daily Care

A vital function of the family is to provide the elements of daily care, including meals, clothing, maintaining the home, health care, and keeping children safe. The greatest stress for families with a son or daughter with a disability is likely to be simply the amount of work and vigilance required. Medical tasks such as tube feeding or catheterization make daily demands on time and energy. The watchful eye required for a child with hyperactivity or the extra study time and parental help needed by an adolescent with a learning disability, although they may be lovingly given, are time and energy drains. These tasks are superimposed on ordinary tasks such as washing clothes, buying groceries, cleaning the house, and maintaining a yard.

If a physical disability is present, adaptation to the home (e.g., installing ramps) may be a necessary accommodation and an additional expense. Also, some disabilities and medical conditions require special diets (Magol, 1995). Parents then have the challenge of preparing special food and dealing with the child's feelings about it. For example, parents may need to teach their child to cope in circumstances such as a birthday party where he or she is the only child who cannot have ice cream and cake.

An additional task for families is teaching the child with disabilities to participate in his or her own care and, as much as possible, help with the household tasks. This goal was met creatively by Amy's family. Amy, a 12-year-old girl with severe spastic cerebral palsy, had the nightly duty to put the silverware on the table. Her father built her a special silverware tray for her wheelchair and she was able to load the utensils into her tray sections and place it on the table. Her older brother was responsible for putting the silverware into the correct setting because Amy did not have adequate upper extremity control for precise placement (Hallum, 1995, p. 25).

## Recreation

Families need to play together as well. All families face the challenge of carving out playtime from busy schedules and finding activities enjoyable for family members individually and as a group. This challenge is intensified when disability is present. The five hours needed for Dad to play a round of golf or the three hours a week for Mom to attend an aerobics class may simply not be available. The 10-year-old son without disabilities may have to pass up playing on the baseball team because his mother, a single parent, cannot bring his medically fragile younger brother to the game or find suitable child care for him. Lack of community programs, such as summer day camps or swimming programs designed to

---

★ **WINDOW 3.3**

---

## *Kate's Skating Lessons*

BILL WANTED TO HELP HIS 10-YEAR-OLD DAUGHTER, Kate, fulfill her dream of learning to ice skate. Bill knew this would be a challenging task because Kate, like other children with Williams syndrome, had coordination difficulties and problems with "motor planning"—the ability to get one's body to move in the complex ways necessary for activities such as skating. On the other hand, Bill knew that a strong sense of rhythm and love of music were characteristics also associated with Williams syndrome. This gave him an idea about how to approach the task. Bill and Kate hit the ice rink armed with a tape recorder and cassettes of Kate's favorite music. Using the rhythm of the music, Bill was able to help Kate learn to perform the smooth movement sequences the activity required. Those "skating lessons" with Dad paid off. Kate, now 16, is an enthusiastic recreational skater who regularly participates in a sport she can enjoy for many years to come.

*Source:* Reprinted with the expressed consent and approval of *Exceptional Parent*, a monthly magazine for parents and families of children with disabilities and special health care needs. Subscription cost is $32 per year for 12 issues; Call 1-800-247-8080. Offices at 555 Kinderkamack Rd. Oradell, N.J. 07649.

---

include young people with disabilities, is another dilemma that families face. Family vacations may also be difficult because of the importance of a predictable routine for the brother with emotional problems or the importance of being able to access the physician of the sister with a seizure disorder.

Some families, however, have managed creative solutions to these problems such as a family camp with activities for parents, siblings, and children and adolescents with disabilities that utilizes college students majoring in special education as counselors (Berry & Becker, 1981). Another creative recreational opportunity is Camp CAMP (Children's Association for Maximum Potential), an away-from-home camp designed for children with disabilities and special health-care needs (Holmstrand, 1996). Perhaps best of all are the everyday approaches families use to create recreational opportunities and develop recreational skills (Window 3.3).

## Socialization

The family is the arena for developing social relationships and making connections with peers of both the children and the parents. These social relationships provide social skill development for the child or adolescent, support in parenting, and fun for everyone. Families with a son or daughter with disabilities may be socially isolated because of the child's medical needs or the parents' reluctance to venture into a social arena where their child may not be accepted.

Recreation can be a means of socialization for children and adults with disabilities just as it is for people without disabilities. Programs such as Special Olympics (which includes children and adults with developmental disabilities) and Challenger Little League serve this dual purpose, to the delight of the participants and their families. Patty's mother, Marjorie Burke, told about her ball-playing daughter who happens to use a wheelchair.

> Patty has seen enough of team sports to last a lifetime. But it was, of course, always for others. Now, for the first time, the question "Does Patty have a game tonight?" was music to our ears and a symphony to hers! Patty was a team member complete with uniform, team schedule and team photo! She relished every minute of being an active, participating member of the Challenger Division. Most of all, it afforded her that special feeling of belonging, which was a terrific boost for her self-esteem. (Therrien, 1992, p. 21)

Families play an important role in the social development of all children, but for children with disabilities, creative solutions to social challenges may be needed. For example, medical-care needs and socialization needs may not be compatible. Jennifer Titrud's daughter, Laura, who has serious medical problems, wanted to go on a sleepover. By experimenting with her medical-care regime, Mrs. Titrud was able to prepare Laura for an event that was a developmental milestone for both of them. Mrs. Titrud admitted, "the sleepover was probably a much-needed break from an overprotective mother. I did stop by twice that evening to check on her, and I phoned at eight the next morning, but otherwise, I restrained myself admirably" (Titrud, 1995, p. 29).

The parents of adolescents and adults with disabilities must expand the support they give their sons and daughters in terms of socialization and friendships to issues of dating and sexuality. The challenge for parents of teaching their sons and daughters about sexuality involves examining their own values, finding materials appropriate to physical and mental developmental levels that may not be in synch, teaching socially appropriate behavior, and addressing difficult issues such as sexual molestation. Some excellent advice for parents and professionals is offered by Barnes (1982a&b, 1984) and by Ikeler (1990).

The needs of their sons and daughters may limit social opportunities for parents, but this circumstance may also introduce parents to rewarding social contacts when they make connections with other parents of children with disabilities. These connections can provide both social interaction and ongoing support. Jan Spiegle-Mariska (1993), mother of Sara who has Down syndrome, shared these thoughts:

> I have gotten to know many families of children with disabilities. All of them have this unique sense about them. They were ordinary people who faced extraordinary problems. They did so with tears and anger at first, with fists raised to the heavens asking "Why me?" But they have come through it in triumph. They have grown in courage, self-worth, sensitivity, understanding and sharing. Without Sara, I would not have known them, would not have their friendship, a friendship that I cannot now imagine being without. The

depth of sorrow that we have known and shared has somehow made us each a part of the other. In my soul, I will treasure these people forever. (p. 50)

## Affection

The family is the setting to learn to love and be loved. Although families with a child with disabilities share warm examples of love given and received, stress, frustration, and fatigue may make intimacy and loving interactions more complicated among all family members, but they may also be more meaningful. Bud Mariska (1993) wrote of his love for his daughter, Sara, who has Down syndrome, and of her love for him, especially her ability to cheer him up after a stressful day. "She . . . gives me hugs and tells me that she loves me, all the while patting me on the shoulder . . . she starts to do funny tricks until I smile. With that task completed, she goes on to her next 'happiness assignment'" (p. 43).

## Self-Definition

The family plays a part in establishing self-identity for all family members. This, too, can be affected by the presence of disability. The limitations imposed by the disability as well as societal attitudes can have a negative influence on the child's self-definition. The family, however, can have a buffering effect by emphasizing strengths and providing or acquiring help for areas of need. Tom Hershey (1995), at age 32, gave his parents credit for helping him achieve his considerable success when he said, "My disability . . . gets more attention from other people than it does from me. My parents taught me not to be afraid of the unknown and to be inventive about creating ways to be self-sufficient" (p. 20). The self-definition of Mom and Dad as parents is also vulnerable. For example, parents of an infant who is difficult to feed and difficult to console may define themselves as inadequate parents, or the parents of a teenager who is teased may feel frustrated and helpless.

Research in issues concerning self-esteem and development of self-identity for children and adults with disabilities and their parents is quite limited. The impact of inclusion (school and recreational programs that serve children and adolescents with and without disabilities together) on self-esteem has been targeted as an important area for research by Stainback et al. (1994). These authors stress the need for choice concerning friendships and group affiliations, with positive outcomes available both through mainstream opportunities and through association with others with disabilities.

## Educational/Vocational

For all children, the family is the training ground for developing beliefs and values as well as for learning life skills. The family has primary responsibility for early learning and the skills that lead to increasing independence, such as helping children learn to feed and dress themselves. The family also influences early cognitive, motor, and social development. As the child gets older, the family shares the responsibility for teaching with the educational system. As the child becomes an adolescent and then an adult, the family provides advice on areas of study and career choice.

For a child with a disability, these direct and supportive roles are even more important. The child may enter the formal educational system shortly after birth, and parents may continue to provide advice and assistance even after their adult son or daughter is successfully employed. This can be a demanding, frustrating, rewarding, and sometimes humorous role, as reported by Josh's mother, Lynn Fay (Window 3.4). Parental involvement in education is a role that clearly predicts improved outcomes for their sons and daughters with disabilities (Berger, 1995).

The preceding discussion of family functions suggests ways in which families who are rearing a child with disabilities may need understanding and support. Referrals to agencies providing financial assistance and/or child care is sometimes appropriate. Professionals can also help by providing information about or helping to create recreational opportunities that include children with and without disabilities, especially because recreational programs can foster socialization and self-esteem. It is important to keep in mind the heterogeneity of families. Some may need help in several areas, others in only a few. A particular family may need a great amount of help at one point in time and less help later. In addition, a family crisis may mean that a family which was meeting family needs very well suddenly is not.

---

★ **WINDOW 3.4**

## *Academic Enlightenment*

WHEN JOSH WAS ABOUT FOUR, he finally learned to count to twenty. We were *really* proud of him. All those hours of hard work had finally paid off. He could read those numbers in any order, and counting was one of his favorite pastimes.

One night, all our friends had gathered in our home for a formal holiday dinner party. It had been a pleasant evening. The kids had cooperated, and chaos had been kept to a minimum. As we enjoyed a final cup of coffee around the big harvest table, Josh climbed up on to my lap and gave me one of his big sloppy kisses. As a lull in the conversation occurred, Josh pointed to my chest. "One! Two!" he counted proudly and loudly. When the laughter subsided, and all eyes were wiped dry, my husband sweetly remarked that not only was Josh extraordinarily brilliant, but his eyesight must be much better than we had previously assumed! All in all, I couldn't be *too* upset. Hey the kid was learning!

*Source:* Reprinted with the expressed consent and approval of *Exceptional Parent*, a monthly magazine for parents and families of children with disabilities and special health care needs. Subscription cost is $32 per year for 12 issues; Call 1-800-247-8080. Offices at 555 Kinderkamack Rd. Oradell, N.J. 07649.

## FAMILIES OVER THE LIFESPAN

**⊕   FOCUS 4**

*What is the purpose of studying families that include a member with disabilities in terms of the family life cycle?*

Just as each individual has a life cycle, the family can be studied in terms of a family life cycle (Carter & McGoldrick, 1989). This approach provides a framework for predicting family roles, functions, and goals at various times as well as for delineating family transition points. For example, the family with a newborn infant has different goals and strategies for reaching those goals than the family that is launching its youngest daughter to live on her own. The life cycles of individual family members, including physical and cognitive development as well as the achievement of developmental tasks (Erikson, 1963), take place within the framework of the family life cycle. For example, at a given point the family may be experiencing the growing independence of adolescent children, the midlife crisis of a parent, and the fragile health of elderly grandparents.

Families that include a member with a disability have different needs and strengths at various points in the family life cycle. Several authors (Eisenberg, Sutkin, & Jansen, 1984; Gath, 1993; Lesar, Trivette, & Dunst, 1996; Orr et al., 1993) have addressed the impact of a family member with disabilities on the family life cycle. They stress the importance of a perspective that focuses on the age of the family member with disabilities, the developmental tasks of that age, and the impact of disability on the individual life cycles of each family member and on the family life cycle. The work of psychological theorist Erik Erikson (1963) provides a framework for studying psychosocial development from infancy to adulthood. We use this framework in the next section to describe the impact of disability on child and family development over the lifespan (Table 3.1).

**TABLE 3.1**    *Erikson's Eight Stages of Development*

| Developmental Period | Psychosocial Task |
| --- | --- |
| 1. Infancy | Trust vs. mistrust |
| 2. Early childhood | Autonomy vs. shame and doubt |
| 3. Preschool age | Initiative vs. guilt |
| 4. School age | Industry vs. inferiority |
| 5. Adolescence | Identity vs. role confusion |
| 6. Young adulthood | Intimacy vs. isolation |
| 7. Adulthood | Generativity vs. stagnation |
| 8. Senescense | Ego integrity vs. despair |

*Source:* Adapted from Erikson (1963).

---

### ⊕     FOCUS 5

*Identify the developmental tasks of infancy through adulthood and the impact of disability on these tasks.*

## Infancy, Early Childhood, and Preschool

According to Erikson, the developmental task of the first year of life is the development of trust. The developmental task of the second and third years of life is autonomy, followed by initiative in the fourth and fifth years. The quality of the relationship between the infant and the parents predicts the child's sense of the world as an essentially secure place where basic needs will be met.

If this trust is established, the toddler can begin to move away from the parents and gain a sense of autonomy and self-sufficiency in activities such as walking, talking, feeding, toileting, and exploring. Then the preschool child will initiate activities with confidence and find pleasure in achievement. This trust relationship during the first year leads to parent-infant attachment, and secure attachment in the 1-year-old predicts a more socially competent 3-year-old (Berger, 1994). This developmentally competent 3-year-old then has the developmental base for growth in physical, cognitive, and psychosocial domains.

Attachment is an affectional tie between parent and child that binds them together and endures over time. Infants show attachment by "proximity-seeking" behaviors such as following the parent or climbing up onto his or her lap and "contact-maintaining" behaviors such as resisting being put down. Parents show attachment by keeping a watchful eye and by responding affectionately, sensitively, and appropriately to the baby (Ainsworth & Bell, 1970).

Medical problems that impose both separation between parent and baby and rigorous and exhausting care needs can place attachment at risk. The anxiety that parents experience in these situations can undermine self-esteem and the parents' trust in their abilities to parent, thereby interfering with the baby's development of trust. In addition, parental depression can interfere with responsiveness and the development of synchrony between parent and infant (Field, 1987). For infants, development of the central nervous system, vision, and hearing are important for responding socially to their parents. Impairment in any or all of these areas can disturb this synchronized parent–child "dance." For example, one way that parent and baby bond is by gazing at one another, which can be disrupted by a baby's visual impairment. The feeding experience is also a key component of parent–infant bonding and may be disrupted when a child is difficult to feed (Gath, 1993). Neurological impairment can cause infants to be difficult to hold or resistant to being held or touched, which can be extremely confusing and disheartening to parents. The baby's developmental delays in smiling and vocalizing can leave the parents "dancing" alone.

A baby who is insecurely attached may be delayed in the development of autonomy. This baby may be reluctant to explore and overly dependent on the parents. Of course, motor and cognitive developmental delays can also limit independence. Furthermore, parents can be confused about when to expect developmental independence and when to protect. Parents of a medically fragile infant may find it difficult later not to hover over their energetic 2-year-old or to allow their 4-year-old to attend preschool.

Professionals can support parents by respecting the difficult start in life that has occurred not only for the child, but for the parents. This child will need appropriate medical care and developmental interventions, perhaps for the rest of his or her life. But another lifelong need is for the parents to fall in love with the baby and to find joy and satisfaction in this parenting role. The need for professional support that strengthens parent–child relationships was addressed by Bernstein, Hans, and Percansky (1991), who stressed the importance of mutual competence, or increasingly effective interaction between the parent and the infant. This competence mediates risk for both parent and child. Early intervention programs that focus on the physical, cognitive, and social development of the child are particularly valuable in supporting child autonomy and initiative. Programs that stress parent training and value parent input promote this development as well as the parent–child bond.

## Middle Childhood

For all children during middle childhood, the world further expands beyond the family. The child's increasing competence and independence means the child can have school, neighborhood, social, and athletic experiences with peers as well as with teachers, coaches, and other adults outside the family. The developmental task at this stage is industry, which means mastery of skills ranging from academic to athletic. It is typically a smooth developmental phase; however, school and friendships are extremely important and school failure or rejection by peers can seem crushing (Berger, 1994).

Children with disabilities are vulnerable to both school failure and peer rejection. Coordinated support from family and school is vital to achieving industry rather than inferiority. Families can work with the school system to design and implement programs in which the child will experience success, not just academic success, but progress in adaptive behaviors and personal-social relationships. Indeed, parents' satisfaction with school programs has been shown to correspond with student progress in self-sufficiency and personal-social responsibility (Saint-Laurent & Fournier, 1993). Furthermore, social, rather than physical, problems were found to be most stressful for both children and their mothers (Tackett, Kerr, & Helmstadter, 1990).

Parents face difficult decisions concerning the balance between challenge and stress when their son or daughter participates in school, athletic, and social activities with peers without disabilities. When their children participate in challenging school and social activities, families can provide the safety zone for their children—the place to turn to for advice and support or to dry tears when failure or teasing occurs. Professionals can assist families in this role by helping them to become advocates for their children, intervening between the child and the broad world beyond the family. Professionals can also help parents help their sons and daughters begin the role of self-advocate so they will have skills and strengths in situations in which their families are not immediately available (Alper, Schloss, & Schloss, 1996).

## Adolescence

Adolescence is a time of rapid physical and social change. The developmental task of adolescence is identity. Adolescents must form their own identity, distinct from their parents, in order to accomplish the task of separation from the family at the end of adolescence. The adolescent will test his or her autonomy and seek emotional independence and an orientation toward the future. This task is accomplished, in part, through greater involvement with and dependence on peers. Self-esteem for the adolescent is contingent on positive comparisons between self and peers.

Lowered self-esteem and anxiety concerning body image may be major problems for adolescents with disabilities and concerns for their parents. These adolescents may worry their parents further by resisting medical compliance (e.g., taking medication, following a special diet) because it sets them apart from their peers.

Another challenge, faced by all families of adolescents, but with particular saliency for families with adolescents with disabilities, is deciding how much autonomy is appropriate. These parents are faced with the dilemma of a son or daughter who has needed extra protection and parental involvement and now needs more independence to form his or her own identity (Barnes, 1982b). They are also faced with issues such as providing sex education for a son or daughter who may have a grownup body, but limited ability to understand the physical changes taking place. Other concerns expressed by parents of adolescents with disabilities include lack of community-based supports, lack of social opportunities for their sons and daughters, how to prepare for the transition from school to adult life, and future work opportunities (Brandt & Berry, 1991; Lehman & Roberto, 1996; McNair & Rusch, 1991).

Families may need a great deal of support during this developmental stage. Guidance in determining what is appropriate involvement and what is overprotection is important for many families. Other complicated issues that may be faced by some families include behavior problems of the adolescent with disabilities, which are made more challenging by hormonal changes and increased physical strength. Or an adolescent sibling without disabilities may express embarrassment or rejection toward a brother or sister with disabilities (Tolmas, 1986). Families may also profit from support that helps them learn to listen to their adolescent sons and daughters and involve them in decision making. It is encouraging that research which asked adolescents with disabilities about family involvement during transition to adult life indicates that family involvement is important and valued (Morningstar, Turnbull, & Turnbull, 1996).

## Adulthood

Families typically weather the storm of adolescence and form new adult-to-adult relationships with their sons and daughters. These adults now encounter the developmental tasks of forming intimate relationships with spouses, friends, and their own children and generativity or productivity through work and caring for or giving to others. Adulthood typically involves living apart from the family of origin and becoming financially independent through employment.

Disability complicates the achievement of the developmental tasks of adulthood and complicates family relationships at this lifespan stage. Families are faced with the dilemma of letting go but staying involved (Mitchell, 1981). Issues faced by adults with disabilities and their families include determining appropriate living arrangements and levels of independence, family support for adult social relationships that may involve dating and marriage, and employment and financial arrangements. Some adults with disabilities need relatively little support. For example, adults with learning disabilities may need emotional and academic support from their families as they negotiate college and job applications or financial help for tutoring or therapy (Greenbaum, Graham, & Scales, 1995). Other adults may need 24-hour care, which may be provided by the family or by an agency.

If the family continues to provide care for an adult with disabilities, professionals can help with issues of stress and burnout as well as with long-range planning including financial and care arrangements for the time when parents are no longer able to provide care (Brunetti, 1995; Smith, Tobin, & Fulmer, 1995). These families may also need help accessing community programs for recreation and socialization for their sons and daughters. If care is provided by an agency, family input and family advocacy is still important, and professionals should seek ways to facilitate this involvement (Baker & Blacher, 1988; Berry, 1995; Blacher & Baker, 1992). Siblings may play more active roles at this point in both direct care and as advocates for their sister or brother, or they may not, leaving these responsibilities to aging parents or to agencies within the community. Recent research indicates that affective relationships are likely to be strong and close between nondisabled siblings and their brothers and sisters with disabilities; however, functional assistance provided by these siblings is minimal (Pruchno, Patrick, & Burant, 1996). These research findings imply that sibling roles in later years should be addressed earlier as care plans are developed.

Parents can have a role in employment of their adult sons and daughters as well. Parental attitudes and expectancies are important for vocational success (Turnbull & Turnbull, 1988) so parent involvement and advocacy in all steps of the vocational process is vital. Parents can help with planning and preparation, which should begin in adolescence. They can share their knowledge of their son or daughter in terms of abilities and preferences during the job selection and training process, and they can help with skill development.

For a person with a disability, the family will typically be the most important life influence day by day and the only constant over time. Organized support for families is more likely to be available for parents of young children with disabilities and tends to decrease as the children grow older. Professionals have the challenge of responding to the needs of the individual with disabilities and his or her family throughout the lifespan. We address disability and family dynamics in depth at each lifespan stage in Chapters 7 through 10.

# REVIEW

*FOCUS 1: What are the feeling states typically experienced by parents?*

- Parents experience the loss of the child they expected to have or a "shattered dream."
- Feelings about the loss of the expected child are superimposed on the day-to-day tasks of caring for the real child.
- Parents are likely to experience feelings of denial, anxiety, fear, guilt, depression, and anger.

*FOCUS 2: What is meant by the reoccurrence of feeling states and the impact of societal attitudes?*

- Parents are vulnerable to recurrent sorrow about their child's disability.
- This sorrow may occur at predictable developmental points or at totally unexpected times.
- Negative attitudes and experiences with society can contribute to the distress experienced by parents.

*FOCUS 3: Identify seven family functions affected by a family member with a disability.*

- The care needs of the child with disabilities may make economic demands on a family as well as limit their economic opportunities.
- Providing daily care for a son or daughter with disabilities can be a source of stress because of the amount of work and vigilance required.

- Recreational outlets are important for all family members, but may be difficult to achieve due to lack of resources.

- Socialization of both children and parents may be limited by the social isolation imposed by the disability.

- Giving and receiving affection is as important for these families as for any others, but may be made more difficult by stress, frustration, and fatigue.

- Limitations imposed by the disability and negative societal attitudes can have a negative influence on the self-definition of the child and other family members.

- Supporting their child's educational/vocational training is a demanding but rewarding role for these parents. Parental involvement in this area is predictive of improved outcomes for their sons and daughters.

*FOCUS 4: What is the purpose of studying families that include a member with disabilities in terms of the family life cycle?*

- Family stress and family support can be addressed from a perspective that focuses on the age of the child and the developmental tasks of that age.

- The impact of disability can be assessed in terms of the life stage of the family member with a disability and the life stage of other family members.

*FOCUS 5: Identify the developmental tasks of infancy through adulthood and the impact of disability on these tasks.*

- The developmental task of the infant is trust, for the toddler, autonomy, and for the young child, initiative.

- Disability may interfere with parent-infant attachment. Delays in motor and cognitive development, limited opportunities for socialization, and parental tendencies to overprotect may influence the development of independence.

- The developmental task of middle childhood is industry.

- During middle childhood, vulnerability to academic problems and rejection by peers may result in lowering of self-esteem.

- The task of adolescence is formation of identity leading to separation from family.

- Issues of body image and need to conform to peers may trouble the adolescent with disabilities. Decisions about autonomy may be troubling to parents.

- The developmental tasks of adults include the formation of intimate relationships outside of the family of origin and the achievement of generativity through vocational and avocational activities and service to others.

• Disability and society's response to disability may limit the achievement of these tasks. Lack of opportunities for independent or supported living and employment are particularly problematic.

## REFERENCES

Ainsworth, M. D. S., & Bell, S. M. (1970). Attachment, exploration, and separation: Illustrated by the behavior of one-year-olds in a strange situation. *Child Development, 41*, 49–67.

Alper, S., Schloss, P. J., & Schloss, C. N. (1996). Families of children with disabilities in elementary and middle school: Advocacy models and strategies. *Exceptional Children, 62*, 261–270.

Baker, B. L., & Blacher, J. (1988). Family involvement with community residential programs. In M. P. Janicki, W. W. Krauss, & M. M. Seltzer (Eds.), *Community residences for persons with developmental disabilities: Here to stay* (pp. 173–188). Baltimore: Brookes.

Barnes, K. (1982a, February). Life with our changing teenager. *Exceptional Parent*, pp. 37–39.

Barnes, K. (1982b, December). Mother to daughter: Woman to woman talks. *Exceptional Parent*, pp. 47–49.

Barnes, K. (1984, December). Sex education. Let's not pretend. *Exceptional Parent*, pp. 43–44.

Beckman, P. J. (1991). Comparisons of mothers' and fathers' perception of the effect of young children with and without disabilities. *American Journal on Mental Retardation, 95*, 585–595.

Berger, E. H. (1995). *Parents as partners in education* (4th ed.). Englewood Cliffs, NJ: Merrill.

Berger, K. S. (1994). *The developing person through the life span* (3rd ed.). New York: Worth.

Bernstein, V. J., Hans, S. L., & Percansky, C. (1991). Advocating for the young child in need through strengthening the parent-child relationship. *Journal of Clinical Child Psychology, 20*, 28–41.

Berry, J. O. (1995). Families and deinstitutionalization: An application of Bronfenbrenner's social ecology model. *Journal of Counseling and Development, 73*, 379–383.

Berry, J. O., & Becker, M. A. (1981, April). Family camping. *Exceptional Parent*, pp. S15, S18–S19.

Berry, J. O., & Jones, W. H. (1995). The Parental Stress Scale: Initial psychometric findings. *Journal of Personal and Social Relationships, 12*, 463–472.

Berry, J. O., & Zimmerman, W. W. (1983). The stage model revisited. *Rehabilitation Literature, 44*, 275–277, 320.

Blacher, J. (1984). Sequential stages of parental adjustment to the birth of a child with handicaps: Fact or artifact? *Mental Retardation, 22*, 55–68.

Blacher, J., & Baker, B. L. (1992). Toward meaningful family involvement in out-of-home placement settings. *Mental Retardation, 30*, 35–43.

Brandt, M. D., & Berry, J. O. (1991). Transitioning college bound students with LD. *Intervention in School and Clinic, 26*, 297–301.

Breslau, N. (1983). Care of disabled children and women's time use. *Medical Care, 21*, 620–629.

Breslau, N., Staruch, K. S., & Mortimer, E. A. (1982). Psychological distress in mothers of disabled children. *American Journal of Diseases of Childhood, 136*, 682–686.

Bruce, E. J., Schultz, C. L., Smyrnios, K. X., & Schultz, N. C. (1994). Grieving related to development: A preliminary comparison of three age cohorts of parents of children with intellectual disability. *British Journal of Medical Psychology, 67*, 37–52.

Brunetti, F. L. (1995, December). Getting started. *Exceptional Parent*, pp. 41, 43–44.

Carter, B., & McGoldrick, M. (1989). *The changing family life cycle*. Boston: Allyn & Bacon.

Crnic, K. A., & Greenberg, M. T. (1990). Minor parenting stresses with young children. *Child Development, 54*, 209–217.

Davis, B. H. (1987). Disability and grief. *Social Casework, 68*, 352–357.

Eisenberg, M. G., Sutkin, L. C., & Jansen, M. A. (Eds.). (1984). *Chronic illness and disability through the life span*. New York: Springer.

Erikson, E. H. (1963). *Childhood and society* (2nd ed.). New York: Norton.

Fay, L. K. (1994, April). Sense of humor required. *Exceptional Parent*, pp. 34–36.

Featherstone, H. (1980). *A difference in the family*. New York: Basic.

Field, T. M. (1987). Affective and interactive disturbances in infants. In J. D. Osofsky (Ed.), *Handbook of infant development* (2nd ed.) (pp. 972–1005). New York: Wiley.

Gath, A. (1993). Changes that occur in families as children with intellectual disability grow up. *International Journal of Disability, Development and Education, 40*, 167–174.

Greenbaum, B., Graham, S., & Scales, W. (1995). Adults with learning disabilities: Educational and social experiences during college. *Exceptional Children, 61*, 460–471.

Hallum, A. (1995). Disability and the transition to adulthood: Issues for the disabled child, the family, and the pediatrician. *Current Problems in Pediatrics, 25*, 12–46?

Hershey, T. (1995, July). Role models: My family was a team. *Exceptional Parent*, pp. 16, 18, 20.

Holmstrand, K. E. (1996, March). Camp CAMP: A camping experience for every child. *Exceptional Parent*, pp. 66, 68–71.

Ikeler, B. (1990, July/August). Teaching about sexuality. *Exceptional Parent*, pp. 24–26.

Johnson, D. L. (1993). Grieving is the pits. In G. H. S. Singer & L. E. Powers (Eds.), *Families, disability, and empowerment* (pp. 151–154). Baltimore: Brookes.

Kopp, C. B., & Kaler, S. R. (1989). Risk in infancy: Origins and implications. *American Psychologist, 44*, 224–230.

Kubler-Ross, E. (1969). *On death and dying*. New York: Macmillan.

Kupfer, F. (1982). *Before and after Zachariah*. New York: Delacorte.

Lehman, J. P., & Roberto, K. A. (1996). Comparison of factors influencing mother's perceptions about the futures of their adolescent children with and without disabilities. *Mental Retardation, 34*, 27–38.

Lesar, S., Trivette, C. M., & Dunst, C. J. (1996). Families of children and adolescents with special needs across the lifespan. *Exceptional Children, 62*, 197–199.

Levine, K. (1995, October). Beyond labels: How to use information about specific diagnoses. *Exceptional Parent*, pp. 38–40, 43.

Magol, M. (1995, August). Food for thought: Helping your child on a special diet eat right. *Exceptional Parent*, p. 52.

Mariska, B. (1993). Daddy, phone's busy. In J. A. Spiegle & R. A. van den Pol (Eds.), *Making changes: Family voices on living with disabilities* (pp. 42–45). Cambridge: Brookline.

McNair, J., & Rusch, F. R. (1991). Parent involvement in transition programs. *Mental Retardation, 29*, 93–101.

McPhee, N. (1982, June). A very special magic: A grandparent's delight. *Exceptional Parent*, pp. 13–16.

Mitchell, C. (1981, December). Separating from our children. *Exceptional Parent*, pp. 15–19.

Moore, A. (1990). *Broken arrow boy*. Kansas City: Landmark.

Morningstar, M. E., Turnbull, A. P., & Turnbull, H. R. (1996). What do students with disabilities tell us about the importance of family involvement in the transition from school to adult life? *Exceptional Children, 62,* 249–260.

Morton, K. (1985). Identifying the enemy—A parent's complaint. In H. R. Turnbull and A. P. Turnbull (Eds.), *Parents speak out: Then and now* (pp. 143–147). Columbus: Merrill.

Moses, K. (1991). *Shattered dreams and growth: Loss and the art of grief counseling.* Evanston: Resource Networks.

Moses, K. (1987, Spring). The impact of childhood disability: The parent's struggle. *Ways,* pp. 6–10.

O'Halloran, J. M. (1993). Welcome to our family, Casey Patrick. In A. P. Turnbull, J. M. Patterson, S. K. Behr, D. L. Murphy, J. G. Marquis, & M. J. Blue-Banning (Eds.), *Cognitive coping, families and disability* (pp. 19–29). Baltimore: Brookes.

Olshansky, S. (1962). Chronic sorrow: A response to having a mentally defective child. *Social Casework, 43,* 190–193.

Orr, R. R., Cameron, S. J., Dobson, L. A., & Day, D. M. (1993). Age-related changes in stress experienced by families with a child who has developmental delays. *Mental Retardation, 31,* 171–176.

Pruchno, R. A., Patrick, J. H., & Burant, C. J. (1996). Aging women and their children with chronic disabilities: Perceptions of sibling involvement and effects on well-being. *Family Relations, 45,* 318–326.

Saint-Laurent, L., & Fournier, A. L. (1993). Children with intellectual disabilities: Parents' satisfaction with school. *Developmental Disabilities Bulletin, 21,* 15–33.

Searl, S. J. (1978, April). Stages of parent reaction. *Exceptional Parent,* pp. 27–29.

Seligman, M. (1991). Grandparents of disabled grandchildren: Hopes, fears, and adaptation. *Families in Society, 72,* 147–152.

Smith, G. C., Tobin, S. S., & Fulmer, E. M. (1995). Elderly mothers caring at home for offspring with mental retardation: A model of permanency planning. *American Journal on Mental Retardation, 99,* 487–499.

Spiegle, J. A., & van den Pol, R. A. (1993). *Making changes: Family voices on living with disabilities.* Cambridge: Brookline.

Spiegle-Mariska, J. A. (1993). It's OK because she's Sara. In J. A. Spiegle and R. A. van den Pol (Eds.), *Making changes: Family voices on living with disabilities* (pp. 46–52). Cambridge: Brookline.

Stainback, S., Stainback, W., East, K., & Sapon-Shevin, M. (1994). A commentary on inclusion and the development of a positive self-identity by people with disabilities. *Exceptional Children, 60,* 486–490.

Tackett, P., Kerr, N., & Helmstadter, G. (1990, July/August/September). Stresses as perceived by children with physical disabilities and their mothers. *Journal of Rehabilitation,* pp. 30–34.

Therrien, V. (1992, April/May). Challenger little league: It's a hit! *Exceptional Parent,* pp. 20–22.

Titrud, J. (1995, November). The first sleepover. *Exceptional Parent,* pp. 28–29.

Tolmas, H. C. (1986). Adolescent disability and family dynamics. *International Journal of Adolescent Medicine and Health, 2,* 197–209.

Trainer, M. (1991). *Differences in common: Straight talk on mental retardation, Down syndrome, and life.* Rockville, MD: Woodbine.

Turnbull, A. P., Summers, J. A., & Brotherson, M. J. (1984). *Working with families with disabled members: A family systems approach.* Lawrence: University of Kansas, Kansas University Affiliated Facility.

Turnbull, A. P., Summers, J. A., & Brotherson, M. J. (1986). Family life cycle: Theoretical and empirical implications and future directions for families with mentally retarded members. In J. J. Gallagher & P. Vietze (Eds.), *Families of handicapped persons* (pp. 45–66). Baltimore: Brookes.

Turnbull, A. P., & Turnbull, H. R. (1985). *Parents speak out: Then and now* (2nd ed.). Columbus: Merrill.

Turnbull, A. P., & Turnbull, H. R. (1988). Toward greater expectations for vocational opportunities: Family-Professional Partnerships. *Mental Retardation, 26,* 337–342.

Voydanoff, P. (1993). Work and family relationships. In T. H. Brubaker (Ed.), *Family relations: Challenges for the future* (pp. 98–111). Newbury Park, CA: Sage.

Wikler, L., Wasow, M., & Hatfield, E. (1981). Chronic sorrow revisited: Parent vs. professional depiction of the adjustment of parents of mentally retarded children. *American Journal of Orthopsychiatry, 51,* 63–70.

# CHAPTER FOUR

# Stress, Coping, and Family Support

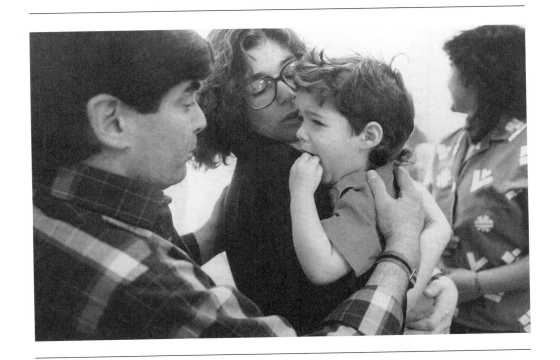

---

★ **WINDOW 4.1**
_____

### *Laura and Her Mother*

SOMETIMES I WONDERED IF I WAS REALLY OF HELP TO LAURA in her moments of extreme
fear or anguish. One unforgettable, touching moment gave me my answer.

Laura's legs were in casts from toes to knees after the surgery; the doctors had allowed room in the casts for swelling, but Laura's feet and legs, despite being elevated,
began to swell far more than expected. The pain woke her out of her morphine sleep; she
began to whimper and then to scream. The puffy toes peeping out of the cotton began
to turn bluish. The nurse ran for the phone. When the breathless resident rushed in, she
took one look and muttered, "I wish they had told me to bring a cast saw," and hurried
out to find one.

(The minutes of waiting were endless. I had never seen Laura in such overwhelming
pain. The screams were literally ripped out of her as the pressure increased; she was so
in the grip of pain that it was as if she had been transported beyond my reach. I tried to
encircle her with my arms, saying over and over, "Mommy's here; mommy's here. The
doctor is hurrying." She seemed not to hear me.)

Now cast saws were chief among Laura's true hates; the noise had always frightened
her out of her wits, and no amount of demonstrating had ever assured her that she
would not be hurt by the blade. I braced myself for a grim scene as the resident plugged
in the saw. I brought my face in front of Laura's and told her, "Honey, the doctor must
cut the casts to give your legs room and stop the squeezing and bad hurting. You *absolutely must* hold still, but you can scream as much as you need to, and you can hold my
hands as tight as you want to, as long as you don't move your legs."

White and sweating, Laura took my hands and gasped, "Thanks; it's good to have a
friend like you."

*Source:* Copyright © 1992 by Brookline Books.

---

THE BIRTH OF A CHILD WITH DISABILITIES, or later diagnosis of disability or illness,
produces stress associated with the life change this event brings to the family.
The perpetual process of meeting the needs of this child contributes to stress as a
dynamic state that involves an ongoing relationship between the organism—in
this case Mom, Dad, and other family members—and the environment (Lazarus
& Folkman, 1984). This environment includes the child's needs (which may be
extensive), balancing those needs with the needs of the rest of the family, and interactions with the community beyond the family. The topic of stress experienced by caregiving families has gained attention during the last decade because
of the increased focus on normalization for families (Winkler, 1988). Evidence of
this normalization is shown by nationwide closure of institutions for persons
with mental retardation and other disabilities and development of community-
based living and employment services. Further evidence is found in the expansion
of educational services, including ages served, types of services available, and eli-

gibility for services. Increased family care and family involvement—although a laudable accomplishment—can mean increased family stress. An understanding of the nature of this stress, the coping abilities or resilience of families, and how to best support families is crucial for professionals providing services for individuals with disabilities and their families. This chapter focuses on a theoretical and demographic view of what constitutes stress, how families respond to stress, and how professionals can help families cope.

## UNDERSTANDING STRESS

⊕ **FOCUS 1**

*Identify frameworks for studying stress as experienced by families with a member with disabilities.*

### Stress, Appraisal, and Coping

The work of Lazarus and his colleagues has made and continues to make a major contribution to the formulation of stress theory. Three major types of stress, or stressors, have been delineated (Lazarus & Cohen, 1977): (1) major changes affecting large numbers of people, such as war or natural disasters such as floods or earthquakes; (2) major changes affecting one or a few people; and (3) daily hassles. Numbers 2 and 3 are particularly relevant for families that include a member with disabilities because disability brings about major change for the family system and increased (sometimes enormously increased) daily responsibilities for the caregivers within the family.

Lazarus and Folkman (1984) further defined stress as follows: "Psychological stress is a particular relationship between the person and the environment that is appraised by the person as taxing or exceeding his or her resources and endangering his or her well-being" (p. 19). Cognitive appraisal of what is stressful is vital to understanding family stress and helping families cope with stressful situations. Coping involves managing the demands of the person-environment relationship that are appraised as stressful and dealing with emotions that occur in this stressful situation (Lazarus & Folkman, 1984).

### ABCX Models

The original ABCX family stress model was developed by Hill (1949, 1958). In this model, A was the stressor event, B was the family's resources to meet the crisis, and C was the family's definition of the event (appraisal). In Hill's model, C interacted with A and B to produce X, the crisis. For example, the birth of a child with a cleft palate would be A, the stressor event, which would include both normative stress (the family transition involved in the birth of a child) and nonnormative stress (the medical and specialized care needs of this infant). Family resources (B) would include availability of medical care and health insurance. The definition or appraisal by the family (C) might be that this situation is terrible because funds are not available to provide the complete medical and cosmetic interventions the child needs. This would produce X, the crisis.

McCubbin and Patterson (1982, 1983a, 1983b) focused on appraisal and expanded Hill's work in their theoretical work on stress involving families of children with disabilities or chronic illness. In the McCubbin and Patterson double ABCX model, the C factor is expanded (cC) and defined as "the family's perception of the original stressor event, plus the pile-up of other stressors and strains ('aA' factor), plus its perception of its resources ('bB' factor)" (Patterson, 1993, p. 224). This allows for both primary appraisal of the stressfulness of the event and secondary appraisal of capacities for managing the stress and strain (demands) stemming from the event. This model addresses cognitive appraisal of the event, behavioral action that might be taken in response to the event, and coherence. The family's sense of coherence is the "ability to balance control and trust—that is, knowing when to take charge and when to trust in or believe in the authority and/or power of others" (Patterson, 1993, p. 224).

If this model is applied to the example of the family with a baby born with a cleft palate, the family may already be under stress because the parents are unemployed (aA). They may, however, be able to appraise (cC) not just their own limited financial resources, but their capacity for problem solving (bB). The mother might remember that a social worker came to speak to her parenting preparation class and told of community resources available to children and families. The cognitive appraisal of the situation as very difficult then combines with a belief in problem-solving ability and the designation of an action that can be taken to secure assistance. This results in coherence between personal control and the power or ability of others to provide help.

### FAAR Model

Another model useful in understanding family stress is the family adjustment and adaptation response model (FAAR) (Patterson, 1988, 1989), which emphasizes family adaptation over time. It also supports the idea of positive outcomes or the salutogenic perspective. This perspective comes from the work of Antonovsky (1979, 1993) and means constructive processes or positive responses as opposed to pathogenic.

The FAAR model, like the double ABCX model, emphasizes cognitive appraisal or the meanings that families use in adapting to rearing a child with disabilities. Both situational meanings and global meanings are considered. Situational meanings refer to how the family defines the demands of the situation and their capacity to meet the demands. Global meanings go beyond the immediate situation. They are a more stable set of cognitive beliefs about relationships within the family and relationships between the family and the broader community and are referred to as "family schema" (Patterson, 1993, p. 225).

This model includes the adjustment phase during which families respond to crisis by making minor, or first-order, changes that will reduce demands and/or increase capabilities to meet demands so balance can be achieved. These changes may be real and objective, such as hiring someone to provide child care each afternoon so the mother of an irritable newborn can take a nap. They may also be subjective or involve appraising the situation differently. An example might be a mother who says she does not mind being up at night because she likes to watch old movies on television while she rocks and pats the fussy baby.

When crisis continues and imbalance persists, second-order change is needed. During this adaptation phase, restructuring of the family system occurs, including changes in boundaries, rules, and roles. For a family with a child with disabilities, the child's irritability and feeding problems may persist long after early infancy. Mom may no longer have the positive attitude toward sleep deprivation or the financial resources to hire the amount of help needed. This family might adapt by making major role changes. For example, Mom might take a part-time job to get both some time away from child care and some additional income to use to hire help with child and home responsibilities. Dad might decrease his employment hours or develop a more flexible work schedule and increase his responsibilities for child care and night feedings.

As families find ways to reduce stress and adapt, they are better able to draw on positive cognitive perceptions of the situation (salutogenesis). These perceptions—in and of themselves—can reduce stress and promote adaptation. Patterson, based on research findings (Patterson & Leonard, 1993, p. 227), provided the following summary of positive aspects of having a child with intense medical needs, as reported by parents:

- the child's warmth and responsiveness
- the tenacity and perseverance of the child to endure, which made the parents want to invest more of their effort
- the closeness felt in the family unit by pulling together to manage
- the assertiveness and skill that they as parents developed in response to caring for the child, as well as learning to deal with multiple providers and third-party payers
- the growth in empathy and kindness in their other children.

Patterson referred to these examples of positive attributions as "situational meanings about capabilities" (p. 227). These meanings benefit parents by helping them form positive perceptions of a situation that they cannot change, and as Moses (1987) noted, form new dreams (see Chapter 3).

In terms of global meanings, the family develops shared beliefs, values, and purposes. For example, if a child with delayed motor development falls and has to have stitches in the emergency room, the family may be able to approach this situation calmly. They draw from their experience of having been there before as well as from their beliefs in their ability to communicate with the service delivery system and their ability to gather needed supports quickly (e.g., calling on a neighbor to stay with their other children so both parents can go to the hospital). The family consensus about what needs to be done and how to coordinate to achieve this purpose is an adaptive response on the part of the family system that facilitates coping.

The emergency room example also demonstrates the relationship among cognitions, behaviors, and emotions. The parents' cognitive belief in their competence to manage the crisis with their child allowed them to take the appropriate actions of going to the hospital and getting care for their other children. They still experienced anxiety about the child's injury and the treatment regime, but they were not incapacitated by this anxiety. The positive impact of cognitions on actions and emotions is even more important for the protracted circumstance of caring for a child with disability or chronic illness than it is for managing a short-term crisis such as the emergency room.

## STRESS AND COPING: FAMILY CHARACTERISTICS

### ✠ FOCUS 2

*What family characteristics are associated with stress and coping?*

### Demographics of Stress and Coping

Winkler (1988) reviewed studies that addressed family resources and family perceptions as related to stress in families with a son or daughter with mental retardation. These studies, published between 1954 and 1983, indicated that child characteristics such as caregiving demands, behavior problems, and lack of ability to show affection contribute to stress, especially for mothers. Lower IQ of the child was also associated with increased stress. These families were more socially isolated and engaged in fewer social outings and vacations. Financial resources, as well as access to and skill in negotiating the service delivery system, were higher for parents of higher social class. Parents without these resources relied more on informal support networks, such as extended family. Frequency of church contacts and intensity of personal belief were also associated with less stress. Finally, more educated parents had more difficulty adjusting to their child's mental retardation, which they perceived as a tragedy.

More recent and, for the most part, better designed studies support and expand these findings. In studies that compared parents of children with disabilities with parents of children with typical development (Beckman, 1991; Dyson, 1991), disability was associated with more stress and greater caregiver demands (particularly for mothers), and these finding were stable when families were studied longitudinally (Dyson, 1993).

Several more recent studies have addressed the impact of different types of disability on family stress. Sloper and Turner (1993) studied parents of children with severe physical disabilities and found high levels of psychological distress, especially for mothers. Noh and colleagues (1989) found similar levels of stress for mothers and fathers, but differences were related to the type of disability. Parents experiencing the most stress had children with conduct disorders or autism; stress experienced by parents of children with Down syndrome was similar to that of parents of children with typical development. Behavior problems of their children with disabilities were associated with increased parental stress for mothers of children in middle childhood and adolescence studied by Orr et al. (1993).

Parents of 1,726 children receiving special education services were interviewed by Palfrey et al. (1989). Types of disabilities represented included communication disorders, learning disabilities, emotional disturbance, mental retardation, sensory impairment, and physical/multiple disabilities. Overall, 28 percent of these parents indicated a stressful impact of the child's disability on their daily lives (jobs, housing, friendships, marital harmony) with the figure rising to 60 percent for families of children with physical/multiple disabilities. This study also supported the finding reported by Winkler (1988) that higher maternal education was related to increased stress. This was true in all disability groups studied.

Additional findings reported by Winkler (1988) are supported in more recent studies, including increased stress with lower financial resources (Bradley et al., 1991) and decreased stress with greater emphasis on religious beliefs (Dyson, 1991). In addition, Beckman (1991) found more stress for single mothers; Trute and Hauch (1988) found less stress in two-parent families; and Beavers et al. (1986) found less stress in families that included two adults (not necessarily a mother and father). Fathers of young children reported more stress related to the child's temperament and the parent–child relationship, whereas mothers were more stressed by the demands of the parenting experience (Krauss, 1993). Furthermore, mothers expressed more needs than fathers, with needs for family and social support, help in explaining to others, and child care being particularly important for mothers (Bailey, Blasco, & Simeonsson, 1992).

Demographics are helpful in understanding family stress, but it takes the words of a parent to paint a picture of how stressful it can be to see a child suffer and wonder how to help. Such a picture is provided by Laura's mother in Window 4.1 on page 72.

## Stress, Coping, and Family Functioning

The preceding demographics point to increased stress for families that include a child with disabilities. Also, more severe disability and the presence of behavior problems as well as increased involvement in caregiving are associated with increased stress. However, the literature also provides a picture of families that include a child with disabilities as functioning competently (e.g., Kazak, 1992a). It is, therefore, important to study family adaptation (Crnic, Freidrich, & Greenberg, 1983) or resilience (Patterson, 1991) in order to determine what contributes to successful coping.

One component of resilience or effective coping appears to be how well the family functions as a system. Dyson (1991) found families of children with disabilities to enjoy as much positive family interaction as families of children with typical development, and this finding was consistent over time (Dyson, 1993).

Schwab's (1989, p. 112) research addressed perceptions of strengths of families that include a member with a disability. Strengths endorsed by at least 75 percent of the respondents included the following:

- individual commitment to the family
- commitment to the family member having a disability
- support of family when member with a disability has a problem
- concern of family for promoting welfare and happiness of member with disability
- commitment of husband and wife to each other.

Trute and Hauch (1988) also studied family strengths. They found that positive family adaptation was related to the functioning of the parental subsystem as well as to the skills of the parents in utilizing family and friend network resources.

However, in a study comparing parents of children with disabilities with parents of children with typical development, Margalit and Ankonina (1991) found less emphasis on interrelational aspects within the family, fewer opportunities for personal growth, more negative affect, and more usage of avoidant coping strategies. Patching and Watson (1993) found consensus among the parents they studied about concern for the future of the child with disabilities, concern for the parents' own future, and concern for their own emotional health or that of their partner. These findings suggest families at risk. They also suggest the need to understand coping strategies that can build on the strengths of the family system and help families access and use these strategies.

## COPING RESPONSES AND FAMILY ADAPTATION

⊕     **FOCUS 3**

*What coping responses contribute to family adaptation?*

### Assigning Meaning

Stress can be reduced when potentially stressful events are appraised as challenges, rather than threats. Taylor (1983) developed a theory of cognitive adaptation to crisis that included three adjustment themes: (1) searching for meaning of the event; (2) increasing self-esteem; and (3) establishing mastery over the event and one's life more broadly. Interest in cognitive coping has grown from insights from both professionals and parents concerning the disability/stress paradox. Both the research literature and accounts by parents documented the reality of stress, caregiving demands, and grief responses in families that included a member with disabilities. Yet there was also ample evidence, again in both research and personal accounts, of families doing well (Turnbull et al., 1993). A positive attitude appears to be an important component of effective coping. Specifically, families who cope well look for ways to accept aspects of their lives that cannot be changed, gain as much control over their complicated lives as possible, and assign positive meanings to the reality of their daily lives. Furthermore, improved overall well-being has been shown, through research studies, in parents who were able to move beyond asking "Why me?" (Shapp, Thurman, & Ducette, 1992).

Life crises can be opportunities for personal growth, and cognitive coping skills can help people focus on beneficial aspects of the crisis (Schaefer & Moos, 1992, p. 153). Three major types of positive outcomes of crisis were delineated by Schaefer and Moos: (1) enhanced social resources; (2) enhanced personal resources; and (3) development of new coping skills. All of these have been embraced in the writings of parents and siblings of persons with disabilities.

Enhanced social resources for families that include a member with a disability include positive relationships with professionals, care providers, extended family members, and, frequently, other parents or siblings of children with disabilities. Enhanced personal resources include increased self-reliance, maturity, empathy, and altruism as well as changes in values and priorities. Finally, these families value their coping abilities, including taking pride in their problem-solving and help-seeking skills and expressing confidence that these skills will help them with future challenges (Powell & Gallagher, 1993; Singer & Powers, 1993; Spiegle & van den Pol, 1993; Turnbull et al., 1993). This positive perspective does not discount the reality of a situation that is frequently demanding or resources which are frequently scarce; it means, rather, that cognitive reframing occurs, allowing families to emphasize what is "good" or "right" about their lives.

Cognitive coping should not be confused with wishful thinking, which has been found to be ineffective in reducing stress (Olin, 1995). Family members who engage in cognitive coping do not focus on wishing their situation was different, but look for positive aspects and meanings in the situation as it is. For example, they value a sense of humor, which is frequently cited by parents as one of their most prized coping strategies. Sue Wilson (1993), the mother of a son with multiple disabilities, had this to say:

> Humor has been the most important tool that we have had. Believe it or not, we laugh a lot! Granted, the jokes are sometimes slightly warped. Although it seems obvious, it took us a while to learn that laughter can see you through rough spots. We know that there is a time to cry, but there is also a time when grief becomes debilitating. Overall, humor can make you much more productive. I have a newfound ability to find something good in something bad. Sometimes you just have to look harder and wait longer. (p. 29)

In Window 4.2, Claire's mother, Marianne Jennings, presents a humorous picture of looking on the bright side.

### Increasing Self-Esteem

For parents, self-esteem is tied to how well they parent and how well their children are doing. For parents of a child with a disability or chronic illness, three different scenarios may threaten self-esteem and increase parental stress. In the first scenario, the parents may be parenting effectively and yet their son or daughter may not be doing well because of the nature of the developmental and/or health problems. In the second circumstance, the parents may not be parenting that well because they do not have the skills or resources required for their challenging parental responsibilities. In the third circumstance, parenting may be adequate but be perceived by society in a negative way because the child looks different or has behavior problems.

Enhancing self-esteem can facilitate effective coping. One means of enhancing self-esteem is through parental empowerment. Empowerment was described by Dunst, Trivette, and Deal (1988) as involving three conditions: (1) a proactive stance on the part of professionals who believe in parental competence or the capacity of parents to become competent; (2) provision of enabling experiences or opportunities for competence to be displayed; and (3) the attribution of success by the parent to his or her own actions. These conditions provide the sense of control necessary for empowerment (p. 4).

Empowerment is contrasted to the sense of powerlessness that parents may feel when faced with the needs of their child and problems—including pain and

---

★ **WINDOW 4.2**
_____

## *Learning to See the Bright Side*

I HAVE DISCOVERED THAT THE JOYS OF RAISING A CHILD with disabilities can outweigh the challenges. In fact, raising a child with disabilities offers some of life's greatest moments and sweetest rewards. I begin with the obvious—we get the world's best parking spaces. They are extra wide, thus helping us avoid the "door-ding elves" who occupy all parking lots. Claire brings us valet-quality parking without the requisite tip.

Then there are the airplane trips. We will always pre-board, qualifying under that airplane lingo of "passengers needing extra assistance in boarding." In fact, we are always first—even the passengers with small children allow us to go first. The passengers who need assistance assist us. I feel like royalty when we travel with Claire.

Then there's that door-to-door school bus service. No waiting in the rain. No scrambling to find a seat. No worries for me about the walk between the bus stop and home. It's as close to a limo as we'll come. Royalty again.

We sit in the shade and comfort waiting our turn at Disneyland while other families stand in line and struggle in the hot sun. At school, Claire has an individual study plan. It's like a private education without the tuition.

And then there's Claire. She's the only one of my three children who has never argued about what she's wearing. She always looks picture-perfect. There's no back talk, no whining and the only food she's ever turned down is crumbled bacon—a healthy choice. Sometimes I find myself saying to my other children, "Why can't you be more like Claire?"

The best part of Claire is that she has brought a perspective and a sense of priorities to me and our family. Claire has taught me to cope graciously with life's challenges.

*Source:* Reprinted with the expressed consent and approval of *Exceptional Parent*, a monthly magazine for parents and families of children with disabilities and special health care needs. Subscription cost is $32 per year for 12 issues; Call 1-800-247-8080. Offices at 555 Kinderkamack Rd. Oradell, N.J. 07649.

---

suffering—which he or she may face. Parents are confronted with problems that they cannot fix or cure and even improvement is dependent, at least to some extent, on others. Empowerment gives parents ways to help their children, with increased parental self-esteem an additional benefit (see Window 4.1 on page 72).

Kroth (1985), with his mirror model of parental involvement, suggested looking at levels of parental involvement or advocacy as parental strengths, with these strengths tied to enhanced self-esteem. According to the mirror model, all parents can share their special knowledge about their son or daughter. Most parents can work with professionals to learn ways to assist with developmental skills, homework, or skills related to vocational achievements. Some parents can use their abilities in a leadership capacity by volunteering to help other children and families and by serving schools and other agencies in an advisory capacity. A few parents can extend their advocacy efforts to program development and political advocacy. At the first two levels, parents reduce stress and become empowered by helping their own children. At the next two levels, parents are further empowered and self-esteem is enhanced by being able to help other children with disabilities and their families. Professionals who respect and acknowledge these efforts contribute to positive self-esteem, stress reduction, and empowerment.

Parents can also be encouraged to develop self-esteem through means other than parenting their child with disabilities. Their work, their hobbies, abilities such as cooking, gardening, or woodworking, and their activities with their children without disabilities are all important sources of self-esteem. Professionals can help families by nurturing and encouraging these activities and praising the outcomes of these endeavors. Being a helpful and caring brother or sister can be a source of self-esteem for siblings of persons with disabilities, but their own achievements in school, work, sports, and personal relationships deserve respect and recognition as well. Delanie Baker (1993), the mother of 20-year-old Austin, who has autism, wrote about her struggles, her successes, and Austin's influence on her personal growth:

> All these things leave me today feeling proud to have survived. I have a sense of well-being and self-confidence. Austin has given me a voice, a connection to the world, and a compassion has grown in me that serves me well in my nursing and teaching careers. Though the road I traveled has been fraught with detours and obstacles, I am who I am today because of having traveled the path. Yes, I would do it all over again. (p. 105)

### Establishing Mastery

If stress occurs when environmental demands are perceived as exceeding response capabilities, improving one's ability to meet demands or exert control over challenges can reduce stress. Mastery involves acquiring needed information, developing communication and problem-solving abilities, and developing skills specific to the tasks involved. Mastery also involves achieving a sense of control (McKinney & Peterson, 1987) and being able to make choices.

For families with a child with a disability or illness, mastery starts with understanding the diagnosis and learning how the child can be helped and who the helpers will be (Vincent, 1990). Unfortunately, this can also be the starting place for learned helplessness, or the assumption of inability. As professionals prescribe medical treatment regimes and educational and therapy programs, parents may feel overwhelmed. They may believe that only the professionals can care for and educate their child. Efforts on the part of professionals to provide reassurance of parents' primary role in this collaborative effort need to be early and ongoing.

Mastery for parents is a skill that varies with the life stage of the child. Need for mastery may begin at the time of the child's birth if the infant requires intensive medical care. These babies need extensive care that can only be provided by physicians, nurses, and other specialists. But they also need their parents. Hospital protocols are increasingly designed with both needs in mind. Flynn and McCollum (1989) described hospital intensive care for newborns that involves parents at every step. Then at the time of the child's discharge, parents are ready to assume daily care with backup support from professionals.

For parents of young children in early intervention programs, professionals can foster a sense of control and mastery by teaching parents the skills they need to care for and instruct their children. This strategy involves giving parents choices, whenever possible, regarding treatment. For example, parents could choose to carry out the home physical therapy program themselves or to have the therapist train the babysitter to carry out the program, thereby allowing for more parent–child playtime when the parents get home from work.

Communication and problem-solving skills are important components of mastery for parents at all child ages, but particularly so at school age and beyond. Their sons and daughters are now spending significant time away from them at school or at work, and parent involvement and participation, as well as the sense of control in their children's lives, greatly depends on effective communication with the service delivery system and proficiency in problem solving if conflicts occur. Parental self-esteem and the sense of mastery regarding their ability to parent their children can be important to helping their sons and daughters develop positive self-esteem and independence as well (Todis et al., 1993).

Mastery also involves gaining the skills and capabilities needed to parent the child. Parents can benefit from training specifically designed to teach them child-care skills (feeding, toileting), play skills, or behavior management. Training in life skills can also be valuable. Kirkham (1993) developed a life skills training program for mothers of children with developmental disabilities that could be implemented by teachers and other professionals. This skills-building intervention included coping and communication skills, problem-solving and decision-making techniques, and skills to manage and control the social network. This program was successful in reducing stress and depression and improving coping skills for the participant mothers, and the improvements were maintained at a follow-up assessment two years later.

Improving communication skills can be particularly meaningful for parents. A sense of mastery depends on being able to communicate effectively with professionals in order to gain needed information and make appropriate choices. Communication skills are vital within the family as well, especially in light of research evidence that relates stress reduction to shared parenting between spouses (McKinney & Peterson, 1987; Willoughby & Glidden, 1995). Effective functioning within the family system involves balancing the needs of all family members, and communicative skill in expressing needs and feelings is crucial. Both the ability to balance family needs and communicative competence are characteristics of resilient families (Patterson, 1991).

Professionals can also help parents realize that they have at least some control over the social environment in which they live and the social interactions with others, which can sometimes be stressful and even hurtful. Nan Nelson (1993), the mother of Annie, who was born prematurely and continued to be small for her age, shared her views on this issue.

> I don't care to discuss the subject with anyone, particularly strangers, ever again. This means that when we are at the supermarket and someone asks me how old she is, I will say she is five, almost six, and that's all I will say. . . . And then Annie and I will continue on our way. (p. 85)

Professionals can also guide parents in helping their sons and daughters, particularly adolescents and adults, increase their control over their treatment regimes and other aspects of their lives. This may involve addressing the issue of overprotection. Adults with chronic illness and disability were found, in several studies, to be more depressed and to have a decreased sense of control when they felt they were being overprotected by family members (Thompson, 1993). Specific techniques can be used by professionals and parents to increase a sense of control for children as well. Adam Moore (1990), an 8-year-old, described this event from one of his multiple hospitalizations:

> One day a special nurse came in to talk with me. She brought a puppet and let me stick an IV into its arm. That was fun. You can bet, I poked it real hard. Then, for a change, my nurse let me take her blood pressure. And she gave me some shot needles of my very own to play with. I gave shots to some balloons. POP! POP! POP! Now that was more like it! I began to feel in charge. (p. 24)

Brown's (1993) thoughts on coping provide a fitting summary for this section:

> A positive attitude toward the self, a belief in one's ability to master environmental events, and the conviction that the future will be bright and rosy can reduce stress by: (1) leading individuals to appraise negative events in terms of challenge rather than threat, (2) fostering active attempts to alter stressful situations, (3) promoting the effective use of cognitive reinterpretation in which individuals are able to construe stressful events in a manner that renders them less threatening, and (4) helping individuals to manage emotional distress. (p. 129)

## RESOURCES TO FACILITATE COPING

### ⊕ FOCUS 4

*What resources facilitate coping?*

### *Resources for Stress Reduction*

Resources that support coping and reduce stress include financial resources, spiritual beliefs, health, and activities which promote relaxation and taking a temporary break from problems and responsibilities. Parents of children with disabilities may have both greater need for these resources and more limited access to them. In addition to the financial drain imposed by the expenses of the disability or illness, parents may be limited in employability and flexibility of work arrangements because of the care needs of their child. Spiritual beliefs are very personal, but parents who wish and would profit from involvement in the religious community may be limited by the needs of the child and, in some cases, a religious community that is not welcoming to individuals with disabilities and their families (Thornburgh, 1993). Activities that promote health and relaxation, such as exercise, sports, hobbies, social activities, or just time to rest, may be severely limited by family responsibilities. For example, Barnett and Boyce (1995) found that mothers and fathers of children with Down syndrome spent more time on child care and less time on social activities than parents of children with typical development. And Kathy McGlynn, the mother of a son with a seizure disorder, had this to say about fatigue:

> I'm so tired I barely have the strength to hold him anymore. I got less than two hours sleep again last night. I can't think; I can't react. I just spent half an hour reading the front page of the newspaper, but I don't remember any of it. (McGlynn & Dodd, 1993, p. 67)

Professionals can help these families in a variety of ways. An understanding of family vulnerability to stress is the starting point, along with respect for the importance of physical and emotional well-being and utilitarian resources (Crnic, Friedrich, & Greenberg, 1983). Professionals can monitor programming suggestions for the child to make sure they do not increase stress or overload limited resources, especially time and energy. Professionals can also help families find ways to increase resources and reduce stress. For example, helping families find appropriate and dependable child care can meet family needs ranging from holding a job to attending an exercise class.

Respite care is another valuable resource for families. Respite care involves giving families a brief time-out from their responsibilities—an evening, a weekend, a week—in which they can get caught up with other responsibilities and/or do something relaxing, such as go to a movie or take a short trip. Respite care programs have been shown to reduce stress for families (Sherman, 1995). However, families are only going to be able to relax and enjoy their time away from caregiving if they know their children are safe. Respite care providers must receive appropriate training to deliver quality services (Neef & Parrish, 1989).

Parents can also profit from programs designed to teach stress management techniques (Hawkins & Singer, 1989). It is important to remember that these families also have ordinary everyday stress that is superimposed on the stress involved in responsibilities related to the family member with disabilities. Sometimes these daily hassles can be the final straw. Stress management programs include a focus on lifestyle alteration such as diet and exercise. They can teach behaviors such as relaxation, imagery, and cognitive reframing. Learning assertiveness skills can be a means of accessing needed supports, such as encouraging a church to include children with disabilities in their programming. In addition, these training programs can serve as forums for reminding parents that caring for themselves is not only okay, it is essential for effective parenting. This premise is supported by research findings that link active involvement with the family member with a disability and involvement with multiple service providers to caregiver burnout (Heller, 1993). A mother, Valerie Bateman (1993), adds this advice, "Get away from everything, alone or with a friend, for a few minutes a day, a week or whatever you feel is best for you. You'll be surprised at how it will change your perspective on caring for your child." (pp. 257–258)

## Social Support

A vital resource for all families, but particularly for families that include a member with a disability, is social support. Social support includes emotional, informational, and material support received from friends, relatives, or others that a person can turn to in times of both day-to-day need and crisis. The impact of social support networks has received considerable attention in the psychological literature (e.g., Sarason & Sarason, 1985), and social support has been shown to be linked to positive personal and family outcomes. In fact, "the stress-buffering and health-promoting influences of social support have been so well documented that it is now almost axiomatic to state that social support both enhances well-being and lessens the likelihood of emotional and physical distress" (Dunst et al., 1989, p. 124).

Social support has also received attention in research focusing on individuals with disabilities and their families. Research studies by Dunst and his colleagues of social support in families that include a member with disabilities support the mediating influences of social support. Results of these studies indicated that more supportive social networks are associated with enhanced parent and family well-being, positive caregiving, positive attitudes of parents, positive parent-child interaction, and better child behavior (Dunst et al., 1989). However, families with a member with disabilities may be at risk for social isolation. Singer and Irvin (1991, p. 289) suggested reasons why families might experience social isolation:

- They are fatigued from caregiving.
- They have limited opportunities for leisure time because of the difficulty in obtaining child care.
- They encounter misunderstandings and, sometimes, negative reactions from others regarding their relative with severe handicaps.
- Their children with handicaps are excluded from the normal social institutions that allow social networks to form.

An additional problem may be that these families are unable to participate in the easy give-and-take of families with children with typical development. They need too much and can repay too little. So they exhaust their resources and feel inadequate (Hobfoll & Lerman, 1988). Also, issues unrelated to disability influence access to and utilization of social support such as the parents' relational competence (Hansson, Jones, & Carpenter, 1984).

Studies that have compared the social support networks of families of children with disabilities with the networks of families with children with typical development suggest that the type and circumstance of the disability play a role in network size and density. In separate studies, Kazak (1992a, 1992b) compared parents of children with typical development with parents of children with spina bifida, PKU, and mental retardation (institutionalized adolescents). Smaller and more dense (more associations among network members) social support networks were found for the parents of children with spina bifida, but not for the other disability groups. In another study, mothers of hearing impaired children (Quittner, 1992) reported significantly smaller social support networks than mothers of hearing children. As an explanation for her findings and those of Kazak, Quittner suggested that spina bifida and profound deafness are publicly observable and, therefore, stigmatizing conditions. PKU, in contrast, is not observable, and the institutionalized adolescents did not interact directly with their parents' social support networks.

Interestingly, Quittner (1992) found no significant differences between the groups (mothers of children with and without severe hearing impairment) on measures of perceived support. The explanation for these findings appeared to be that the mothers of children with hearing impairment listed professional service providers in their social support networks. So professionals play a vital role in the provision of social support for parents of children with disabilities, both directly and indirectly. Professionals are valued by parents not only for the services they provide, but also for their friendship. The indirect professional role in social support may involve linking parents with child-care services so they can spend time with friends and linking parents with other parents of children with disabilities, both individually and through support groups (Smith et al., 1994). This parent-to-parent linkage was endorsed by a parent, Mary Pielaet (1993), as the best social support of all: "Nothing helps more than finding someone else who has stood in our shoes, particularly if they have gone on to lead accepting, productive and happy lives" (p. 41).

### Collaborative Relationships with Professionals

A special kind of resource for parents, which combines social support and tangible help, is a strong, collaborative relationship with the professionals providing services for their son or daughter. There is enormous potential for professionals to be strong sources of support for parents. As a means of supporting families, Power and Bartholomew (1987) advocated collaboration or reciprocal involvement between professionals and parents in a working alliance. Dunst and Paget (1991) recommended professional responses that promote parental independence and empowerment. Janet Vohs (1993), a mother, reminded professionals of the power of both negative and positive attitudes. She also suggested the need for ideas and stories that can help and empower.

One such idea has a lifespan focus and stems from the research of Behr and Murphy (1993). In addressing stress experienced by parents of children with disabilities, they found age of the child to be an important variable. Specifically, parents of younger children reported higher levels of stress and lower perceptions of some kind of positive contribution from the child. They stated that "these differences were robust, even when the severity of the disability was taken into account" (p. 157). These findings combined with the comments of parents suggest that professionals could support parents by linking parents of younger children with parents who are further along the lifespan and who have developed more effective coping responses. Evelyn and Charles Lusthaus (1993), the parents of 13-year-old Hannah, who has developmental disabilities, had this to say: "As the years pass, we are learning to reframe our fear of Hannah's future into a recognition that she is able to cope with her life and its hardships" (p. 47). Virginia DeLand (1993), the mother of Lisa, a young adult with developmental disabilities, adds this thought: "I would never have believed in 1970, as a devastated parent in the doctor's office, that there would be a day when I could say, with honesty, that I had been blessed, but it's true" (p. 95).

Finally, Cohen et al. (1989) remind professionals that family support cannot be separated from advocacy. Professionals can advocate for persons with disabilities in the agencies in which they work, in the communities in which they live, and through their volunteer efforts and political choices, every single day. These advocacy efforts by professionals are valued, even cherished, by families.

# SOURCES OF FAMILY SUPPORT

⊞ **FOCUS 5**

*What types of formal and natural supports benefit families?*

## Formal Support

Families of children with disabilities must access service systems beyond the family in order to receive the support needed to care for their children. Different families need different types and levels of support, but most need help from medical and educational systems, and many need help from professionals providing psychosocial and habilitative/rehabilitative services. As their children grow older, vocational services may be added, and at various lifespan points many families need financial assistance.

Formal supports also include state and federal program mandates and funding allocations for programs and for families. Cohen et al. (1989) delineated emerging service themes of formal support to families as follows: "(1) families should receive the supports necessary to maintain their children at home; (2) family supports should support the entire family; and (3) family supports should maximize the family's control over the services and supports they receive" (p. 159). Currently 34 states have adopted legislation mandating family support services, and 27 states offer some form of cash assistance to families to allow them to purchase needed services and items such as adaptive equipment (Agosta & Melda, 1996).

Formal supports are essential, and families express appreciation for them while working to expand and improve needed services. However, the literature documents problems in availability, delivery, and coordination of services that can impede support for families. Problems include professionals perceiving families as satisfied with services when in fact they are not satisfied (Spaniol & Zipple, 1988), professionals (in this case, pediatricians) who overestimate the negative impact of the child on the family (Sloper & Turner, 1991), and discrepancies between what families need and what they actually get (O'Connor, 1992).

Also, problems can stem from the quantity of service providers and lack of coordination of services. Families studied by Sloper and Turner (1992) had been in contact with an average of ten different professionals during the past year, yet only 55 percent of these families had a professional to help them link and coordinate these services. In spite of this high number of professionals in the lives of the families studied, these researchers found evidence of considerable unmet need, particularly in the provision of information to families.

Patterson and Geber (1991) stressed the importance of coordination of care and offered the following suggestions:

[E]fforts must be directed so that care is (a) coordinated across the many disciplines involved through the use of care coordinators; (b) continuous across settings; (c) continuous across stages of a child's development; (d) collaborative among family members and professionals; (e) organized around the family's needs, concerns, and aspirations . . .; (f) sensitive and responsive to racial and ethnic variability; and (g) based in the community, where the child can be integrated as completely as possible into family and neighborhood environments. (p. 157)

### Informal/Natural Support

The goal of community-based living and care and the concept of normalization for all family members have heightened interest in informal or natural supports for families. These supports are provided by the family members themselves in conjunction with friends, neighbors, and the community. However, there is overlap between formal and informal support. This was demonstrated graphically by Patterson and Geber (1991) (Figure 4.1).

In addition to their role in providing formal support, professionals can assist in the acquisition and implementation of informal supports. One way professionals can help is by aiding families in identifying, not only their needs, but their

**FIGURE 4.1**    *Formal and Informal Supports*

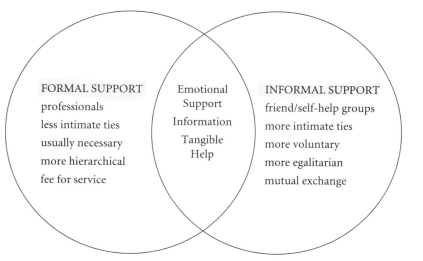

FORMAL SUPPORT
professionals
less intimate ties
usually necessary
more hierarchical
fee for service

Emotional Support
Information
Tangible Help

INFORMAL SUPPORT
friend/self-help groups
more intimate ties
more voluntary
more egalitarian
mutual exchange

*Source:* Reproduced with permission of the Association for the Care of Children's Health, 7910 Woodmont Avenue, Suite 3000, Bethesda, Maryland 20814, from *Children's Health Care*, Summer 1991, Vol. 20, No. 3, pp. 150–161.

strengths (Dunst et al., 1989). For example, a single mother might need more financial resources. Although she has marketable skills, she might be unable to secure employment because her job skills are not up to date. A professional could help her determine that family support funds could be used for short-term child care, and link her to a facility providing such care, so she could take a job training course. Professionals can also develop programs that help parents help each other, such as support groups or opportunities for the parents of a newborn with Down syndrome, for example, to meet and talk with parents of an older child with Down syndrome.

An example of a unique program that combines professional leadership, community involvement, and parental needs and strengths is the Building Community Resources Project (Umstead, Boyd, & Dunst, 1995). This program supports participation of children with disabilities and their families in the full range of programs available in a community. Most communities have a rich array of programs such as library story hour, swimming lessons, day camp, various sports and scout troops, as well as facilities such as parks, pools, recreation centers, child-care centers, churches and synagogues. The goals of the Building Community Resources project are to identify available programs and activities, to enhance the capacity of the programs to involve community members with disabilities, and to foster enjoyable family participation. The obvious benefit of involving children with disabilities and their families in the community is paired with the benefit of giving the community the chance to know these children and families and to experience the similarities between children with and without disabilities. The project staff develops strategies around the needs and strengths of the particular family. "Strategies may focus on sharing information about the child, ensuring safety, building friendships, making physical adaptations or securing funding" (Umstead, Boyd, & Dunst, 1995, p. 37).

Natural supports hold the key to stress reduction and positive coping for families because they enhance self-esteem and mastery through social support and community inclusion. Natural supports combine collaborative relationships with professionals and family empowerment. Furthermore, they help families see their sons and daughters as having what one mother, Judy O'Halloran (1993, p. 20), termed "difabilities," or differences that may need certain accommodations, but need not be isolating or stigmatizing (see Window 3.1, on page 48).

Cooley (1994) adds these final thoughts:

> A life-span perspective for individuals and families acknowledges that fluctuating needs are a natural expectation. The primary goal of family support is to help individuals with disabilities and their families find balance and nourishment sufficient for them to feel fully included as citizens of their communities. (p. 119)

# REVIEW

*FOCUS 1: Identify frameworks for studying stress as experienced by families with a member with disabilities.*

- The work of Lazarus and his colleagues defines stress as a relationship between the person and the environment which is appraised as stressful, that is, exceeding the resources available to the person.
- ABCX models identify X (the crisis) as the result of A (the stressor), B (the resources), and C (the appraisal).
- The family adjustment and adaptation response model (FAAR) emphasizes family adaptation over time.

*FOCUS 2: What family characteristics are associated with stress and coping?*

- The presence of disability, particular types of disability (severe disability, behavior problems), and increased caregiver demands are associated with greater stress. Financial and spiritual resources and the presence of more than one adult in the family are associated with more effective coping.
- Improved family functioning stems from an emphasis on positive family interaction and family strengths.

*FOCUS 3: What coping responses contribute to family adaptation?*

- Families can cope by searching for meaning in their situations, adopting positive attitudes, and viewing their situations as challenges, rather than threats.
- The child's disability may have a negative impact on parental self-esteem, but increasing self-esteem through efforts such as parental empowerment can enhance coping.
- Mastery is an effective coping response that involves acquiring needed information, developing communication and problem-solving abilities, and developing skills specific to the tasks involved.

*FOCUS 4: What resources facilitate coping?*

- Resources that support coping and reduce stress include financial resources, spiritual beliefs, health, and activities which promote relaxation and taking a temporary break from problems and responsibilities. Parents of children with disabilities may have both greater need for these resources and more limited access to them.
- For families that include a child with a disability, more supportive social support networks are associated with better family outcomes.

- A strong, collaborative relationship with professionals is a resource for parents that combines social support and tangible help.

*FOCUS 5: What types of formal and natural supports benefit families?*

- Families require a variety of formal supports based on their particular needs. The best ones foster empowerment, rather than dependency.
- Natural supports combine professional leadership, community inclusion, and family empowerment.

## REFERENCES

Agosta, J., & Melda, K. (1996). Supporting families who provide care at home for children with disabilities. *Exceptional Children, 62,* 271–282.

Antonovsky, A. (1979). *Health, stress and coping.* San Francisco: Jossey-Bass.

Antonovsky, A. (1993). The implications of salutogenesis: An outsider's view. In A. P. Turnbull, J. M. Patterson, S. K. Behr, D. L. Murphy, J. G. Marquis, and M. J. Blue-Banning (Eds.), *Cognitive coping, families, and disability* (pp. 111–122). Baltimore: Brookes.

Bailey, D. B., Blasco, P. M., & Simeonsson, R. J. (1992). Needs expressed by mothers and fathers of young children with disabilities. *American Journal on Mental Retardation, 97,* 1–10.

Baker, D. (1993). The decision for out-of-home placement. In J. A. Spiegle and R. A. van den Pol (Eds.), *Making changes: Family voices on living with disabilities* (pp. 96–105). Cambridge: Brookline.

Barnett, W. S., & Boyce, G. C. (1995). Effects of children with Down syndrome on parent's activities. *American Journal on Mental Retardation, 100,* 115–127.

Bateman, V. (1993). A new beginning. In G. H. S. Singer & L. E. Powers (Eds.), *Families, disability, and empowerment: Active coping skills and strategies for family interventions.* Baltimore: Brookes.

Beavers, J., Hampson, R. B., Hulgus, Y. F., & Beavers, W. R. (1986). Coping in families with a retarded child, *Family Process, 25,* 365–378.

Beckman, P. J. (1991). Comparison of mothers' and fathers' perceptions of the effect of young children with and without disabilities. *American Journal on Mental Retardation, 95,* 585–595.

Behr, S. K., & Murphy, D. L. (1993). Research progress and promise: The role of perceptions in cognitive adaptation to disability. In A. P. Turnbull, J. M. Patterson, S. K. Behr, D. L. Murphy, J. G. Marquis, & M. J. Blue-Banning (Eds.), *Cognitive coping, families, and disability* (pp. 151–163). Baltimore: Brookes.

Bradley, R. H., Rock, S. L., Whiteside, L., Caldwell, B. M., & Brisby, J. (1991). Dimensions of parenting in families having children with disabilities. *Exceptionality, 2,* 41–61.

Brown, J. D. (1993). Coping with stress: The beneficial role of positive illusions. In A. P. Turnbull, J. M. Patterson, S. K. Behr, D. L. Murphy, J. G. Marquis, & M. J. Blue-Banning (Eds.), *Cognitive coping, families, and disability* (pp. 123–133). Baltimore: Brookes.

Cohen, S., Agosta, J., Cohen, J., & Warren, R. (1989). Supporting families of children with severe disabilities. *Journal of the Association for Persons with Severe Handicaps, 14,* 155–162.

Cooley, W. C. (1994). The ecology of support for caregiving families. *Developmental and Behavioral Pediatrics, 15,* 117–119.

Crnic, K. A., Friedrich, W. N., & Greenberg, M. T. (1983). Adaptation of families of mentally retarded children: A model of stress, coping, and family ecology. *American Journal of Mental Deficiency, 88*, 125–138.

DeLand, V. (1993). One bite at a time. In J. A. Spiegle & R. A. van den Pol (Eds.), *Making changes: Family voices on living with disabilities* (pp. 90–95). Cambridge: Brookline.

Dunst, C. J., & Paget, K. D. (1991). Parent-professional partnerships and family empowerment. In M. J. Fine (Ed.), *Collaboration with parents of exceptional children* (pp. 25–44). Brandon, VT: Clinical Psychology Publishing.

Dunst, C. J., Trivette, C. M., & Deal, A. G. (1988). *Enabling and empowering families.* Cambridge: Brookline.

Dunst, C. J., Trivette, C. M., Gordon, N. J., & Pletcher, L. L. (1989). Building and mobilizing informal family support networks. In G. H. S. Singer & L. K. Irvin (Eds.), *Support for caregiving families: Enabling positive adaptation to disability* (pp. 121–141). Baltimore: Brookes.

Dyson, L. L. (1991). Families of young children with handicaps: Parental stress and family functioning. *American Journal on Mental Retardation, 95*, 623–629.

Dyson, L. L. (1993). Response to the presence of a child with disabilities: Parental stress and family functioning over time. *American Journal on Mental Retardation, 98*, 207–218.

Flynn, L. L., & McCollum, J. (1989). Support systems: Strategies and implications for hospitalized newborns and families. *Journal of Early Intervention, 13*, 173–182.

Hansson, R. O., Jones, W. H., & Carpenter, B. N. (1984). Relational competence and social support. In P. Shaver (Ed.), *Review of personality and social psychology. Vol. 5: Emotions, relationships, and health* (pp. 265–284). Beverly Hills, CA: Sage.

Hawkins, N. E., & Singer, G. H. S. (1989). A skills training approach for assisting parents to cope with stress. In G. H. S. Singer & L. K. Irvin (Eds.), *Support for caregiving families: Enabling positive adaptation to disability* (pp. 71–83). Baltimore: Brookes.

Heller, T. (1993). Self-efficacy coping, active involvement, and caregiver well-being throughout the life course among families of persons with mental retardation. In A. P. Turnbull, J. M. Patterson, S. K. Behr, D. L. Murphy, J. G. Marquis, & M. J. Blue-Banning (Eds.), *Cognitive coping, families, and disability* (pp. 195–206). Baltimore: Brookes.

Hill, R. (1949). *Families under stress.* New York: Harper.

Hill, R. (1958). Generic features of families under stress. *Social Casework, 49*, 139–150.

Hobfoll, S. E., & Lerman, M. (1988). Personal relationships, personal attributes, and stress resistance: Mothers' reactions to their child's illness. *American Journal of Community Psychology, 16*, 565–589.

Jennings, M. M. (1993, July/August). Learning to see the bright side. *Exceptional Parent,* pp. 16–18.

Kazak, A. (1992a). Family systems, social ecology, and chronic pediatric illness: Conceptual, methodological, and intervention issues. In T. J. Akamatsu, M. A. P. Stephens, S. E. Hobfall, & J. H. Crowther (Eds.), *Family Health Psychology* (pp. 93–110). Washington, DC: Hemisphere.

Kazak, A. (1992b). The social context of coping with childhood chronic illness: Family systems and social support. In A. M. La Greca, L. J. Siegel, J. L. Wallander, & C. E. Walker (Eds.), *Stress and coping in child health* (pp. 262–298). New York: Guilford.

Kirkham, M. A. (1993). Two-year follow-up of skills training with mothers of children with disabilities. *American Journal on Mental Retardation, 97*, 509–520.

Krauss, M. W. (1993). Child-related and parenting stress: Similarities and differences between mothers and fathers of children with disabilities. *American Journal on Mental Retardation, 97*, 393–404.

Kroth, R. L. (1985). *Communicating with parents of exceptional children* (2nd ed.). Denver: Love.

Lazarus, R. S., & Cohen, J. B. (1977). Environmental stress. In I. Altman & J. F. Wohlwill (Eds.), *Coping and adaptation*. New York: Basic.

Lazarus, R. S., & Folkman, S. (1984). *Stress, appraisal, and coping*. New York: Springer.

Leff, P. T., & Walizer, E. H. (1992). *Building the healing partnership*. Cambridge: Brookline.

Lusthaus, E., & Lusthaus, C. (1993). A "normal" life for Hannah: Trying to make it possible. In A. P. Turnbull, J. M. Patterson, S. K. Behr, D. L. Murphy, J. G. Marquis, & M. J. Blue-Banning (Eds.), *Cognitive coping, families, and disability* (pp. 43–50). Baltimore: Brookes.

Margalit, M., & Ankonina, D. B. (1991). Positive and negative affect in parenting disabled children. *Counseling Psychology Quarterly, 4*, 289–299.

McCubbin, H. I., & Patterson, J. M. (1982). Family adaptation to crises. In H. I. McCubbin, A. E. Cauble, & J. M. Patterson (Eds.), *Family stress, coping, and social support* (pp. 26–47). Springfield, IL: Thomas.

McCubbin, H. I., & Patterson, J. M. (1983a). Family stress and adaptation to crises: A double ABCX model of family behavior. In D. Olson & B. Miler (Eds.), *Family studies review yearbook* (pp. 87–106). Beverly Hills, CA: Sage.

McCubbin, H. I., & Patterson, J. M. (1983b). The family stress process: The double ABCX model of family adjustment and adaptation. *Marriage and Family Review, 6*, 7–37.

McGlynn, K., & Dodd, B. (1993). Dispensing more than drugs. In J. A. Spiegle & R. A. van den Pol (Eds.), *Making changes: Family voices on living with disabilities* (pp. 65–69). Cambridge: Brookline.

McKinney, B., & Peterson, R. A. (1987). Predictors of stress in parents of developmentally disabled children. *Journal of Pediatric Psychology, 12*, 133–149.

Moore, A. (1990). *Broken arrow boy*. Kansas City: Landmark.

Moses, K. (1987, Spring). The impact of childhood disability: The parent's struggle. *Ways*, pp. 6–10.

Neef, N. A., & Parrish, J. M. (1989). Training respite care providers: A model for curriculum design, evaluation, and dissemination. In G. H. S. Singer and L. K. Irvin (Eds.), *Support for caregiving families: Enabling positive adaptation to disability* (pp. 175–188). Baltimore: Brookes.

Nelson, N. D. (1993). Meet my daughter, Annie. In G. H. S. Singer and L. E. Powers (Eds.), *Families, disability and empowerment: Active coping skills and strategies for family interventions*. Baltimore: Brookes.

Noh, S., Dumas, J. E., Wolf, L. C., & Fishman, S. N. (1989). Delineating sources of stress in parents of exceptional children. *Family Relations, 38*, 456–461.

Olin, K. (1995). Perceived caregiving burden as a function of differential coping strategies. *The Family Psychologist, 11*, 17–20.

O'Connor, S. (1992). Supporting families: What they want versus what they get. *OSERS News in Print, 5*, 7–11.

O'Halloran, J. M. (1993). Welcome to our family Casey Patrick. In A. P. Turnbull, J. M. Patterson, S. K. Behr, D. L. Murphy, J. G. Marquis, and M. J. Blue-Banning (Eds.), *Cognitive coping, families, and disability* (pp. 19–29). Baltimore: Brookes.

Orr, R. R., Cameron, S. J., Dobson, L. A., & Day, D. M. (1993). Age-related changes in stress experienced by families with a child who has developmental delays. *Mental Retardation, 31*, 171–176.

Palfrey, J. S., Walker, D. K., Butler, J. A., & Singer, J. D. (1989). Patterns of response in families of chronically disabled children: An assessment in five metropolitan school districts. *American Journal of Orthopsychiatry, 59*, 94–104.

Patching, B., & Watson, B. (1993). Living with children with an intellectual disability: Parents construct their reality. *International Journal of Disability, Development and Education, 40,* 115–131.

Patterson, J. M. (1988). Chronic illness in children and the impact on families. In C. Chilman, E. Nunally, & F. Cox (Eds.), *Chronic illness and disability* (pp. 69–107). Newbury Park, CA: Sage.

Patterson, J. M. (1989). A family stress model: The Family Adjustment and Adaptation Response. In C. Ramsey (Ed.), *The science of family medicine* (pp. 95–117). New York: Guilford.

Patterson, J. M. (1991). Family resilience to the challenge of a child's disability. *Pediatric Annals, 20,* 491–499.

Patterson, J. M. (1993). The role of family meanings in adaptation to chronic illness and disability. In A. P. Turnbull, J. M. Patterson, S. K. Behr, D. L. Murphy, J. G. Marquis, & M. J. Blue-Banning (Eds.), *Cognitive coping, families, and disability* (pp. 221–238). Baltimore: Brookes.

Patterson, J. M., & Geber, G. (1991). Preventing mental health problems in children with chronic illness or disability. *Children's Health Care, 20,* 150–161.

Patterson, J. M., & Leonard, B. J. (1993). Caregiving and children. In E. Kahana, D. E. Biegel, & M. Wykle (Eds.), *Family caregiving across the lifespan* (pp. 133–158). Newbury Park, CA: Sage.

Pielaet, M. (1993). Untold diagnosis. In J. A. Spiegle & R. A. van den Pol (Eds.), *Making changes: Family voices on living with disabilities* (pp. 33–41). Cambridge: Brookline.

Powell, T. H., & Gallagher, P. A. (1993). *Brothers & sisters: A special part of exceptional families* (2nd ed.). Baltimore: Brookes.

Power, T. J., & Bartholomew, K. L. (1987). Family-school relationship patterns: An ecological assessment. *School Psychology Review, 16,* 498–512.

Quittner, A. L. (1992). Re-examining research on stress and social support: The importance of contextual factors. In A. M. La Greca, L. J. Siegel, J. L. Wallander, & C. E. Walker (Eds.), *Stress and coping in child health* (pp. 85–115). New York: Guilford.

Sarason, I. G., & Sarason, B. R. (1985). *Social support: Theory, research and applications.* Boston: Martinus-Nijhoff.

Schaefer, J. A., & Moos, R. H. (1992). Life crises and personal growth. In B. N. Carpenter (Ed.), *Personal coping* (pp. 149–170). Westport, CT: Praeger.

Schwab, L. O. (1989). Strengths of families having a member with a disability. *Journal of the Multihandicapped Person, 2,* 105–117.

Shapp, L. C., Thurman, S. K., & Ducette, J. P. (1992). The relationship of attributions and personal well-being in parents of preschool children with disabilities. *Journal of Early Intervention, 16,* 295–303.

Sherman, B. R. (1995). Impact of home-based respite care on families of children with chronic illness. *Children's Health Care, 24,* 33–45.

Singer, G. H. S., & Irvin, L. K. (1991). Supporting families of persons with severe disabilities: Emerging findings, practices, and questions. In L. H. Meyer, C. A. Peck, & L. Brown (Eds.), *Critical issues in the lives of people with severe disabilities* (pp. 271–312). Baltimore: Brookes.

Singer, G. H. S., & Powers, L. E. (Eds.). (1993). *Families, disability, and empowerment: Active coping skills and strategies for family intervention.* Baltimore: Brookes.

Sloper, P., & Turner, S. (1991). Parental and professional views of the needs of families with a child with severe physical disability. *Counseling Psychology Quarterly, 4,* 323–330.

Sloper, P., & Turner, S. (1992). Service needs of families of children with severe physical disability. *Child Care, Health and Development, 18,* 259–282.

Sloper, P., & Turner, S. (1993). Risk and resistance factors in the adaptation of parents of children with severe physical disability. *Journal of Child Psychology and Psychiatry, 34,* 167–188.

Smith, K., Gabard, D., Dale, D., & Drucker, A. (1994). Parental opinions about attending parent support groups. *Children's Health Care, 23,* 127–136.

Spaniol, L., & Zipple, A. M. (1988). Family and professional perceptions of family needs and coping strengths. *Rehabilitation Psychology, 33,* 37–45.

Spiegle, J. A., & van den Pol, R. A. (Eds.). (1993). *Making changes: Family voices on living with disabilities.* Cambridge: Brookline.

Taylor, S. E. (1983). Adjustment to threatening events: A theory of cognitive adaptation. *American Psychologist, 38,* 1161–1173.

Thompson, S. C. (1993). Individual and interpersonal influences on the use of cognitive coping. In A. P. Turnbull, J. M. Patterson, S. K. Behr, D. L. Murphy, J. G. Marquis, & M. J. Blue-Banning (Eds.), *Cognitive coping, families, and disability* (pp. 165–172). Baltimore: Brookes.

Thornburgh, G. (1993, October). For the love of Peter. *Guideposts,* pp. 2–5.

Todis, B., Irvin, L. K., Singer, H. S., & Yovanoff, P. (1993). The self-esteem parent program: Quantitative and qualitative evaluation of a cognitive-behavioral intervention. In G. H. S. Singer & L. E. Powers (Eds.), *Families, disability, and empowerment* (pp. 203–229). Baltimore: Brookes.

Trute, B., & Hauch, C. (1988). Building on family strength: A study of families with positive adjustment to the birth of a developmentally disabled child. *Journal of Marital and Family Therapy, 14,* 185–193.

Turnbull, A. P., Patterson, J. M., Behr, S. K., Murphy, D. L., Marquis, J. G., & Blue-Banning, M. J. (1993). *Cognitive coping, families, and disability.* Baltimore: Brookes.

Umstead, S., Boyd, K., & Dunst, C. (1995, July). Building community resources. *Exceptional Parent,* pp. 36–37.

Vincent, K. R. (1990). Coping with disability: The individual or a family member's. *Social Behavior and Personality, 18,* 1–6.

Vohs, J. (1993). On belonging: A place to stand, a gift to give. In A. P. Turnbull, J. M. Patterson, S. K. Behr, D. L. Murphy, J. G. Marquis, & M. J. Blue-Banning (Eds.), *Cognitive coping, families, and disability* (pp. 51–66). Baltimore: Brookes.

Willoughby, J. C., & Glidden, L. M. (1995). Fathers helping out: Shared child care and marital satisfaction of parents of children with disabilities. *American Journal on Mental Retardation, 99,* 399–406.

Wilson, S. (1993). Letter to a friend. In J. A. Spiegle & R. A. van den Pol (Eds.), *Making changes: Family voices on living with disabilities* (pp. 25–30). Cambridge: Brookline.

Winkler, L. M. (1988). Family stress theory and research on families of children with mental retardation. In J. J. Gallagher and P. M. Vietze (Eds.), *Families of handicapped persons: Research, programs, and policy issues* (pp. 167–195). Baltimore: Brookes.

# CHAPTER FIVE

# The Family within the Community and Broader Social Environment

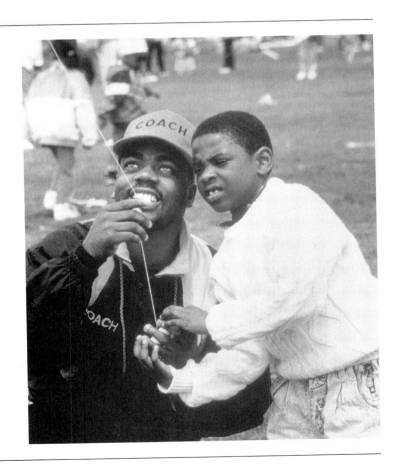

---

★ **WINDOW 5.1**

---

## The Birthday Invitation

Picking up Sara from her class, I found in her locker a birthday party invitation. She had, of course, been to parties before, for her sisters and a couple of neighborhood friends. This was different. Her sisters had no choice but to include her. The neighbors had been good friends of ours before Sara's birth, and had worked hard to fit our special child into the neighborhood. But this was an invitation that Sara had earned on her own. It came from Zach, a little boy I knew only in passing. It came from a mom I really didn't know at all. I had nothing to do with it.

I had not cried in a long, long time, but as I stood reading the colorful dinosaur birthday card inviting my daughter to a "real world" birthday party, tears flowed. Feeling elated and very silly, I retreated to the car, Sara demanding all the way to know why I was crying, and me at a total loss for words. How could I explain that this simple invitation meant more to me than one engraved in gold? How could I explain that it meant the risks were well worth taking? How could she know that, for me, the card symbolized hope in its purest form? Hope that acceptance, not just from me or people close to us, but from regular people in the "real world," was not just a dream, but an attainable goal.

*Source:* Copyright © 1993 by Brookline Books.

---

To understand and help children with disabilities, we must understand families, how families work, and the stress experienced by families. But it is also necessary to understand these caregiving families in terms of the broader social network in which they exist. According to Cooley (1994), "the success of family caregiving is dependent upon a web of factors including the family's past experience, its members' coping skills, the caregiving demands, and the ways in which society values and supports this important family activity" (p. 117).

Theories of socialization address the nature/nurture controversy (the impact of heredity and biological predisposition vs. the impact of the environment) on human development. This controversy is being resolved through research in developmental psychology that supports the contributions of both nature and nurture and the interplay of these influences. Both Erik Erikson's psychosocial theory and Jean Piaget's cognitive theory present stage models of human development that respect the biological endowment of the individual. However, both view children and adults as active learners and active participants in their environmental settings. Furthermore, Albert Bandura's social learning theory espouses a continuing state of reciprocal interaction between the person and the environment (Shaffer, 1994). Jacobs (1994) summarized developmental perspectives as follows:

> Child development was once viewed as the inevitable unfolding of innate temperament and inherited capacity. It is now increasingly understood as a

complex interaction between a child's natural endowments and constitu-
tion, and multiple forces in the environment. The most intimate and powerful context affecting children is the family; others include neighbors and
community members, formal and informal community organizations and
institutions . . . and ultimately, government policies. (p. 21)

How the broad and complex social environment influences and is influenced by
families that include a member with a disability is the focus of this chapter.

## THE ECOLOGICAL SYSTEM

⊕　　**FOCUS 1**

*Identify the four systems included in Bronfenbrenner's social ecology model.*

Relations between the developing person and the environment are reflected in the
work of Urie Bronfenbrenner (1979), who provided a framework, or model, for
understanding societal values and supports as they apply to families. This framework, which applies to all families, is particularly useful for families that include a
member with a disability (Bernier & Siegel, 1994; Berry, 1995; Kazak, 1986, 1989).
Bronfenbrenner focuses on the developing person as part of the broader social environment and on the interaction between the person and the environment. This
social ecology system resembles the family system in the sense that change in one
part of the system affects other parts of the system and the system as a whole.
　　According to Bronfenbrenner (1979), the ecological environment "is con-
ceived as a set of nested structures, each inside the next, like a set of Russian dolls"
(p. 3). This systems model moves beyond the family system to encompass other
systems that make demands, produce stress, or provide support for families. Bronfenbrenner believes that the way parents view both their child and their own capacity to function in the parental role are influenced by these external factors.
Bronfenbrenner termed these systems, in order of increasing distance from the individual, the microsystem, the mesosystem, the exosystem, and the macrosystem.
　　The microsystem is the immediate system within which the individual exists.
For children, this is the family. As children grow older, additional microsystems
are added, such as school and peers. The term *mesosystem* applies to linkages or
relationships between microsystems. The child does not actually participate in exosystems (the next system), but exosystems can still influence his or her development. For example, the mother's or father's workplace, which is a microsystem
for that adult, is an exosystem for the child. The child does not directly participate
in the parent's workplace, but that system can influence the child. The overarch-
ing system surrounding these other systems is the macrosystem. Macrosystems
are the broad ideological patterns of a particular culture. The macrosystem is the

"blueprint" for the ecology of human development, reflecting "shared assumptions about 'how things should be done'" (Garbarino & Abramowitz, 1992, p. 27).

Garbarino and Abramowitz (1992) present an ecological map for studying Bronfenbrenner's model (Figure 5.1). They stress the importance of viewing this system in terms of both opportunities and risks for the child. The Individuals with Disabilities Education Act (IDEA) provides an example of interconnections among these systems. Viewed from the outside in, at the macrosystem level, IDEA is a federal law reflecting a shared value within the culture of the United States

**FIGURE 5.1**    *The Ecology of Human Development*

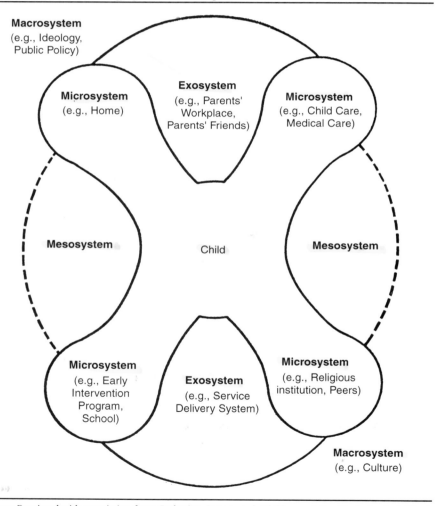

*Source:* Reprinted with permission from Garbarino, James, et al. *Children and Families in the Social Environment.* 2nd edition. (New York: Aldine de Gruyter). Copyright © 1992 Walter de Gruyter, Inc. New York.

that all children should receive free and appropriate education. At the exosystem level, state plans are developed and local school boards design systems for implementing IDEA. Individualized education programs (IEPs) are designed for children, and mesosystem connections between home and school microsystems become vital for optimal implementation of these plans. This same example can be applied from the other direction. Federal education laws are relatively recent and reflect microsystem needs expressed by parents for educational opportunities for their sons and daughters with disabilities, and the lack of such opportunities. Parental desire for educational opportunities resulted in some school programs for some children. Parents had to advocate at the exosystem level (sometimes joined by service provider advocates) to expand services and, finally, at the macrosystem level to assure universal services. Clearly, the system affects the child and family, but the child and family also affect the system.

A paradox for families with a member with disabilities is that they face both social isolation, due to care needs of the child and societal stigma as well as accelerated social involvement. An important difference between families of children with and without disabilities is that the needs associated with the disability quickly move the family beyond the home microsystem. Branching out to other systems is necessary to secure services, but it is not without stress. Communication and strong interconnections between systems become vitally important for these children and their families. We use the ecological map (Garbarino & Abramowitz, 1992; Figure 5.1) to demonstrate the social ecology of these families.

## MICROSYSTEM AND MESOSYSTEM CONNECTIONS

### ⊞ FOCUS 2

*How are microsystem and mesosystem connections influenced by disability?*

### The Home Microsystem

The most important microsystem for a young child with a disability, or for any child, is the home. As children grow older, additional microsystems are added, until the adult leaves the home of origin to create a new system, which still includes the family. The home microsystem is the family system. This system is the primary source of nurturing, caregiving, and support for the person with a disability until adulthood, and perhaps even then. At the mesosystem level, the family interacts with all other systems important to the child. Frequency of interaction, quality of communication, and shared values all influence outcomes for the child. Garbarino and Abramowitz (1992) stated that "a rich range of mesosystems is both a product and cause of development. A well-connected child's competence increases, and increases her or his ability to form further connections" (p. 26).

Families of children with disabilities are as varied as the children themselves. Fish (1991) addressed parenting a child with disabilities in nontraditional families, including single-parent and stepparent families, foster and adoptive parents, and families in which the parents have disabilities. She stressed the importance of considering the unique characteristics of these families. Another family structure that is increasingly prevalent is children being raised by their grandparents (Bell & Smith, 1996). Circumstances such as substance abuse on the part of the parents, which in some cases led to grandparents assuming the parenting role, are also risk factors for developmental problems for the children. These varying family configurations present unique strengths and needs. For example, parents who have disabilities themselves and are rearing a child with special needs are considered at risk. However, they must be considered individually. Some function well with minimal supports, others are not able to care for their children at all, and many fall somewhere in between these two points (Ray, Rubenstein, & Russo, 1994).

Some families, for a variety of reasons, are unable to care for a son or daughter with disabilities and must seek temporary or permanent out-of-home care through foster care or institutional placement. In these situations, positive and productive interactions between home settings—that is, the residence of the child with disabilities and the family of origin—support improved outcomes for the child. The same is true for interactions between families and community living situations for adults with disabilities (Berry, 1995; Blacher & Baker, 1992).

### The School Microsystem

School is a critical microsystem, and all children benefit from strong mesosystem connections between home and school (Berger, 1995). For a child with disabilities, the addition of the school microsystem may start early. The introduction to formal education may start with an early intervention program for an infant or toddler with developmental disabilities. This experience may be followed by preschool, elementary, middle and secondary programs, and finally, postsecondary programs ranging from vocational to college. Although close communication and reciprocal interaction between home and school are stressed for optimal outcomes for any child, it can be crucial for a child with disabilities. Laws mandating parent involvement in special education programs recognize the importance of this home-school connection and provide a structure for its occurrence.

Ideally, parental involvement in education follows a developmental course throughout the lifespan of the child (Hardman, Drew, & Egan, 1996). Parents incorporate teaching and therapy into play and caregiving routines of infants and young children. As older children spend more time in formal educational settings, the parental role becomes less direct but no less important. Parents can be involved in planning and goal setting, in helping with assessment, and in providing additional learning opportunities beyond the classroom. Parents can ask teachers and therapists for suggestions and help as well as share ideas and successes. As their son or daughter enters adolescence, parents can work with the school for future planning. For example, a young person with a learning disability may be able to attend college with appropriate support from the educational system and the family (Brandt & Berry, 1991). Another young person may need vocational skill training in the transition from school to supported employment (McDonnell, Wilcox, & Hardman, 1991), and parents can assist in the design and implementation of these programs.

Although education is a critical support for children and adolescents with disabilities and their families, it can also be a source of stress and disappointment. School may be the setting in which the child's disability is first diagnosed. It can also be a setting of anxiety and frustration for the parents and of social isolation for the child. A sibling shared this story about his parents and his brother Marc, who has autism, from a time when disability meant exclusion from school. "My mother often told me how devastated she felt bringing Marc home after they had dropped me off at school. Watching other children his age getting dropped off with their siblings reinforced this pain" (Siegel & Silverstein, 1994, p. 8).

Jan Spiegle-Mariska (1993), in contrast, tells a positive story about her daughter Sara's success in an inclusive (students with and without disabilities) school setting (Window 5.2). She also tells of her own anxiety about this change for Sara.

---

★ **WINDOW 5.2**
_____

### *Educating Sara*

EDUCATIONALLY, I KNEW IT [A CHANGE TO AN INCLUSIVE SCHOOL SETTING] was the right thing to do. Intellectually, I was extremely pleased that she was ready for such a step. Emotionally, I was scared to death. What if the children made fun of her inadequacies? What if the other parents objected to her presence? What if she wet her pants (a rare, but still possible occurrence)? How would they handle her sometimes noncompliant behavior? What if the teachers found the situation unworkable? In short, what if the transition failed?

Knowing it was important to take the risk, I did place her. The first few weeks were difficult for me; I had a smile tattooed on my face and great fear in my heart. Sara, on the other hand, was doing beautifully. She delighted in being with the (developmentally) older children in [sister] "Susan's school." She was tired of teachers and aides monitoring her every move, and relished the freedom of the less restrictive setting. Aided by support staff in both the sending and receiving schools, she was getting along quite well, although she did wet her pants one day as she played at the "water trough." Some children did give her a wide berth, bewildered by her speech, or her different appearance. Others were intrigued by her differences. She spoke often and enthusiastically of playing with Zach and Maia, Sarah Lynn and Jillian. Eventually (much later than Sara), I began to see that the change had been exactly right for her. I was then able to smile genuinely and feel more at ease within the classroom.

*Source:* Copyright © 1993 by Brookline Books.

## The Religious Microsystem

The place of worship is a microsystem for many children and the connection between their family, and this system is, again, influenced by the child's disability. The presence or absence of religious faith and the level of involvement in formalized religion are likely to be reassessed by parents with a child with a disability. Some research (Stubblefield, 1965) indicates that the birth or diagnosis of a child with disabilities can precipitate a theological crisis for parents. They may reexamine their beliefs and may move closer to or further away from both their beliefs and organized religion.

Some evidence ties greater religious faith and involvement to both acceptance of the child and improved coping (McHale & Gamble, 1987; Zuk et al., 1961). However, there is also evidence of parents, as well as adults with disabilities, being disappointed and even angry with the lack of understanding and lack of support received from organized religion. Ginny Thornburgh (1993) realized that the church which was so important to the rest of her family had little to offer her son, Peter, who has severe mental retardation:

> Peter was six and a half when our fourth son, Bill, was born. Until then we always had a babysitter at home for Peter when we went to church. Now with Bill home too, members of the congregation asked, "When are we going to see that beautiful new baby of yours in the nursery?" *What about Peter?* I thought. *Why don't they ask about Peter?* (pp. 2–3)

Her experiences led to the development of a program designed to teach churches how to welcome and help people with disabilities and their families (Thornburgh, 1994).

## The Peer Microsystem

Peers provide fun, learning experiences, and developmental models for all children. This microsystem takes on increasing importance as children grow older. Interactions among young children, structured primarily through play, provide the basis for social development. In middle childhood, children begin to spend time with peers away from parents, and adolescents turn to peers to achieve separation from parents. For adults with disabilities, peers are vital for the achievement of the developmental tasks of identity, intimacy, and generativity.

Peers are also important for children with disabilities and their parents, but achieving peer interactions can be problematic. Young children's first peers tend to be cousins, neighbor children, and the children of their parents' friends. When a young child has a disability, this important social introduction to the community beyond the family may be limited. A child who is medically fragile will not be able to go out into the community and interact with others. Threat of illness may inhibit participation in the church nursery or a mother's day-out program. Babysitting trade-offs may be limited as well. The parents of the child with disabilities may not feel secure leaving their child, and the friend or neighbor may not feel able to care for the child, especially while caring for his or her own children. Interactions with cousins and friends' children may be limited by lack of acceptance by the adults or the hurt experienced by the parents as they compare the development of their child with that of their niece, nephew, or friend's child. The mother of an infant with severe disabilities told of isolating her baby and herself: "I cut myself off from all my friends, especially those that had babies my son's age . . . I just couldn't bring myself to go to any of the young mothers' groups and see kids Stuart's age toddling about" (Kupfer, 1982, p. 97). With a teenage son, however, Jan Moss sought to teach him ways to cope and be included (see Window 5.3 on page 108).

When children enter school, opportunities for peer interaction increase. These peer interactions are a critical part of social development for all children. Children with disabilities are at risk for limitations in experiences with peers. A school experience that separates students with disabilities from students without disabilities can decrease or even prevent social interactions with peers without disabilities. The social modeling of peers is important for development of communication and other cognitive skills. It is also important for learning appropriate behavior in various social contexts (Hardman & McDonnell, 1995). Furthermore, these peer interactions can provide fun for the children and adolescents and be "normalizing" for parents, as illustrated by Spiegle-Mariska (1993) (see Window 5.1 on page 100).

As children enter adolescence and establish independence from parents, peers assume increasing importance as social models and for advice. Opportunity to participate in activities beyond the school setting, such as sports and social clubs, may be limited. These limitations may be because of the disability, but they may also be due to negative attitudes. Just playing with friends in the neighborhood, which most children and their parents take for granted, may be inhibited by physical limitations, attitudes, or the level of supervision needed by the child. For adults with disabilities, the distressing statistic of limited employment (only 34 percent of those of working age are employed full time) means more than the obvious consequences of lack of financial independence and lowered self-esteem. It also means limited access to peers. The Americans with Disabilities Act has increased employment opportunities, but people with disabilities may still encounter negative attitudes in the workplace that inhibit peer interactions (Berry & Meyer, 1995).

Organized programs that promote peer interaction can be particularly valuable for social development and just for fun, especially those which include a lifespan focus such as Special Olympics. This program provides athletic training, participation, and competition for children and adults with developmental disabilities. Children are typically introduced to this program through their schools, but can continue to participate as adolescents and adults. Interactions with peer participants and community volunteers take place at local, state, national, and international athletic events. Some adult participants also assume roles as coaches

## Learning the "Ability Words"

TALKING TO JASON ABOUT HIS DISABILITIES came out of other people talking *about* Jason. Like in the grocery store, after Jason made a particularly loud remark about whether or not fish pass gas, a woman came up to me and said, "I know just what you're going through. We had one like him in our family too."

Later, Jason asked me, "Does that woman have a little boy like me? What does she mean? Like me, how?"

These situations were only compounded by educational and medical situations in which Jason was referred to as moderately retarded, visually-impaired, hyperactive, dysmorphic, seizure-disordered, multi-handicapped, even "syndromy." I had to ask myself, "What's a fella to think about himself while dodging all these 'diagnoses?'"

I didn't feel fully prepared to tackle this ever-increasing army of adjectives aimed at Jason. So, over a period of time, I began asking everyone involved with Jason to tell me how they saw him, without naming one thing having to do with his disabilities.

I heard things like, "He's a hoot, a very funny kid; he's so observant—notices the smallest things; his sense of smell is uncanny; he has remarkable recall; he has such curiosity; he makes me laugh." To me, these things were so much more Jason, and so much more important for Jason to learn about himself. My plan was taking shape—I wanted to start talking to Jason about his abilities, not just his diagnoses.

We began in the Wal-Mart parking lot, actually. While walking from the car to the store, Jason began his litany of smells—nose down, sniff, sniff—"I smell diesel, road tar, oil, gas."

I replied, "Yes, you do smell them, Jason. You have a great gift of smell. Did you know that about yourself?"

Time after time, I identified Jason's abilities for him. I explained how these "ability words" were not in his diagnosis, and how the words that labeled him were not adequate to tell *who* he was but just said things *about* him.

The terrible taunts—called "teasing" by the people who do it—have been the hardest thing for me to help Jason deal with. It became my goal to disarm these labels and insults. "Some people only know the diagnosis words," I told Jason, "labels like 'retarded.' They haven't learned the other words that tell about you. You will have to be smarter than they are and learn the ability words."

And so, at a neighborhood Christmas party, as the adults gathered in the kitchen, we heard a child's voice from the den, "What's the matter with you? Are you a retard or something?"

The adults fell silent. Husbands and wives looked at each other, wondering whose child had slung the "R-word" at Jason.

But Jason was equipped to handle the situation. We heard him reply, "Retard, yes, absolutely. And I smell real good, too."

A roar of laughter arose from the den and spread through the kitchen. I did not attempt an explanation; it wasn't necessary. I thought to myself, "Jason is a hoot, a very funny kid—he makes us laugh."

*Source:* Reprinted with the expressed consent and approval of *Exceptional Parent*, a monthly magazine for parents and families of children with disabilities and special health care needs. Subscription cost is $32 per year for 12 issues; Call 1-800-247-8080. Offices at 555 Kinderkamack Rd. Oradell, N.J. 07649.

and volunteers. Another program that promotes social development through peer interaction is Best Buddies. This program pairs a young adult with developmental disabilities with a college student "buddy" for social activities that are mutually rewarding and enjoyable.

## The Child-Care Microsystem

Children with disabilities whose parents are employed outside the home may have an additional microsystem: child care. This may be a babysitter or a child-care center. Acquiring appropriate child care is a dilemma faced by many employed parents (Voydanoff, 1993), which may be especially challenging for parents of children with disabilities because of additional care or supervision needs (Greater Minneapolis Day Care, 1993) and because care, in many cases, continues to be needed for adolescents and adults with disabilities. Again, negative attitudes may make this challenging task more difficult. JoEllen Barnhart and her husband, Dave, employed parents of a baby with Down syndrome, encountered people who saw caring for a baby with special needs as an opportunity to charge a higher fee. JoEllen stated, "It seemed they were mostly interested in the money. We didn't like their attitudes, and we couldn't afford their fees anyway" (Cartwright, 1995, p. 26). Parents of adolescents and adults with disabilities may find securing care for their son or daughter while they work or for social outings an even greater challenge (with no end in sight), especially in the circumstance of physical or behavioral problems.

An additional challenge is linking the child-care microsystem with the school or early intervention microsystem, and parents often have to take the lead in facilitating this linkage. The early intervention or school team may have suggestions for a home program that will need to be carried out by the child-care provider. The parents will need to convey information between these two systems and arrange meetings, which can be quite complicated. Parents of adolescents and adults may turn to an agency (through a state-level department of human services, for example) for help in caring for their son or daughter. Establishing relationships, providing training, and negotiating with the care providers themselves and the agency system will be necessary. This may be made more challenging by frequent turnover of care providers. Also, parents may find themselves in the position of trading valued privacy and autonomy in their homes for needed support services.

## The Medical-Care Microsystem

Medical care for a child with disabilities can be a microsystem in which the child spends a large amount of time. The mesosystem connections between this microsystem and the family can be critically important (Ahmann, 1994; DePompei, Whitford, & Beam, 1994). For children born prematurely or with other special needs, their first home is the hospital, and their first caregivers are physicians and nurses, with parents playing a crucial supporting role. Other children may require intermittent, but prolonged periods of hospitalization. Still others may be able to receive services as outpatients but are linked to medical-care providers in a more frequent and more intense manner than children without disabilities.

The medical-care microsystem is complex and seems to be growing more complex through programs such as HMOs and managed care. This complicated microsystem is one of the most challenging for parents to understand and negotiate successfully. Fern Kupfer (1982) shared a story from the early days of involvement with the medical system treating her son Zach:

> It took me a while to catch on to the game at the teaching hospital. Different doctors at different times would come in and start asking me questions about my family history, the pregnancy, was Zach ever dropped on his head, etc. I kept thinking that each was *the* doctor, but no, then he or she would gather up the notes, and minutes later a new person would appear. "Look," I said impatiently after the third one. "Why do I have to keep repeating this same story: why don't you get together with this?" What I didn't understand then was that all these people were medical students, interns, residents; Zach was part of their curriculum. So, of course, they didn't answer any of my questions. They were interested in asking their own. (p. 37)

The research literature documents the stress experienced by families of hospitalized children (Alexander, White, & Powell, 1986; Satterwhite, 1978) and the disruption of family life experienced when a child is hospitalized (Johnson, 1990). The importance of general and crisis specific social support for these families was documented in research by Hobfoll and Lerman (1988). Also, both formal and informal support provided by hospital personnel has been demonstrated empirically by Flynn and McCollum (1993), who stress the need for a support system that "depends on understanding and acknowledging the perspective of individual parents" (p. 35). Additional research findings (Berman, 1991) indicate, however, that stated support for the concept of family-centered medical care may not be borne out by actual beliefs and practices of medical personnel. Strong mesosystem connections between home and medical care are important not only to child health, but for prevention of secondary mental health problems (Patterson & Geber, 1991). Furthermore, connections between the medical-care system and the school and other community resources are needed to promote optimal child and family outcomes (Stuart & Goodsitt, 1996).

## Mesosystem Connections

The success of mesosystem connections among home, school, place of worship, peers, child care, and medical care depends on both the skills of the parents in negotiating the system and how user friendly the system is for families. For parents, communicative and cognitive abilities, self-confidence, personality, and ability to handle stress all play a part in the success or lack of success of the mesosystem relationships and interconnections. How open or closed the family system is may also be relevant. Specifically, a more open family will be more comfortable sharing needs and receiving supports.

Professionals need to keep in mind that these parents already have full plates caring for their child with disabilities and other family members, dealing with their feelings concerning their child, and carrying out other responsibilities such as employment and household tasks. So professionals need to seek ways to establish welcoming relationships, facilitate communication, and provide support. This is especially important in light of research findings in which families reported dissatisfaction with services while professionals reported that families were satisfied with these same services (Spaniol & Zipple, 1988).

## THE EXOSYSTEM

### ⊞  FOCUS 3

*How does the exosystem function as a source of opportunity and risk for families that include a family member with a disability?*

Children do not participate directly in the exosystem and, in many cases, neither do their parents. These settings, however, can have tremendous power and influence over a child's life. According to Garbarino and Abramowitz (1992), the child is vulnerable to risk from the exosystem in two ways. The first risk comes when the exosystem exerts influence in a way that impoverishes parental behavior toward the child at the microsystem level, for example, stress experienced by the parent in the workplace. A second type of risk results when decisions made in the service delivery component of the exosystem adversely affect the child, such as a decision to reduce funding for special education services. The exosystem can also be a source of opportunity for children and families. Empowering parents to exert influence at the exosystem level is an important component in improving outcomes for children.

### The Parent's Workplace

The workplace is a microsystem for the individual parent and an exosystem for the child. The workplace provides resources such as money and medical insurance for the family as well as social support for the parents, all of which can benefit the child. However, the workplace creates responsibilities and demands on parents that may conflict with the care needs of the child. This workplace/family conflict is an issue for many parents (Voydanoff, 1993) that may be exacerbated for families of children with disabilities. Potential conflicts between home and workplace for these families include school conferences and IEP meetings held during work hours, a work transfer that takes the family away from a valued service delivery system, or meeting work responsibilities at a time of high demand from the child, such as surgery. Single-parent and dual-earner families are especially vulnerable to these stresses. Dual-couple earners may also be vulnerable to conflict between the two parents concerning division of responsibilities (Berry, Meyer, & Reed, 1994). Benefits such as parental leave and flexible work schedules may be extremely important for these families, but they may not be available.

Research addressing employed parents of children with special needs is sparse, but compelling. Studies of employed caregivers (Fernandez, 1990) found that 10 percent of the study population cared for children with disabilities. These studies, as well as additional work (Freedman, Litchfield, & Warfield, 1995; Krauskopf & Akabas, 1988; Zigler & Lang, 1991), present a picture of parents experiencing increased stress and more difficulty finding appropriate child care. In addition, the parents studied reported problems with missing work, arriving late, and leaving early. Yet these parents may have increased needs for employment, in terms of finances and health insurance and as a means of social support.

## The Service Delivery System

Other exosystems exclude the child and exclude or have very limited participation from parents, and yet they have enormous influence on child and family outcomes. Examples include school boards, departments of human services, local governments, medical-care systems, and health insurance programs. Decisions of school boards concerning delivery of educational services impact the child and parents directly, as well as the mesosystem connection between home and school. For example, a teacher may agree with a parent about how best to serve the child but may still be restricted in implementation by school rules. The health insurance system may impose limits on both the patient and the physician or therapist. A positive example of exosystem influence would be a city park and recreation department that stresses inclusion of children and adolescents with disabilities in summer day camp programs and provides supports needed for success.

When the service structure at the exosystem level and the needs of individuals with disabilities do not mesh, advocacy efforts are appropriate. An advocate is an "informed friend" or a person who pleads the case of a person with disabilities (Heward & Orlansky, 1988, p. 117). Both service providers and family members can be advocates. But exosystem level advocacy is not for everyone.

All parents should be supported as advocates for their sons and daughters through interactions with teachers, therapists, physicians, and others at the mesosystem level. Exosystem-level advocacy seems to require higher levels of confidence and self-esteem and resources such as time, energy, and money. The pay-off, however, can be extremely rewarding. At the level of the individual, research has shown that parents of children with disabilities who score higher on a measure of parental advocacy have lower scores on a measure of parental stress (Patterson & Berry, 1997). In terms of the service delivery system, federal legislation, including the Individuals with Disabilities Education Act (IDEA) and the Americans with Disabilities Act (ADA), began with advocacy efforts at the exosystem level on the part of individuals with disabilities and their families. Major changes at the exosystem level because of advocacy by front-line professionals such as teachers and nurses have also occurred. Change in hospital policy concerning parental access to hospitalized children is a good example (Flynn & McCollum, 1993; Klaus & Kennell, 1982).

Just as exosystem-level advocacy is not for everyone, it is not for anyone all the time. Darling (1988) presented the idea of parental entrepreneurship, which includes "(1) seeking information, (2) seeking control, and (3) challenging authority in order to secure services to meet the needs of the disabled child" (p. 142). Parental entrepreneurship is framed in terms of "career paths of parents of disabled children" (p. 157). This is not a static model but instead includes times of greater or less advocacy involvement depending on the needs of the child and parental resources, as well as "turning points" based on both need and opportunity. Successful advocacy at the exosystem level can be highly reinforcing because these parents see positive changes, not only for their child, but for other (in some cases *many* other) children as well. These parents are likely to continue to be advocates, but they may experience periods of exhaustion and burnout. They may also curtail advocacy efforts if they find they are spending too much time on activities *for* their child and too little time *with* their child (Turnbull, 1985).

Another important advocacy effort is self-advocacy for adults with disabilities. These programs empower adults with disabilities while providing social interaction, peer support, and extensive opportunities for advocacy. The disability rights movement, which brought positive changes for people with disabilities at all ages, came about through the advocacy efforts of adults with disabilities (Shapiro, 1994).

Additional examples of exosystem effects on individuals with disabilities and their families include media influence and decisions about how programs are staffed and financed and how professionals are trained. The media is a part of the exosystem that may be a source of stress or support, information or confusion, for families (Rankin & Phillips, 1995). A newspaper article depicting a child with disabilities as a subject of pity may be distressing to parents. However, publications such as *Exceptional Parent* can serve as a source of both information and support for families and can foster advocacy efforts. The popular media can and does influence attitudes in both positive and negative directions.

## Parents' Friends

The social support that parents receive from their friends can reduce stress and enhance coping, and friendships with other parents in similar circumstances are particularly valued. A turning point that often leads parents in the direction of increased well-being and increased advocacy is getting to know other parents of children with disabilities. These parents can provide friendship, support because of mutual problems, and advice about child development. This developmental advice is particularly important because it often cannot be found through interaction with parents of children with typical development or through reading material on child development that focuses on typical development. This parent-to-parent support system decreases risk for children.

From the standpoint of advocacy, linkages with these parents can lead to increased empowerment through greater numbers of consumers seeking systems change. Also, other parents can be a source for learning advocacy skills. Buscaglia (1983), a special education professional, tells this story about the evaluation of a series of parent education programs:

> One of the evaluation questions was "What *one* thing did you find *most valuable* in this experience?" I was certain it would be one of my pearls of wisdom, or that of one of my illustrious colleagues. Much to my surprise, over 85 percent of the responses suggested that the most valuable experience was learning that there were so many other parents who had children who were disabled like their own! I am wiser for the experience, too! (p. 108)

## THE MACROSYSTEM

**⊞   FOCUS 4**

*How does the macrosystem influence the family microsystem?*

The macrosystem includes the cultural and ideological values of society as a whole. The macrosystem is also politics and policies. It is the arena in which a society's values become government policy and are financed accordingly. Government philosophy leads to legislation that leads to policies for administering and funding particular programs. The decisions regarding special education, medical care, and social welfare made at the macrosystem level have critical consequences for the family microsystem. For example, the decision of Congress in 1990 to expand IDEA to include infants and toddlers has had a direct impact on the lives of thousands of infants and toddlers and their families.

## Ideology

Although politicians love to speak of family values, U.S. society has an ideological pattern of macrosystem risk for children. Data presented by Jacobs (1994) bear this out:

> Of eight indicators used by the Center for the Study of Social Policy to determine national and state trends in child well-being, two have changed for the better since the 1980s: infant mortality and child death rates. The others—the percent of low birth-weight babies, of all births that are to single teens, of youths graduating high school, of children living in poverty, of children living in single-parent households, and teen violent death rate—have changed for the worse. (p. 20)

Today's children are vulnerable to what has been termed a "litany of modern social woes" (Horowitz & O'Brien, 1989, p. 444). This litany includes teenage pregnancy, domestic violence, and substance abuse. Any of these circumstances may play a role in causing a child's disability. The result is a child at risk being cared for by parents at risk.

Families that include a child with a disability are at particular risk when vulnerabilities converge. For example, it is more difficult for these parents to acquire the supports needed for their child and family if poverty is part of the picture. The combination of cultural diversity, poverty, and disability portends both risk for the child and family and the potential for alienation from the service delivery system (Harry, 1992). Similarly, all children and families are affected negatively by societal prejudice in the form of racism and sexism. Persons with disabilities and their families are likely to encounter handicapism—prejudice based on the disability—as well. Ideology that values and supports children and families is important for all families, but particularly when disability is part of the picture.

## Culture and Diversity

Culture is the collective beliefs of a society and the impact of those beliefs on social behavior. U.S. society is multicultural. African, Asian, Hispanic, and Native Americans constitute approximately one-third of the U.S. population, with projections for increased representation. Furthermore, students with multicultural backgrounds comprise approximately 15 percent of school populations (Misra, 1994). These statistics, as well as the troubling data that reveal overrepresentation of multicultural students classified as disabled, have important implications for professionals working with families. American society also includes broad variability in socioeconomic status, which has been found to be more important than race in shaping parental values (Scanzoni, 1985). Furthermore, socioeconomic needs can add another governmental system to a family's life—the welfare system.

Empirical evidence supports the potential for conflict between service providers and families in a multicultural society (Westbrook & Legge, 1993). Harry (1996) identified five areas of potential dissonance between families from culturally diverse backgrounds and the professionals who provide services to these families: (1) interpretations of the meaning of disability; (2) concepts of family structure and identity; (3) goals of education; (4) parent–child interaction; and (5) communication style. Effectively bridging these differences requires both sensitivity and professional competence. McCubbin and his colleagues (1993) offered this advice, which was directed toward medical professionals but has broad application for professionals providing services to families and children:

> Cultural sensitivity and competence to deal with ethnicity can prevent health care professionals from unintentionally alienating parents or families through miscommunication or what the family considers inappropriate and unacceptable suggestions or behavior. Since such misunderstandings could result in the child's receiving inadequate medical attention, particularly if the family feels hesitant about placing trust in someone who so clearly does not understand their values, it is vital that practitioners remain aware of the cultural context within which the family is operating. (p. 1068)

## Public Policy

Cooley (1994) discussed problems faced by families that include a member with disabilities in terms of issues and troubles. Troubles are faced by families and by individuals within families as personal matters, but issues are matters of public policy. All parents face limits in what they, as individuals, can provide for their sons and daughters. That is why families turn to schools, religious institutions, medical establishments, and other systems for support in caring for, teaching, and nurturing their children. For parents of children with disabilities, these support systems are likely to be both needed more and less available.

However, there are some encouraging trends of direct and indirect impact of public policy on families. The Americans with Disabilities Act (ADA) prohibits discrimination on the basis of disability for child-care programs (with the exception of church-operated programs). Child-care programs must now make needed changes (reasonable accommodations) to provide services to children with disabilities (Gil de Lamadrid, 1996). In addition to these legal rights, it is encouraging to see articles on how to achieve success in inclusive child care in publications intended, not for special educators, but for regular educators (e.g., Leister, Koonce, & Nisbet, 1993).

A minister, Bill Gaventa (1994), credits ADA and other legislation with helping religious denominations and faith groups develop resources to stimulate and encourage religious congregations to include children and adults with disabilities. He defined these resources as follows:

> Models of congregational ministry and services include both specialized and inclusive religious education programs, creative ways to facilitate participation in worship, congregational respite care, group homes run by religious groups, disability awareness materials, daycare, camps and congregation-based circles of support. (p. 22)

Also important for families are state initiatives designed to provide families with a variety of supportive goods and services, including cash subsidies that families can use for goods and services of their choice (Agosta & Melda, 1995; Herman, 1991; Herman & Thompson, 1995). Families use these funds to purchase clothing, toys, and diapers, to acquire professional services for the child, for adaptive equipment (including creative problem solving such as renting a motorized wheelchair on a trial basis), and for obtaining child care (both to give the parents a break and so parents can seek employment).

As discussed in Chapter 1, public policies concerning persons with disabilities are the consequence of historical processes. Newman (1987) studied public policy with respect to persons with disabilities and stated that "the issues involved in those policies are complex, changing, and highly politicized" (p. 41). This is reflected currently as IDEA is under scrutiny for change and possible reduction at a time when more students than ever need services. Specifically, from the 1992–1993 school year to the 1993–1994 school year there was an increase of 4.2 percent in students served, which represents the largest increase since the inception of IDEA in 1976 (Seventeenth Annual Report to Congress, 1995).

Ideology and culture influence public policy and, happily, sometimes this influence comes full circle, with service recipients as policymakers, as was the case with Greg:

> Greg is a young attorney. He does some work for a Washington-based association. California Governor Pete Wilson recently named him to a state advisory panel.
>
> This might be the story of just another ordinary up-and-comer, except that Greg was diagnosed with cerebral palsy in infancy. His lack of muscle control slows his speech; he needs a motorized wheel-chair to get around and uses a computer to write.
>
> Greg's success would not have been possible without the Individuals with Disabilities Education Act, or IDEA, which mandated and financially supported his education. In generations past, Greg probably would have been institutionalized. (Cunningham, 1995, p. 46)

Although our society has moved in a positive direction of more humanitarian treatment and inclusive involvement of persons with disabilities and their families, these positive changes require constant vigilance on the part of families and service providers, at all system levels, for maintenance and growth.

# REVIEW

*FOCUS 1: Identify the four systems included in Bronfenbrenner's social ecology model.*

- The microsystem is the immediate system in which the individual exists.
- The mesosystem involves linkages or relationships between various microsystems.
- The exosystem involves settings in which the individual does not participate, but that exert influence over his or her life.
- Macrosystems are broad ideological patterns of a particular culture.

*FOCUS 2: How are microsystem and mesosystem connections influenced by disability?*

- The home microsystem is the primary source of nurturing, caregiving, and support for the person with a disability until adulthood, and perhaps even then.
- School involvement follows a developmental course for the child, but close communication and reciprocal interaction between home and school is important for optimal outcomes for the child at all ages.
- The religious microsystem is a source of support for some families, but can also be a source of disappointment.
- Peers are important for persons with disabilities and their families, but achieving peer interactions can be problematic.
- The child-care microsystem can be challenging for children with disabilities and their parents because of the care and supervision needs of the child and negative attitudes.
- The medical-care microsystem is one of the most complex systems experienced by children and parents, and mesosystem connections are crucial for positive outcomes.

*FOCUS 3: How does the exosystem function as a source of opportunity and risk for families that include a family member with a disability?*

- The workplace provides financial and other resources such as medical insurance. However, the workplace creates responsibilities and demands on parents that may be in conflict with the care needs of the child.

- Parents often become advocates to increase services for their son or daughter with disabilities. These advocacy efforts are frequently successful and satisfying, but they are not without stress.

- Relationships with friends, including other parents of children with disabilities, can be particularly important sources of support for parents as individuals and as advocates.

*FOCUS 4: How does the macrosystem influence the family microsystem?*

- Ideological patterns in our society place many children at risk. This risk is likely to be magnified for children with disabilities.

- Cultural diversity affects social policy and is a source of potential conflict between service providers and families.

- Public policy affects provision of services, which has a direct impact on persons with disabilities and their families.

## REFERENCES

Agosta, J., & Melda, K. (1995). Supporting families who provide care at home for children with disabilities. *Exceptional Children, 62*, 271–282.

Ahmann, E. (1994). Family centered care: The time has come. *Pediatric Nursing, 20*, 52–53.

Alexander, D., White, M., & Powell, G. (1986). Anxiety of non-rooming in parents of hospitalized children. *Children's Health Care, 15*, 14–19.

Bell, M. L., & Smith, B. R. (1996). Grandparents as primary caregivers. *Teaching Exceptional Children, 28*, 18–19.

Berger, E. H. (1995). *Parents as partners in education* (4th ed.). Englewood Cliffs, NJ: Merrill.

Berman, H. (1991). Nurses' beliefs about family involvement in a children's hospital. *Pediatric Nursing, 14*, 141–153.

Bernier, J. C., & Siegel, D. H. (1994). Attention-deficit hyperactive disorder: A family and ecological systems perspective. *Families in Society, 75*, 142–150.

Berry, J. O. (1995). Families and deinstitutionalization: An application of Bronfenbrenner's social ecology model. *Journal of Counseling and Development, 73*, 379–383.

Berry, J. O., & Meyer, J. A. (1995). Employing people with disabilities: Impact of attitude and situation. *Rehabilitation Psychology, 40*, 211–222.

Berry, J. O., Meyer, J. A., & Reed, C. N. (1994, October). *Combining employment and care of a young child with special needs: A special balancing act.* Paper presented at the meeting of the Oklahoma Federation of the Council for Exceptional Children, Tulsa.

Blacher, J., & Baker, B. L. (1992). Toward meaningful family involvement in out-of-home placement settings. *Mental Retardation, 30*, 35–43.

Brandt, M. S., & Berry, J. O. (1991). Transitioning college-bound students with LD. *Intervention in School and Clinic, 26*, 297–301.

Bronfenbrenner, U. (1979). *The ecology of human development: Experiments by nature and design.* Cambridge: Harvard University Press.

Buscaglia, L. (1983). *The disabled and their parents: A counseling challenge* (2nd ed.). Thorofare, NJ: Slack.

Cartwright, C. (1995, May). What love can teach. *Working Mother*, pp. 26, 28.

Cooley, W. C. (1994). The ecology of support for caregiving families. *Developmental and Behavioral Pediatrics, 15*, 117–119.

Cunningham, R. (1995, November). "Special ed" deserves special emphasis. *Exceptional Parent*, pp. 46–47.

Darling, R. B. (1988). Parental entrepreneurship: A consumerist response to professional dominance. *Journal of Social Issues, 44*, 141–158.

DePompei, P. M., Whitford, K. M., & Beam, P. H. (1994). One institution's effort to implement family-centered care. *Pediatric Nursing, 20*, 119–121, 204.

Fernandez, J. P. (1990). *The politics and reality of family care in corporate America*. Lexington, MA: Lexington.

Fish, M. C. (1991). Exceptional children in nontraditional families. In M. J. Fine (Ed.), *Collaboration with parents of exceptional children* (pp. 45–59). Brandon, VT: Clinical Psychology Press.

Flynn, L. L., & McCollum, J. (1993). Support for rural families of hospitalized infants: The parents' perspective. *Children's Health Care, 22*, 19–37.

Freedman, R. I., Litchfield, L. C., & Warfield, M. E. (1995). Balancing work and family: Perspectives of parents of children with developmental disabilities. *Families in Society, 76*, 507–514.

Garbarino, J., & Abramowitz, R. H. (1992). The ecology of human development. In J. Garbarino (Ed.), *Children and families in the social environment* (pp. 11–33). New York: Aldine de Gruyter.

Gaventa, B. (1994, December). Religious participation for all. *Exceptional Parent*, pp. 22–25.

Gil de Lamadrid, M. (1996, February). Child care and the ADA: Litigation updates. *Exceptional Parent*, pp. 40–43.

Greater Minneapolis Day Care Association. (1993). *Child care for children with special needs*. [Brochure]. Minneapolis: Author.

Hardman, M. L., Drew, C. J., & Egan, M. W. (1996). *Human exceptionality: Society, school and family* (5th ed.). Boston: Allyn & Bacon.

Hardman, M. L., & McDonnell, A. P. (1995). Family, friends, and society: Supporting people with severe disabilities. In J. J. McDonnell, M. L. Hardman, A. P. McDonnell, & R. Kiefer-O'Donnell (Eds.), *An introduction to persons with severe disabilities* (pp. 47–74). Boston: Allyn & Bacon.

Harry, B. (1992). *Cultural diversity, families, and the special education system: Communication and empowerment*. New York: Teachers College Press, Columbia University.

Harry, B. (1996). Developing cultural self-awareness: The first step in values clarification for early interventionists. *Topics in Early Childhood Special Education, 12*, 333–350.

Herman, S. E. (1991). Use and impact of a cash subsidy program. *Mental Retardation, 29*, 253–258.

Herman, S. E., & Thompson, L. (1995). Families' perceptions of their resources for caring for children with developmental disabilities. *Mental Retardation, 33*, 73–83.

Heward, W. L., & Orlansky, M. D. (1988). *Exceptional children* (3rd ed.). Columbus: Merrill.

Hobfoll, S. E., & Lerman, M. (1988). Personal relationships, personal attributes, and stress resistance: Mothers' reactions to their child's illness. *American Journal of Community Psychology, 16*, 565–589.

Horowitz, F. D., & O'Brien, M. (1989). In the interest of a nation: A reflective essay on the state of our knowledge and the challenges before us. *American Psychologist, 44,* 441–445.

Jacobs, F. H. (1994). Child and family policy: Framing the issues. In F. H. Jacobs & M. W. Davies (Eds.), *More than kissing babies? Current child and family policy in the United States* (pp. 9–35). Westport, CT: Auburn.

Johnson, S. B. (1990). The family and the child with chronic illness. In D. C. Turk & R. D. Kerns (Eds.), *Health, illness, and families: A life-span perspective* (pp. 220–254). New York: Wiley.

Kazak, A. (1986). Families with physically handicapped children: Social ecology and family systems. *Family Process, 25,* 265–281.

Kazak, A. (1989). Families of chronically ill children: A systems and social-ecological model of adaptation and challenge. *Journal of Consulting and Clinical Psychology, 57,* 25–30.

Klaus, M. H., & Kennell, J. H. (1982). *Parent-infant bonding* (2nd ed.). St. Louis: Mosby.

Krauskopf, M. S., & Akabas, S. H. (1988). Children with disabilities: A family/work partnership in problem resolution. *Social Work Papers, 21,* 28–35.

Kupfer, F. (1982). *Before and after Zachariah.* New York: Delacorte.

Leister, C., Koonce, D., & Nisbet, S. (1993). Best practices for preschool programs: An update on inclusive settings. *Day Care and Early Education, 21,* 9–12.

McCubbin, H. I., Thompson, E. A., Thompson, A. I., McCubbin, M. A., & Kaston, A. J. (1993). Culture, ethnicity, and the family: Critical factors in childhood chronic illness and disabilities. *Pediatrics, 91,* 1063–1070.

McDonnell, J., Wilcox, B., & Hardman, M. L. (1991). *Secondary programs for students with developmental disabilities.* Boston: Allyn & Bacon.

McHale, S. M., & Gamble, W. C. (1987). Sibling relationships and adjustment of children with disabled brothers and sisters. *Journal of Children in Contemporary Society, 19,* 131–158.

Misra, A. (1994). Partnership with multicultural families. In S. Alper, P. J. Schloss, & C. N. Schloss (Eds.), *Families of students with disabilities: Consultation and advocacy* (pp. 143–179). Boston: Allyn & Bacon.

Moss, J. (1995, June). Learning the "Ability Words." *Exceptional Parent,* p. 96.

Newman, J. (1987). Background forces in policies for care and treatment of disability. *Marriage and Family Review, 11,* 25–44.

Patterson, J. M., & Geber, G. (1991). Preventing mental health problems in children with chronic illness or disability. *Children's Health Care, 20,* 150–161.

Patterson, L., & Berry, J. O. (1997). *Parental advocacy and child disability: Personal and social characteristics of an advocate.* Poster session presented at the annual conference of the Council for Exceptional Children, Salt Lake City, UT.

Rankin, J. L., & Phillips, S. (1995). Learning disabilities in the popular press: Suggestion for educators. *Teaching Exceptional Children, 27,* 35–39.

Ray, N. K., Rubenstein, H., & Russo, N. J. (1994). Understanding the parents who are mentally retarded: Guidelines for family preservation programs. *Child Welfare, 123,* 725–743.

Satterwhite, B. B. (1978). Impact of chronic illness on child and family: An overview based on five surveys with implications for management. *International Journal of Rehabilitation Research, 1,* 7–17.

Scanzoni, J. (1985). Black parental values and expectations of children's occupational and educational success: Theoretical implications. In H. P. McAdoo & J. L. McAdoo (Eds.), *Black children: Social, educational and parental environments* (pp. 113–122). Beverly Hills, CA: Sage.

*Seventeenth Annual Report to Congress on the Individuals with Disabilities Education Act* (1995). Washington, DC: U.S. Department of Education.

Shaffer, D. R. (1994). *Social and personality development* (3rd ed.). Pacific Grove: Brooks/Cole.

Shapiro, J. P. (1994). *No pity.* New York: Times Books.

Siegel, B., & Silverstein, S. (1994). *What about me?* New York: Plenum.

Spaniol, L., & Zipple, A. M. (1988). Family and professional perceptions of family needs and coping strengths. *Rehabilitation Psychology, 33,* 37–45.

Spiegle-Mariska, J. (1993). The birthday invitation. In J. A. Spiegle and R. A. van den Pol (Eds.), *Making changes: Family voices on living with disabilities* (pp. 53–55). Cambridge: Brookline.

Stuart, J. L., & Goodsitt, J. L. (1996). From hospital to school: How a transition liaison can help. *Teaching Exceptional Children, 28,* 58–62.

Stubblefield, H. W. (1965). Religion, parents, and mental retardation. *Mental Retardation, 3, 4,* 8–11.

Thornburgh, G. (1993, October). For the love of Peter. *Guideposts,* pp. 2–5.

Thornburgh, G. (Ed.). (1994). *That all may worship: An interfaith welcome to people with disabilities.* Washington, DC: National Organization on Disability.

Turnbull, A. P. (1985). From professional to parent—a startling experience. In H. R. Turnbull & A. P. Turnbull (Eds.), *Parents speak out: Then & now* (pp. 127–135). Columbus: Merrill.

Voydanoff, P. (1993). Work and family relationships. In T. H. Brubaker (Ed.), *Family relations: Challenges for the future* (pp. 98–111). Newbury Park, CA: Sage.

Westbrook, M. T., & Legge, V. (1993). Health practitioners' perceptions of family attitudes toward children with disabilities: A comparison of six communities in a multicultural society. *Rehabilitation Psychology, 38,* 177–185.

Zigler, E. F., & Lang, M. E. (1991). *Child care choices: Balancing the needs of children, families, and society.* New York: Free Press.

Zuk, G. H., Miller, R. L., Bartram, J. B., & Kling, F. (1961). Maternal acceptance of retarded children: A questionnaire study of attitudes and religious background. *Child Development, 32,* 525–540.

# CHAPTER SIX

# Communicating and Collaborating with Families

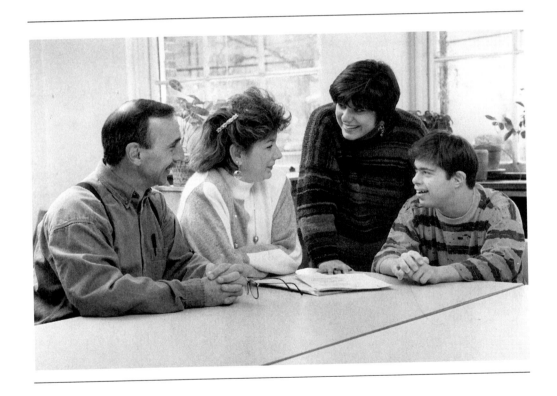

---

✳ **WINDOW 6.1**

---

## You've Got to Have Heart

Joe is 18, and a big, strong, good-looking young man who has mild mental retardation. . . .

Joe's parents wanted to sit down and talk about Joe. They wanted me to know him as a person and to hear his questions. Could he go to a technical college? Could he work in landscaping or carpentry? They wished Joe had more friends and fun things to do. They appreciated his quiet nature and hard working spirit. They primarily wanted to make sure that they knew what options were out there for him and how to feel confident enough to ask.

Parents of young adults with disabilities are often viewed as a barrier or overprotective. Many times I've heard the phrase, "if only we could get rid of the parents, we'd have a good transition plan."

It's difficult, however, for a parent to step back if no one else has shown a genuine caring. As one parent said to me, "This is only about one thing . . . HEART. I just want people to care about my kid."

*Source:* Reprinted with permission from PACER Center, (612) 827-2966.

---

The diagnosis of disability in a son or daughter broadens the social/ecological environment of parents and introduces them to a service delivery system that, although necessary, can be a source of stress as well as a source of support. In order to parent their child effectively, parents must communicate and collaborate with professionals. To better serve the child, professionals must communicate and collaborate with parents. Neither parent nor professional would dispute that successful communication is a vital, ongoing goal of the parent/professional relationship. Yet most would say that this goal is frequently difficult to achieve. Success for parents, and ultimately for their children, as the home mesosystem connects with service delivery mesosystems, or "the parents' journey through the community service maze" (Rubin & Quinn-Curran, 1983, p. 63), depends on effective parent/professional communication and a relationship built on collaboration.

This chapter addresses both information sharing between families and professionals and potential roadblocks to effective communication and collaboration. In addition, we discuss skills needed for successful communication, collaboration, and teamwork. Finally, the chapter suggests ways to prevent and resolve conflict.

## SHARING INFORMATION

### ⊕ FOCUS 1

*What is involved in information sharing between families and professionals?*

Families and professionals come together to share information that will benefit the child or adult with disabilities. This information sharing is a two-way process. Parents know their child best and observe and interact with the child in circumstances in which professionals will never participate, such as when the child awakens from a bad dream in the middle of the night. Even a critically ill newborn, whom everyone is trying to get to know, is observed differently by parents than by professionals, and an adolescent may share some feelings only with Mom or Dad. The parents' unique contribution to the understanding of their child comes both from the greater amount of time the child spends with the parents and from the emotional bond between parent and child.

The starting point of effective relationships between parents and professionals is professional valuing of the information base that families can provide. This information base includes information about the family system and about the child's developmental and health history. Information about the child's personality, behavior, and interests is helpful as well. Information shared by parents is important for young children, but may become even more critical over time as the background and history of services received (e.g., medical, school) becomes lengthy and more complex. As children with disabilities become adolescents and adults, they may be able to participate more directly in the information-sharing process by providing history and by discussing their own dreams and goals and their own preferences for services and modes of service delivery (Kingsley & Levitz, 1994; Pierro, 1996).

Thus the parents' role is to provide information about their son or daughter, and the first role of the professional is to solicit this information and to listen carefully and empathically when it is presented. In addition, professionals have information-sharing roles that relate to the mesosystem connections between the home microsystem and the other microsystems in which the child may participate (e.g., school, hospital, and clinic). These information-sharing roles are related to specific parent needs. Typically, parents need information about (a) the professional assessment and diagnosis; (b) plans and options for intervention and treatment; (c) progress once intervention has begun; (d) parental rights and responsibilities in terms of receiving services for their son or daughter; and (e) options for family support. Sharing information with parents also provides a learning experience for professionals. A health-care professional presented this example:

Mrs. K told me that her family had been great but that she didn't want to burden them with her constant worries and questions. Our time together gave her the opportunity to ask her questions over and over again. She knew that many of her questions had no answers. I listened and learned. (Leff & Walizer, 1992, p. 53)

## Assessment

Assessment information is usually the starting place as well as the focal point for updates between parents and professionals. This may also be the point of parental introduction to the team process. Several professionals may be involved in the evaluation of the child and may then come together to share diagnostic results with one another and with the parents. Providing this information to parents, clearly and thoroughly, is important because assessment is the basis for program planning and goal setting and for referral to additional services.

## Intervention and Treatment

After presenting assessment and diagnostic information, professionals can make recommendations about programming and treatment needs. This usually includes programs that will be carried out by teachers, therapists, and other professionals as well as specific tasks to be carried out by the parents. These tasks range from activities designed to support developmental progress, such as a language stimulation program or tutoring in math, to activities designed to support life, such as a special diet or medication. Ongoing assessment of parental priorities and of parents' willingness and ability to carry out the programs are vital components of the overall intervention process.

## Tracking Progress

After a specialized education and/or therapy program or medical treatment program has started, families and professionals need to meet regularly to share information about progress. This is the time to ascertain if the planned programming is effective. It can also be a time of problem solving. For example, complexities of the broader family system, such as not enough time to carry out a home program for this child and meet the needs of other siblings, may need to be addressed. In some cases, serious family problems may be interfering, not just with programming, but with parenting. Teachers and therapists may need to enlist the help of social workers and other professionals if child abuse or neglect is suspected.

## Parental Rights

Through IDEA, professionals are required to share information with parents about their rights. This includes parental consent to conduct a preplacement evaluation of the child and to place the child in a special education program. Parents also have the right to attend IEP (individual education program) or IFSP (individual family service plan) meetings and to participate in the development of these plans. Parents can request a due process hearing if they disagree with the school, and they can access their child's records (Ordover & Boundy, 1991). This information is vital for parents as they advocate for their children.

## Family Support

Effective parent/professional communication helps professionals provide appropriate programming and support themselves and make timely referrals for these services. Learning parental strengths and needs on an individual basis is vital for helping parents make connections for relevant supports and services (Bailey, Blasco, & Simeonsson, 1992a). For example, many parents are interested in childcare resources to provide a respite from their responsibilities, so this type of referral is often needed. Some parents, however, may have adequate help from family members and friends and therefore do not need this type of help. Still others might like to have a break but do not feel comfortable leaving their child in the care of anyone outside the family. In this case, a referral to an agency providing respite care would not meet the needs of the family. Instead, communication that examines fears about the child's safety and the qualifications of the care providers, as well as a link to another family that has successfully used the child-care program, would be the most supportive type of communication between professional and parent. Parents may also want and need help on how to parent. Fine and Gardner (1991) discuss teaching parenting skills to parents of children with disabilities.

Effective information sharing between parents and professionals can be the key to parental empowerment, that is, helping parents help their children. Information and support offered by professionals become a means of teaching, not only successful parenting, but also productive interaction with the broad service delivery system, both in the present and in the future.

Information sharing is clearly a two-way process between families and professionals, and empowerment can be as well. The experience of seeing families develop proficiency in care provision and in seeking and acquiring needed services can be enormously satisfying and energizing for professionals. In addition, these positive experiences empower professionals to serve families with increasing competence.

# ROADBLOCKS TO EFFECTIVE COMMUNICATION AND COLLABORATION

**⊕   FOCUS 2**

*Identify three common roadblocks to effective communication and collaboration between parents and professionals.*

Effective information sharing between families and professionals provides a base for positive collaborative relationships. However, various barriers can impede this process. Three types of barriers—family, professional, and system—were identified by Bailey et al. (1992b). Their work focused on early intervention programs, but these three barriers can be problematic at any point in the family life cycle.

## Professional Barriers

**Lack of Experience in Working with Families.** Training programs vary in the amount of attention given to learning to work with families. There is a trend toward including this training, with an emphasis on observation and hands-on experiences such as interviewing parents or siblings or helping parents care for their child with disabilities (Berry, 1992). Practicum and intern experiences that allow students to attend team meetings or to observe professionals as they interview or provide feedback to parents are also important additions to class study. New professionals who have limited preparation for working with families and even those with more extensive training often find real-world encounters with families challenging. Mentoring from veteran professionals and inservice training are helpful, but experience and an attitude of openness to learn from families are of even greater importance.

**Attitudes.** Professionals sometimes feel that the parents themselves are a barrier (see Window 6.1 on page 124). Sonnenschein (1984) elaborated on this premise by presenting a list of attitudes on the part of professionals toward parents that can impede effective communication and collaborative relationships. Her list included: (1) *The Parent as Vulnerable Client*, which addressed the natural imbalance between "the helper and the helped, the powerful and the powerless, the expert and the novice" (p. 130). (2) *The Parent and Professional Distance*, which concerned the need on the part of the parents for empathy and the professional reluctance or inability to provide it. (3) *The Parent as Patient*, whose focus was judgments by professionals of parental maladjustment and dysfunction as opposed to seeking and nurturing strengths. (4) *The Parent as Responsible for the Child's Condition*, which addressed blaming the parents for the child's problems. This can be particularly difficult for parents who probably already feel responsible and even guilty. (5) *The Parent as Less Observant, Less Perceptive, and Less Intelligent*, which is another power issue, but also reflects lack of respect for the unique contribution that the parents can make as the experts on their own child. (6) *The Parent as Adversary* describes the adversarial relationships that can result in unrealistic expectations on the part of either parents or professionals. This again points to the need for clear communication. (7) *The Parent as "Pushy," "Angry," "Denying," "Resistant," or "Anxious,"* which addresses concern about labeling parents and letting the labels get in the way of establishing a relationship built on mutual respect. Also, the parent who seems, for example, pushy or anxious may be the parent who is seeking to become more informed and capable. Clearly, none of these reactions are helpful or supportive, and they can serve to increase parental stress and vulnerability and prohibit effective communication.

***Communication Differences.*** Professionals and parents may literally speak different languages, and these language differences and accompanying cultural differences may impose a barrier (Harry, 1992; McCubbin et al., 1993). The education law (IDEA) alerts professionals to the possibility of language barriers to communication. The law requires that information concerning the child's placement and program be provided in the native or primary language of the parents. Also, interpreter services (e.g., Spanish, Italian, Sign) are required for meetings with parents whose native or primary language is different from that of the school personnel providing services (Ordover & Boundy, 1991).

Even situations in which the parents and professionals speak the same language can have language barriers. Common barriers include the use of professional jargon and acronyms or initials. The use of these terms can also interfere with communication among professionals. The use of initials to abbreviate programs and services in medicine and education is a trend that can block effective communication. Although parents can be expected to learn some common abbreviations, such as IEP for individualized education program, the use of initials for numerous programs, personnel categories, and agency names (which is common practice) is extremely confusing to parents and creates distance between professionals who "know the code" and parents who feel they are being served "alphabet soup."

## Family Barriers

***Lack of Knowledge.*** The parents' lack of knowledge about their child's special needs and how to meet them is a common barrier with great individual variation. A child with a disability may have, for example, parents who both have mental retardation or a mother who is a physician and a father who is a physical therapist. The parents with cognitive disability have much to learn about their son's diagnosis and how to care for him. But the parents with the advanced health-care degrees have to learn about their daughter's educational needs. Lack of experience in working with the service delivery system and lack of knowledge and experience in parenting can also create barriers. Also, as we noted in the previous section, professional assumptions about lack of parental knowledge can be a barrier. Professionals are challenged by the need to provide individualized information and instruction patiently to families without overwhelming or patronizing them.

***Lack of Resources.*** Lack of parental resources, particularly time and money, can be a barrier to effective parent–family collaboration. A professional may spend time designing a home therapy program or gathering catalogs featuring specialized toys or equipment for the family to purchase. The professional may then feel frustration toward the family if this professional advice is not followed. The parents may not have the resources available to follow this advice and may not share this fact with professionals because they feel embarrassed or guilty. These emotional responses then compound the resource barrier.

***Emotions.*** Emotions can interfere with effective communication in almost any situation in which people interact with one another. Interactions between parents and professionals are particularly vulnerable to emotions. Parents of newly diagnosed children are grieving, and their emotions can impede the communication process. In fact, emotional reactions at this time can prohibit the giving and receiving of information. Fern Kupfer (1982) described being told for the first time of her son's severe disabilities:

> Something burst in me. Despite the sick feelings of dread that had lain within me in the past few weeks I was still shocked to hear him say the words, to say that there actually could be something wrong. . . . I pounded the wall with my fist, crying and shrieking. (p. 36)

Further down the developmental path, parents still have strong feelings, often focused on the needs of their sons and daughters. Schoeller (1995) provided this example:

> Parents of teenagers have moved through many stages of grieving and many years of gathering information. They have a fierce determination to share this knowledge and experience. They are no longer looking for the "cure" or needing to hear about another IQ/reading level/physical/sensory limitation. They want a "friend" in the case manager or a support in the social worker. They want the world around them to value their kids. (p. 14)

As parents develop a history of interactions with professionals concerning their children, this history has an impact on emotions and expectations. It encompasses the good, the bad, and the ugly of parent–professional relationships. Professionals may increase parents' emotional distress. For example, a mother and father were concerned and puzzled when a noted pediatric neurologist told them that their adored 2-year-old son had a syndrome known medically as FLK. They were deeply hurt and offended when this physician went on to explain that this stood for Funny-Looking Kid. Those parents were wary of physicians, not to mention initials, for a long time after that. On a more positive note, if a home health-care nurse listens empathically when a mother expresses her fears concerning her ability to feed her newborn with cerebral palsy, later this mother will expect that she can tell the physical therapist how upset she feels when her daughter cries during her physical therapy sessions. A father who has been praised for his success in tutoring his son in math will feel pride in his success and look forward to learning future skills of this type from his son's teacher.

### System Barriers

***Policies and Procedures.*** The red tape of the service delivery system, such as the paperwork required by IDEA, Medicaid, and insurance companies, can be frustrating for families and for professionals. Policies and procedures without adequate flexibility can also create barriers, for example, the procedures dictating times and circumstances of meetings and home visits. Not allowing enough time and being unclear about the amount of time scheduled are common problems. Indeed, research by Witt et al. (1984) identified allowing enough time as the most important factor in parent satisfaction with team meetings. IDEA includes provisions for ensuring that parents are given meaningful opportunities to attend meetings and to participate in them. Although the law provides procedural safeguards for minimum criteria interactions, the ongoing meetings and communications between parents and professionals are often scheduled on the basis of what works best for the service delivery system instead of what works best for the family (McBride et al., 1993). Employed parents are particularly vulnerable to restricted interactions with professionals when they are only offered in the framework of a limited number of daytime hours.

These interactions are further restricted when they can only take place in the setting (i.e., school, clinic) that is most convenient for the professional. Also, these settings can be intimidating and confusing for parents. Parents have to find the meeting place, figure out where to park, find the correct office or classroom, and enter a setting of familiarity, control, and power—for the professional. A mother was once observed wandering a hospital corridor holding her screaming baby and looking completely dismayed. When approached by a person offering help, she stated that she had been told to take her baby to X-Ray. She was in the right place, but the sign on the door said Radiology, not X-Ray.

*Lack of Resources.* As we noted earlier, parents may not have sufficient time or money to provide optimally for their sons and daughters. However, this can be true of the service delivery system as well. Medical, educational, and therapeutic services are expensive and service providers are often spread thin. Not being able to procure (parents) or provide (professionals) needed services is a barrier that is troubling for everyone.

## THE PROCESS OF COMMUNICATION AND COLLABORATION

**⊕   FOCUS 3**

*What skills are needed to communicate and collaborate effectively with families?*

Barriers are broken down through respect, trust, skills, experience, and creative problem solving. The following section addresses how to overcome barriers and achieve mutually satisfying relationships that promote success for individuals with disabilities, families, professionals, and the service delivery system.

### Creating a Relationship of Mutual Respect and Trust

Interactions between professionals and families may have a highly formal structure, such as sessions in which professionals share diagnostic or assessment information with families or annual IEP meetings. Interactions may also be informal, such as notes and telephone calls back and forth between a professional and a parent. A session or conference called because either a parent or a professional has a particular concern falls somewhere in between these formal and informal parameters. A relationship built on trust and mutual respect is essential for all these interactions.

Several authors have suggested ways in which professionals can improve their relationship skills. Perl (1995) advocates establishing an atmosphere of genuine caring by monitoring reactions to parents and keeping in mind that some parents will not be easy to like. He suggests to professionals that "your job is to bring out the best in people you work with—to empower them" (p. 29). Simpson (1990) suggests means of developing trust. Parents will be more likely to trust professionals when they feel professionals are committed to their child and will assertively advocate for him or her. He also encourages a positive outlook, sensitivity to needs, and honesty.

Parents also need to feel this sharing situation with professionals is safe—that they will not be judged for feelings they express and that confidentiality will be maintained. Stewart (1986) has suggested that, for parents, being able to express feeling of anger or frustration enhances trust and facilitates moving on to calmer and more effective communication.

---

◆ **POINT OF INTEREST 6.1**
_____

*Beliefs Contributing to Parent–Professional Collaboration*

1. Parents and professionals achieve more constructive outcomes when they work as allies in helping families achieve their goals and developmental potential. Cooperation increases the likelihood of mutually satisfying outcomes.

2. Professionals can offer a variety of constructive roles to family members. Being flexible in accommodating family preferences enhances the helpfulness of professional roles.

3. Professionals can repeatedly seek informed consent for the actions they take to show respect for a family member's autonomy and judgment.

4. Both parents and professionals have unique knowledge and expertise to bring to collaborative relationships. It is a loss if either is expected to ignore or abandon his or her particular expertise.

5. Both parents and professionals are constrained by the systems in which they live and work, whether it be the family system, the school system, or the health care system. It is important to identify and clarify these constraints as part of their partnership and to either accept or overcome them.

6. Professionals increase their helpfulness to families when they value pluralism, that is, when they respect differences in culture, beliefs, class, family structure, and personal styles.

*Source:* From Families, Disability, and Empowerment: Active Coping Skills and Strategies for Family Interventions by G. H. S. Singer and L. E. Powers. Copyright © 1993 by Paul H. Brookes Publishing Co. Reprinted with permission.

---

Walker (1989) stresses the need for a commitment to a cooperative relationship between parents and professionals as opposed to individualistic, or worse yet, competitive relationships. Formation of cooperative relationships is tied to values. Walker and Singer (1993) emphasize "equality, cooperation, partnership, and the incorporation of a family-centered focus in parent–professional relationships" (p. 287). See Point of Interest 6.1 for a summary of their beliefs concerning these relationships.

### Learning to Communicate

Respect and trust are vital to the communication process, but so is skill in how to communicate. Roberds-Baxter (1984) offers this advice: "Regular contact, get-acquainted time, facilitating questions, active listening, and acceptance of grief are all methods for inviting parents to feel respected, wanted, and necessary to the conference procedure" (p. 58). These are also the skills of effective communication.

*Rapport Building.* One of the greatest challenges for rapport building and effective communication for professionals is breaking the news about the child's disability or illness. This is a frequent role for physicians but may also be the responsibility of psychologists, audiologists, teachers, and professional teams. Immediate rapport with families in breaking the news situations is necessary but not easy.

Cooley and Moeschler (1993) present standards of "best practice" for this role that are based not only on professional experience but also on feedback from families, who often express dissatisfaction (e.g., Rees, 1983). Cooley and Moeschler urge the bearer of the diagnostic news to be emotionally prepared, undistracted, and able to answer questions or help find answers. They describe a good bearer of such news as someone who "proceeds with patience and acceptance, with directness and honesty, using understandable language. Listening ability is combined with tolerance both of emotions and of nonacceptance of the news at hand" (p. 160). Joy's mother, Judith Raskin (1993) would add being as positive as possible to that list. Commenting on the physician who diagnosed her daughter's deafness, she said, "I believe we were very lucky, because the physician who gave us the bad news also offered tremendous hope—of what Joy could do" (p. 157).

For teachers, therapists, and other professionals who see children and parents regularly over an extended period of time, rapport can literally be built or nurtured. The first conference with professionals can be stressful for parents, but there are ways of reducing this stress. Professionals can anticipate and prevent barriers by being clear with parents about logistics of the meeting. For example, it is helpful to include, with the meeting notice, directions for finding the office or classroom and information on where to park. The time parameters should also be clearly stated. It is frustrating for parents if they think they have all the time they want and then find the teacher or therapist has another conference scheduled in twenty minutes. It is also frustrating for the professional who is trying to maintain a schedule. Being clear about the length of time allotted and providing options for additional meetings, if necessary, can avert these problems. Also, meeting notices should encourage parents to call and discuss alternative arrangements if the time and place suggested does not work for them.

Meetings should allow for get-acquainted time. Perl (1995) reminds professionals that a school setting may evoke unpleasant memories for some parents. A hospital setting will probably also evoke unpleasant memories for many families. Perl suggests countering these feelings by allowing time for small talk and offering coffee or a soft drink. This is also the time for professionals to introduce themselves and explain their roles and for parents to introduce themselves and anyone accompanying them, such as a grandparent.

A quick, effective, and pleasant way to establish rapport with parents is to share something positive about their son or daughter—an academic accomplishment, a comment on an aspect of the child's personality that is enjoyed, or an account of an enjoyable experience. In other words, show *heart* (see Window 6.1 on page 124). A mother shared a story of how she immediately relaxed, during a rather intimidating team meeting concerning her son's school program, when a school administrator related that she had recently attended a class field trip to the nature center and sat with this mother's teenager on the bus. The administrator told of an enjoyable experience getting to know the young man.

***Regular Contact: Formal and Informal.*** The Individuals with Disabilities Education Act (IDEA) mandates a formal structure for meetings between parents and professionals on an annual basis to create, and later to evaluate and update, the student's individualized education program (IEP). For infants and toddlers, these formal team meetings lead to the creation of an individual family service plan (IFSP). In addition, parents or professionals can ask for a meeting to review these plans at any time. We discuss the team process in the next section.

Another type of formal meeting is the session designed to share information about the child's progress. A single professional, a few professionals, or the entire team may be involved in these meetings along with the parents. Other forms of formal communication include the IEP or IFSP document and written diagnostic and progress reports. Clarity of expression and avoidance of professional jargon and initials are as important in written communication as they are in verbal communication.

These formal meetings are vital for information sharing, goal setting, and accountability of progress. However, research has shown that parents place greater value on informal contacts with professionals (Winton & Turnbull, 1981). Also informal interactions lead to more equal proportions of talk time between parents and professionals (Walker, 1989). Methods of informal communication include brief notes commenting on progress or activities, telephone calls, personal visits, newsletters, and notebooks that travel between home and school. A mother of a son with very limited communication skills sent a small notebook to school each day in his backpack. In this notebook, the teachers and therapists described what happened that day at school and the parents shared what happened at home in the evenings and over the weekend. The mother said she treasured that notebook. After leaving work, picking up her son and coming home, reading the notebook was the first thing she did, even before she kicked off her shoes and shed her panty hose!

Another creative idea is the use of videotape as a way to communicate with parents. Alberto and colleagues (1995) described a communication program using videotape designed for parents of students with severe disabilities. They stated, "Videotapes are picture report cards for parents to view newly acquired skills or procedures the teacher would like the parents to work on at home" (p. 19). Computer-based communication, such as e-mail or the Internet, is an option appropriate for some families (Peters, 1996).

Studies have been conducted to assess the results of training on improving informal communication experiences between parents and professionals. Walker (1989) found increased communication and more positive evaluations of the parent–teacher relationship (by both teachers and parents) following systematic efforts directed at enhancing these skills. Results were similarly positive for Lewis, Pantell, and Sharp (1991) when they provided communication and relationship skill training for physicians.

Walker (1989) suggests training for professionals in perspective taking—understanding of the other person's position; positive reinforcement—expressing appreciation and offering rewards for pleasing behavior; and maintaining frequent contact. Indeed, the key to improving informal communication may be to impose a formal structure. For example, professionals can use a calendar to document informal notes and telephone calls to parents and to post reminders to write or call again. A school principal told of the pleasure he gives and receives when he calls parents to convey good news. When the parents learn who is calling, they automatically tense up and expect that something is wrong. He counters those feelings by telling parents about a particular academic accomplishment or a particularly helpful or kind act by their child. This not only pleases the parents, but it also sets a tone of sharing good news and defuses negative feelings if the principal does have to call and tell the parents that something is wrong.

Flexibility and willingness to operate in a less formal structure can also be important. For example, meetings between parents and professionals do not have to be held at the school, hospital, or clinic. The professional might, for example, arrange to meet the parents at a restaurant during their lunch hour. Or if only one parent can attend a scheduled meeting, the professional might call the other parent at home that evening or e-mail him or her at the office to see if there are questions.

***Active Listening.*** Listening is probably the most important aspect of the communication process. It sounds like it would be the easiest communication skill to achieve, but it may be the most difficult. The barriers to communication we discussed previously can also interfere with effective listening. So can the desire to be a good communicator. The paradox here is that the professional may spend time preparing for the meeting and thinking about what to say and then spend too much of the meeting time saying it and not enough listening to what the parents have to say. One important component of being a good listener is simply to stop talking!

The conference must be planned to include time and opportunity for parents to share information about their son or daughter and about their family system, as well as their feelings about their child and about the program. Simpson (1990) advocates developing a listening environment by preparing materials for the meeting, arranging a private, professional setting, and providing furniture that is comfortable, adult sized, and does not place distance between parent and professional.

However, preparing an atmosphere conducive for listening and allowing time and opportunity for parent participation may not be enough. Parents' lack of experience in communicating with professionals or past negative experience, as well as anxiety about their child or anxiety about what is expected of them, may inhibit their participation. So professionals must engage in specific behaviors designed to encourage parents to share information and feelings about their son or daughter. In addition to sharing something positive themselves, professionals can ask parents to share strengths and positive information about their son or daughter. Meetings with professionals so often focus on "what is wrong" that an opportunity to share family strengths or "what is right" can provide a favorable beginning for everyone involved (Berry, 1983; Krehbiel & Kroth, 1991).

Throughout the team meeting or conference and during informal interactions with parents, empathy (Perl, 1995; Simpson, 1990) or perspective taking (Walker, 1989) is crucial to successful interactions. Attempting to understand how parents feel and what their lives are like is a valuable prerequisite to effective communication, but again, it is not easy. Perl (1995) explains, "Empathy requires carefully attending to speakers' words and nonverbal cues . . . to perceive their feelings and concerns" (p. 30). Perl also encourages reflecting affect, or putting into words the feelings expressed by the parents and using clarifying statements to reduce ambiguity. He advocates practice and self-monitoring of listening skills. "Listening" to nonverbal communication—gestures, facial expression, body language—is important as well. Becoming comfortable with periods of silence is another mark of a good listener (Simpson, 1990). In other words, stop talking!

Mary Ann Duncan is the mother of a son and daughter, now young adults, with multiple developmental disabilities. When asked to describe the most important aspect of the parent–professional communication process, she said, "They listened to me! They listened to me! They listened to me!" (Duncan, 1993).

***Acceptance of Emotion.*** The professional with good listening skills and an empathic approach can break down emotional barriers to parent/professional communication. The atmosphere of the meeting between parents and professionals should be one of psychological comfort for the parents and for the professional (Roberds-Baxter, 1984). Within this atmosphere, parental denial and anxiety will be understood. Furthermore, parents will be able to express frustration and anger without being judged. Allowing parents to express these feelings can be beneficial to understanding how to help the child and the parent. In a case example discussed by Berry (1983), a mother who had been very involved in her daughter's preschool program now seemed disinterested and depressed. A counselor encouraged Mrs. M. to share her feelings about her daughter, Margaret.

> Mrs. M. indicated that she felt very discouraged about Margaret. She stated that she had thought that if she worked hard and followed the suggestions of the various professionals consulted that Margaret would be walking and talking by the time she started public school. Because this had not happened, she felt like a failure and felt that she should turn Margaret's program totally over to "the experts." (p. 422)

Understanding Mrs. M's feelings was key to reinvolving her in Margaret's program.

Professionals who have not been trained as counselors (e.g., teachers, nurses) may need to call on helping professionals (counselors, psychologists, social workers) to assist them in helping parents as well as in providing direct support for parents and for themselves. Walker (1989) suggested that school counselors can help facilitate collaboration between parents and teachers. Berry (1987) designed a program for school counselors to use in teaching counseling skills to special education teachers that included attending to the grieving process, viewing the family as a system, and enhancing parental self-esteem. Sawyer and Sawyer (1981) reported significantly increased learning when teachers were trained to communicate with parents using a microcounseling approach as opposed to didactic lecture.

Professionals have feelings, too. Their emotional responses to the children they work with and the families of these children can enhance or impede parent–professional relationships. Professionals may experience frustration and even anger when parents do not follow through with professional recommendations. These feelings can be positive, however, if not directly aimed at parents. They can lead to a problem-solving approach that addresses understanding of why the follow-through is not occurring. Professionals also experience emotions related to their own abilities to meet the needs of the children and families they serve. Sharon Richardson (1993), a speech/language pathologist, shared these feelings: "More than once I have awakened in the middle of the night with this child on my mind and felt nightmarish panic at the prospect of not succeeding" (p. 144). Experiencing the emotions of caring produces better professionals and better parents. The hard part is learning to understand and accept the emotional responses of others and of ourselves.

Several authors (e.g., Cooley & Yovanoff, 1996; Roberds-Baxter, 1984; Schloss et al., 1983) have addressed the importance of relaxation, time management, and other stress reduction techniques for professionals working with children, adolescents, and adults with disabilities and their families. Self-care is an essential component of being an effective professional. It is particularly needed as a buffer for the emotional component of the parent–professional relationship. Professionals may wish to call on counselors to help them handle negative feelings toward a child or parent (Kroth, 1985) or to help them with emotions experienced while helping families. The story shared by a student training to be a hospital child life specialist (Window 6.2) demonstrates the heavy responsibility of responding to parental feelings. It also shows effective listening skills and acceptance of grief.

---

★ **WINDOW 6.2**
_____

## *Sarah's Mother*

I SAW HER SITTING ALONE ON A BROKEN DOWN WHEELCHAIR left in the hallway as I hurried to do an errand. Afraid to ask, "How's Sarah?" I greeted her. She motioned her head away from the court yard to the purple doors behind me.

"Sarah's in ICU," she said. "I can only stay in there a short time. Then I have to come out. I can't stand it, to see her like that. All those tubes down her nostrils to help her breathe. It just hurts me bad to see her like that." Tears rushed to the surface. She wiped them from her face with a moist and crumpled tissue.

I stared and I held on to my own tears. I couldn't speak.

"I'm sorry to upset you," she said.

"No, no," I said. "Sometimes it's good to cry. I just wish I could do something." The white floor and white windows glared. I felt uncomfortable in my body. I wanted to touch her, to comfort her, but I didn't know how. I became aware that I was standing above her. I sat beside her on the windowsill.

She told me all about Sarah, and several times she said, "She was never sick before this. I never saw her sick before. Sixteen years old and I never had her to the doctor except for her shots, you know. I don't know where this leukemia came from."

She told me how they had discovered that Sarah had leukemia, the exact date that she was diagnosed, and about all that had happened since then. I didn't know what to say. I watched intently.

The social worker approached us with a psychiatrist. Sarah's mom stopped in the middle of her story to respond to them. I didn't want to leave before she had finished. I wanted her to know that I had been listening—not to appease her until someone else came along, but because I cared. At the same time, I felt incapable and embarrassed in front of the social worker and the psychiatrist. I felt awkward and moved myself away from the windowsill. I told them that I had to return to the clinic.

I took a box of tissues from the clinic and brought them to Sarah's mother. I handed them to her, and she continued her story as if we had never been interrupted. Her father had died of leukemia here in this hospital one year ago. She didn't know whether to tell her mother that Sarah had been moved to ICU. "Sarah's my baby—my baby."

*Source:* Copyright © 1992 by Brookline Books.

## BECOMING AN EFFECTIVE TEAM MEMBER

⊕     **FOCUS 4**

*What is involved in successful teamwork?*

A *team* is a number of persons associated together. However, *teamwork* is work done by a number of associates, all subordinating personal prominence to the efficiency of the whole (Berry & Niman, 1979). For children and adolescents with disabilities who receive educational services, IDEA mandates an interdisciplinary team that includes parents. Families are also key members of medical and rehabilitation teams. The task of the educational team is to develop and implement the individualized education program (IEP), the individual family service plan (IFSP) for infants and toddlers or the individualized transition plan (ITP) for adolescents. The teams for these purposes must consist of the student's teacher and an administrative representative qualified in special education. The parents must be invited, and the student may attend if the parents wish. Some or many other professionals (speech/language pathologist, physical therapist, occupational therapist, psychologist, nurse, etc.) are included as needed. Parents can also invite people to attend the meetings. These meetings can be quite large, and the parents are usually greatly outnumbered.

The task for the professional is not only including parents in the team process but working effectively with a variety of other professionals. Bailey (1984) advocates moving these interdisciplinary teams to a transdisciplinary level. Transdisciplinary teams perform services together, use their expertise to train other team members, and practice "role release" (p. 19). Lyon and Lyon (1980) defined the three levels of role release as (1) sharing general information and performance competencies concerning basic concepts, approaches, and practices; (2) sharing informational skills, which includes more detailed information about specific practices, methods, and judgments; and (3) sharing performance competencies, which involves actually training other team members to perform specific interventions. For example, a speech/language pathologist might teach an occupational therapist to incorporate language stimulation into a child's motor development program. With role release, true teamwork can be accomplished and these collaborative relationships will benefit not only children and parents but the professionals themselves (Rainforth, York, & McDonald, 1992).

Professionals have the task of including and encouraging parents, sometimes other family members (siblings, grandparents), and the student or adult with a disability as team members. Professionals have the additional task of working cooperatively and effectively with other professionals on the team. The question then becomes, how do these disparate individuals come together to accomplish teamwork? The answer is through continuing hard work and commitment to the team process. An additional component of effective teamwork is learning what is involved in success.

Huszczo (1990) identified seven components of successful teams. He advised that, "A team should assess itself in seven areas, asking critical questions in each" (p. 38). These are the seven areas: (1) *Goals.* Does the team have a sense of direction? (2) *Talent.* Is talent available to fulfill the team objectives? (3) *Roles.* Does each team member understand his or her role? (4) *Procedures.* Are effective and efficient operating procedures in place? (5) *Interpersonal relations.* Do team members get along with each other? (6) *Reinforcement.* Are team members expressing appreciation to one another for team contributions? (7) *External relations.* Does this team have effective external relations with the broader environment? Positive answers to these questions predict success; negative answers show where additional efforts are needed.

We cannot overemphasize the importance of positive reinforcement for effective team functioning. For adults with disabilities, positive feedback leads to improved self-esteem, which leads to stronger self-advocacy (Pierro, 1995). Parental self-esteem can be enhanced as well when parents are praised for their efforts on behalf of their child and, particularly when they are praised for unique and effective ideas. Parents often provide ideas for working with their child that professionals can share with other parents, and they need to be acknowledged for these efforts. In addition, professionals can let parents know how pleased they are to receive praise from parents, such as that expressed by a mother, Joan Simon: "The joy of the system is observing a teacher who is pure magic with my child: a teacher who knows her craft, who understands a child's strengths and weaknesses; a teacher who gives a child knowledge, love and self-esteem" (Dickman & Gordon, 1993, p. 236). Also important in its own right and as a means of modeling positive behavior for parents is for professionals to praise one another.

Another component of successful team meetings is careful planning (Price & Marsh, 1985). This planning should include clear information for all team members about time, place, and purpose of the meeting. Team meetings can be disrupted and parents can be put off by team members who arrive late, leave early, or seem distracted during the meeting. Also, before the meeting, one team member can be designated as the parent advocate. Research by Goldstein and Turnbull (1982) reported increased parent participation when the school counselor was present as a parent advocate. However, any professional on the team can play this role. The designated advocate greets the parents when they arrive, sits with them, and keeps a close eye on their responses to information shared during the meeting. The advocate can model behavior for the parents. For example, this professional might interrupt the occupational therapist to ask, "What does sensory integration mean?" This gives the parents the message that it is okay not to know all the terms and it is okay to ask questions. If the student attends the meeting, another professional, probably the teacher, can serve as his or her advocate. A mother once stated that team meetings became much better after her teenage daughter with learning disabilities started attending. As the team sought to clarify information to accommodate her daughter, the information-sharing process of the meeting became much more user friendly for the mother.

Lack of attention to the elements of successful teams can result in difficult and dissatisfying meetings and failure in operation of special education or rehabilitation programs or medical protocols. Discouraging results have been found by research efforts in which special educators were surveyed concerning their perceptions of parent involvement in the IEP process. Gerber, Banbury, and Miller (1986) found that only slightly more than 50 percent of the teachers surveyed felt that parent participation in IEP formulation had value, 71 percent advocated waiving the option of parent participation, and 44.3 percent viewed the conference as merely a formality. Research efforts that involved observation of team meetings have also been discouraging. Goldstein and colleagues (1980) found that parents' requests for ideas on how to help their children at home did not result in definitive responses from the team. Ysseldyke, Algozzine, and Mitchell (1982) also observed teams and found deficiencies in stating the goal or purpose of the meeting, defining of roles, and consensus decision making. The observed role of the parents in the decision-making process was particularly troubling. "We evaluated the extent to which parents were asked their understanding of the purpose for the meeting and asked their expectations regarding the meeting. This never occurred" (p. 311).

## PREVENTING AND RESOLVING CONFLICT

⊞  **FOCUS 5**

*What are common causes of conflict between parents and professionals, and how can these conflicts be resolved?*

### Reasons for Conflict

Problems in the team process such as failure to communicate purposes and expectations to families, as we just noted, can set the stage for conflict. Additional sources of conflict between parents and professionals were addressed by Mayer (1994), and her work provides a useful framework for addressing this issue. The first cause of conflict may be *blame*. If parents feel they are being blamed for their child's disability or lack of progress, they may become defensive or avoid professionals whenever possible. Being blamed is also hard on professionals (Kroth, 1979).

The second category contributing to conflict is *stress*. Parents may have little energy and few remaining emotional resources for interactions with professionals because of the demands involved in caring for their child. Professionals also experience stress and burnout (Greer & Wethered, 1984).

A third problem area is *stigma*. Parents may feel battered and have low self-esteem because of experiencing societal stigma. This is especially true if their normal and necessary emotional reactions have been labeled disturbed or dysfunctional. If they sense this same judgment from professionals, conflict may occur.

A fourth area of concern is *lack of understanding*. This is a two-way street. Parents may feel that professionals do not understand what it is like to have 24-hour responsibility for a child with disabilities, and professionals may feel that parents do not understand what it is like to meet the needs of many children with complex problems within a system that may not always be supportive of what they are trying to accomplish.

A fifth situation that may result in conflict is *lack of services*. Parents are rightfully distraught when needed services are unavailable or inappropriate. Professionals may be upset by this as well. Instead of working together to problem-solve, parents may blame professionals, and professionals may become defensive or label parents as unreasonable or even emotionally disturbed.

Finally, *lack of knowledge about services* can lead to conflict. It is highly distressing to families to learn that needed services were available, but they did not receive referral to or information about these services. Furthermore, it is time consuming and frustrating for professionals when they cannot access needed information to make appropriate referrals.

### Managing Conflict

The Individuals with Disabilities Education Act (IDEA) anticipated that parents and professionals would not always agree on what was best for the child. Also anticipated was that professionals would have more power than parents in these situations. Therefore, procedural safeguards were written into the law giving parents the right to dispute resolution beginning with mediation and ending in federal court, if necessary (Ordover & Boundy, 1991). These rights are critical to positive outcomes for children and families; however, the circumstances of exercising these rights can be enormously stressful for everyone involved.

It is far better to anticipate and prevent conflict. Keys to prevention include the issues previously addressed in this chapter: being well informed, supportive, and empowering; expecting and overcoming barriers; creating an atmosphere of respect and trust; and communicating effectively, frequently, and with acceptance. In addition, prevention requires avoiding blame and attempting to reduce stress and stigma. This is a tall order—virtually impossible to achieve with all families all the time.

Simpson (1990) has suggested that when conflict does occur the approaches utilized to resolve the conflict may be avoidance and accommodation. These may defuse a situation on a short-term basis but are not adequate for true problem solving. The first step toward problem solving may require a special kind of listening. When parents direct anger and hostility toward a professional, the best approach is to listen attentively, perhaps write down what they say, and allow them to exhaust their list of complaints. While this is occurring, the professional should avoid arguing, becoming defensive, or minimizing the problems (University of New Mexico Institute for Parent Involvement, 1979). Given a chance to release these feelings, in an atmosphere of acceptance, parents may be able to move on to clarifying or defining the problem.

Defining the problem requires the gathering and sharing of pertinent information (Kroth, 1985; Simpson, 1990). This includes assessment information, student files, and program options that would typically be provided by the professional. Parents could provide pertinent history. For example, parents might be upset because a teaching or behavior management technique was being used when it had failed in the past. The professional might not know about this past history, and upon learning it might discontinue the procedure or discuss with the parents the rationale for believing the technique would now succeed. Professionals can also share information from past experience. For example, if parents are doubting the efficacy of a program, professionals can discuss, or better yet, arrange for observation of the use of this technique with other students. This information sharing can lead to delineation of options to deal with the need or problem.

Parents and professionals may be able to discuss options and agree on a solution, at least on a trial basis. Then monitoring and adjusting the program becomes crucial to accomplishing goals for the child and avoiding further conflict. Fiedler (1991, p. 329) proposed a five-step problem-solving process:

- Define the problem (from both parties' perspective)
- Generate possible solutions
- Choose a solution—weigh possible risks, gains, likelihood of success, costs
- Implement the chosen solution
- Evaluate the solution

In some situations a consensus will not be reached. At this point a mediator might become involved to intervene between parent and professional (Simpson, 1990) or a consultant might be utilized to identify and help resolve issues of concern (Wisniewski, 1994). This consultant may be the one to define the problem as a communication issue or a system issue. If the issue is communication, the consultant might work with all parties involved to improve their communication skills. For parents or siblings, this might mean an introduction to the assertiveness skills important to becoming an effective advocate for their family member with disabilities, both in terms of the present issue and for the future. Parent Betty Pendler (1993) wrote about her introduction to advocacy on behalf of her daughter:

> I began to realize that it was easy to speak up for what I want. After all, when we go shopping at the meat market, and we get a piece of bad meat, we do not hesitate to complain—so why shouldn't I be able to speak up when I am getting bad services for my daughter? (p. 165)

If the problem is with the system or due to a lack of institutional support or flexibility, the mediator can address problem solving on this level. If this is not successful, the mediator can inform the parents of their rights and of their options for achieving systems change and assist them in the course that they choose.

Effective parent–professional communication and collaboration is in the best interest of everyone involved: the parents, the professionals and, most of all, the child, adolescent, or adult with disabilities. Leff and Walizer (1992) provide a particularly appropriate summary statement for this chapter: "The ultimate rewards of rethinking and reformulating the critical role of parents include improved care of children, improved relationships with parents, improved satisfaction with one's challenging, difficult work" (p. 56). We address issues related to effective collaboration for each lifespan stage in Chapters 7–10.

# REVIEW

*FOCUS 1: What is involved in information sharing between families and professionals?*

- Information sharing between families and professionals is a two-way process.
- Parents can share information with professionals about the family system, about their child's developmental and health history, and about the child's personality, behavior, and interests.
- Adolescents and adults with disabilities can participate in the information-sharing process by providing history, their own dreams and goals, and their preferences for services and modes of service delivery.
- Professionals can share information with parents about the professional assessment and diagnosis; plans and options for intervention and treatment; developmental progress; parental rights and responsibilities; and family support services.

*FOCUS 2: Identify three common roadblocks to effective communication and collaboration between parents and professionals.*

- Professional barriers include lack of experience in working with families, attitudes, and communication differences such as language differences and use of technical jargon and initials.
- Family barriers include the family member's lack of knowledge about the disability or illness, lack of family resources for meeting the needs of the family member with disabilities, and emotional reactions.
- System barriers include policies and procedures, the systems' red tape, and lack of system resources.

*FOCUS 3: What skills are needed to communicate and collaborate effectively with families?*

- A relationship of mutual respect and trust can be nurtured by professionals by establishing an atmosphere of caring and by demonstrating commitment to the child.
- Effective communication and collaboration also depend on developing specific skills and strategies including rapport building, regular formal and informal contact, active listening, and acceptance of emotion.

*FOCUS 4: What is involved in successful teamwork?*

- Successful teamwork involves planning and ongoing evaluation to accomplish effective collaboration with parents and with other professionals.

*FOCUS 5: What are common causes of conflict between parents and professionals, and how can these conflicts be resolved?*

- Blame, stigma, and stress can lead to conflict as can lack of understanding, lack of services, and lack of knowledge about services.
- If possible, conflict should be prevented. When conflict does occur, techniques such as problem solving and mediation can be helpful.

## REFERENCES

Alberto, P. A., Mechling, L., Taber, T. A., & Thompson, J. (1995). Using videotape to communicate with parents of students with severe disabilities. *Teaching Exceptional Children, 27*, 18–21.

Bailey, D. B. (1984). A triaxial model of the interdisciplinary team and group process. *Exceptional Children, 51*, 17–25.

Bailey, D. B., Blasco, P. M., & Simeonsson, R. J. (1992a). Needs expressed by mothers and fathers of young children with disabilities. *American Journal on Mental Retardation, 97*, 1–10.

Bailey, D. B., Buysse, V., Edmondson, R., & Smith, T. M. (1992b). Creating family centered services in early intervention: Perceptions of professionals in four states. *Exceptional Children, 58*, 298–309.

Berry, J. O. (1983). Adlerian family counseling: A strengths approach. *Individual Psychology, 39*, 419–424.

Berry, J. O. (1987). A program for training teachers as counselors of parents of children with disabilities. *Journal of Counseling and Development, 65*, 508–509.

Berry, J. O. (1992). Preparing college students to work with children and families with special needs. *Family Relations, 41*, 44–48.

Berry, J. O., & Niman, C. (1979). The road to trust: A team treatment approach for multihandicapped children. In J. D. Anderson, J. O. Berry, & J. A. Miller (Eds.), *Teaching speech and language skills to multihandicapped children: A team approach* (pp. 74–78). Tulsa: University of Tulsa.

Cooley, C. J., & Moeschler, J. B. (1993). Counseling in the health care relationship: A natural source of support for people with disabilities and their families. In G. H. S. Singer and L. E. Powers (Eds.), *Families, disability and empowerment: Active coping skills and strategies for family interventions* (pp. 155–174). Baltimore: Brookes.

Cooley, E., & Yovanoff, P. (1996). Supporting professionals-at-risk: Evaluating interventions to reduce burnout and improve retention of special educators. *Exceptional Children, 62*, 336–355.

Dickman, I., & Gordon, S. (1993). *One miracle at a time: Getting help for a child with a disability.* New York: Simon & Schuster.

Duncan, M. A. (1993). *Parent-professional communication: Advice from a parent.* Unpublished manuscript.

Fiedler, C. R. (1991). Preparing parents to participate: Advocacy and education. In M. J. Fine (Ed.), *Collaboration with parents of exceptional children* (pp. 313–333). Brandon, VT: Clinical Psychology Publishing.

Fine, M. J., & Gardner, P. A. (1991). Counseling and education services for families: An empowerment perspective. *Elementary School Guidance & Counseling, 26*, 33–44.

Gerber, P. J., Banbury, M. M., & Miller, J. H. (1986). Special educators' perceptions of parental participation in the individual education plan process. *Psychology in the Schools, 23*, 158–163.

Goldstein, S., Strickland, B., Turnbull, A. P., & Curry, L. (1980). An observational analysis of the IEP conference. *Exceptional Children, 46*, 278–286.

Goldstein, S., & Turnbull, A. P. (1982). Strategies to increase parent participation in IEP conferences. *Exceptional Children, 48*, 360–361.

Greer, J. G., & Wethered, C. E. (1984). Learned helplessness: A piece of the burnout puzzle. *Exceptional Children, 50*, 524–530.

Harry, B. (1992). *Cultural diversity, families, and the special education system: Communication and empowerment.* New York: Teachers College Press, Columbia University.

Huszczo, G. E. (1990). Training for team building. *Training & Development Journal, 44*, 37–43.

Kingsley, J., & Levitz, M. (1994). *Count us in: Growing up with Down syndrome.* San Diego: Harcourt Brace.

Krehbiel, R., & Kroth, R. L. (1991). Communicating with families of children with disabilities or chronic illness. In M. J. Fine (Ed.), *Collaboration with parents of exceptional children* (pp. 103–127). Brandon, VT: Clinical Psychology Publishing.

Kroth, R. L. (1979). Unsuccessful conferencing (or, we've got to stop meeting like this). *Counseling and Human Development, 11*, 1–11.

Kroth, R. L. (1985). *Communicating with parents of exceptional children* (2nd ed.). Denver: Love.

Kupfer, F. (1982). *Before and after Zachariah.* New York: Delacorte.

Leff, P. T., & Walizer, E. H. (1992). *Building the healing partnership.* Cambridge: Brookline.

Lewis, C. C., Pantell, R. H., & Sharp, L. (1991). Increasing patient knowledge, satisfaction, and involvement: Randomized trial of a communication intervention. *Pediatrics, 88,* 351–358.

Lyon, S., & Lyon, G. (1980). Team functioning and staff development: A role release approach to providing integrated educational services for severely handicapped students. *Journal of the Association for the Severely Handicapped, 5,* 250–263.

Mayer, J. A. (1994, May). From rage to reform: What parents say about advocacy. *Exceptional Parent,* pp. 49–51.

McBride, S. L., Brotherson, M. J., Joanning, H., Whiddon, D., & Demmitt, A. (1993). Implementation of family centered services: Perceptions of families and professionals. *Journal of Early Intervention, 17,* 414–430.

McCubbin, H. I., Thompson, E. A., Thompson, A. I., McCubbin, M. A., & Kaston, A. J. (1993). Culture, ethnicity, and the family: Critical factors in childhood chronic illnesses and disabilities. *Pediatrics, 91,* 1063–1070.

Ordover, E. L., & Boundy, K. B. (1991). *Educational rights of children with disabilities: A primer for advocates.* Cambridge: Center for Law and Education.

Pendler, B. (1993). How my daughter changed my personality and taught me to be an assertive parent. In C. Des Jardins (Ed.), *How to get services by being assertive* (pp. 163–166). Chicago: Family Resource Center on Disabilities.

Perl, J. (1995, Fall). Improving relationship skills for parent conferences. *Teaching Exceptional Children,* pp. 29–31.

Peters, J. (1996, January). The Internet: A valuable resource for parents of children with disabilities. *The Pacesetter,* p. 14.

Pierro, C. (1995, June). Self-esteem leads to stronger self-advocacy. *The Pacesetter,* p. 13.

Pierro, C. (1996, January). IEP: Involving the student is important for a successful plan. *The Pacesetter,* pp. 8–9.

Price, B. J., & Marsh, G. E. (1985, Summer). Practical suggestions for planning and conducting parent conferences. *Teaching Exceptional Children,* pp. 274–278.

Rainforth, B., York, J., & MacDonald, C. (1992). *Collaborative teams for students with severe disabilities.* Baltimore: Brookes.

Raskin, J. (1993). Assertiveness—My legacy to my daughter. In C. Des Jardins (Ed.), *How to get services by being assertive* (pp. 157–162). Chicago: Family Resource Center on Disability.

Rees, S. J. (1983). Families' perceptions of services for handicapped children. *International Journal of Rehabilitation Research, 6,* 475–502.

Richardson, S. (1993). Feelings in a manila folder. In J. A. Spiegle and R. A. van den Pol (Eds.), *Making changes: Family voices on living with disabilities* (pp. 144–145). Cambridge: Brookline.

Roberds-Baxter, S. (1984, Fall). The parent connection: Enhancing the affective component of parent conferences. *Teaching Exceptional Children,* pp. 55–58.

Rubin, S., & Quinn-Curran, N. (1983). Lost, then found: Parents' journey through the community service maze. In M. Seligman (Ed.), *The family with a handicapped child: Understanding and treatment* (pp. 63–95). New York: Psychological Corporation.

Sawyer, H. W., & Sawyer, S. H. (1981). A teacher-parent communication training approach. *Exceptional Children, 47,* 305–306.

Schloss, P. J., Sedlak, R. A., Wiggins, E. D., & Ramsey, D. (1983). Stress reduction for professionals working with aggressive adolescents. *Exceptional Children, 49*, 349–354.

Schoeller, K. (1995, February). Determined spirits needed for successful transition. *The Pacesetter*, p. 14.

Simpson, R. (1990). *Conferencing parents of exceptional children* (2nd ed.). Austin: Pro-Ed.

Sonnenschein, P. (1984). Parents and professionals: An uneasy relationship. In M. L. Henniger and E. M. Nesselroad (Eds.), *Working with parents of handicapped children: A book of readings for school personnel* (pp. 129–139). Lanham, MD: University Press of America.

Stewart, J. C. (1986). *Counseling parents of exceptional children* (2nd ed.). Columbus: Merrill.

University of New Mexico Institute for Parent Involvement. (1979). *Tips for dealing with aggression*. Albuquerque, NM: Author.

Walker, B. (1989). Strategies for improving parent-professional cooperation. In G. H. S. Singer & L. K. Irvin (Eds.), *Support for caregiving families: Enabling positive adaptation to disability* (pp. 103–119). Baltimore: Brookes.

Walker, B., & Singer, G. H. S. (1993). Improving collaborative communication between professionals and parents. In G. H. S. Singer and L. E. Powers (Eds.), *Families, disability and empowerment: Active coping skills and strategies for family interventions* (pp. 285–315). Baltimore: Brookes.

Winton, P., & Turnbull, A. P. (1981). Parent involvement as viewed by parents of preschool handicapped children. *Topics in Early Childhood Special Education, 1*, 11–19.

Wisniewski, L. (1994). Interpersonal effectiveness in consultation and advocacy. In S. Alper, P. J. Schloss, & C. N. Schloss (Eds.), *Families of students with disabilities: Consultation and advocacy* (pp. 205–228). Boston: Allyn & Bacon.

Witt, J. C., Miller, C. D., McIntire, R. M., & Smith, D. (1984). Effects of variables on parental perceptions of staffings. *Exceptional Children, 51*, 27–32.

Ysseldyke, J. E., Algozzine, B., & Mitchell, J. (1982). Special education team decision making: An analysis of current practice. *The Personnel and Guidance Journal, 60*, 308–313.

# CHAPTER SEVEN

# Families and the Early Childhood Years

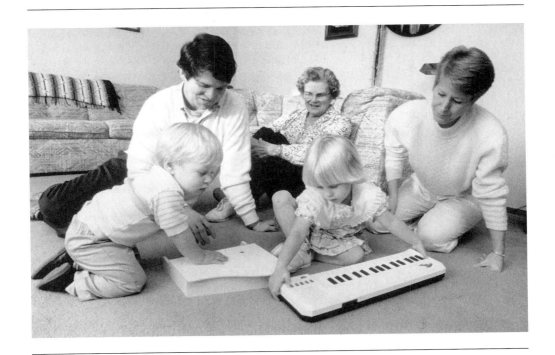

---

✱ **WINDOW 7.1**

---

*Through the Door*

NEARLY EVERY MORNING AT ABOUT BREAKFAST TIME, I walk from the newborn nursery down the hall of the maternity ward to visit the mothers of the newborns I have just examined. What a light step I walk with when I carry good news! What a pleasant way to start the day; to walk into a new mother's room and say, "I have no bad news. There is nothing missing, nothing extra and everything is functioning properly."

On a morning when I must deliver sad news, there is hesitation in every step, in every breath, in every thought and, I think, even in my metabolism itself. The task that is mine, to walk through the door into a new mother's room and give the news that a baby has been born with a permanent defect, is a task that I would do almost anything to be able to wish away. Birth means that now the invisible can be seen, and the promises and hopes are becoming just a memory. The baby that was dreamed of, the toddler, the school child and the teen, doesn't exist anymore. The family's future that was envisioned and hoped for is not to be. My news will replace all of that with shock, helplessness, isolation, emptiness, sadness, and finally, grief. I hope there are family and friends who can be supportive in the right ways and at the right times. At least let there be communication between spouses of strength and love—at least—please.

It doesn't get any easier having done this before. The pain is new each time. Of course, each mother, each family and each support system deals with it differently and in their own way. But, they all want to know "Why?" They want to know what the future will hold. They expect accurate information, although the shock of discovery may not allow them, at first, to comprehend or remember much of what I say.

How can I word my news and my answers to make this traumatic life moment less wrenching? How can I be there enough for this family? How can I help them react? How can I react to their reactions? What can I do that will not only make the news understood, but also start the healing process toward an optimal adjustment. Help me to avoid a word, a phrase, a reaction that will always be looked back upon and remembered with pain or bitterness.

Meanwhile, with each walk down the hall, I confront my own attitudes, emotions, life philosophy and the hollow pit in my gut knowing that I must walk through that door to tell and teach and help and cry.

*Source:* Copyright © 1993 by Brookline Books.

---

WELCOMING A NEW BABY INTO THE FAMILY is an event that combines joy and stress for most families. Families whose babies are born with disabilities or medical problems, like all families, are involved in caring for and forming a relationship with this new little person and integrating him or her into the family.

However, they may also face frightening medical-care situations, difficult decisions, and arduous responsibilities for child care and child development. Their families expand, not just through the addition of this new member, but through an array of professionals whose services are necessary and whose expertise is welcome, but whose presence in their lives can necessitate learning challenging new roles. Our journey through the lifespan begins at the beginning, when a child is born with special needs and then continues into the dynamic preschool period.

For most families, the preschool period is an exciting time of progressive competence for children and parents. Parents have learned the basics of parenting and can relax a little and enjoy a child who is increasingly becoming an individual in his or her own right. The child's developmental growth in skills such as self-help and communication can make the parenting task easier, and development of play skills can make parenting more fun. This rosy scenario may not be in place, however, for parents of children with disabilities or chronic illness. Parents of children diagnosed in infancy may be looking toward a future of slow developmental progress and continuing medical crisis. For other families, the preschool period may be the time of first encountering the possibility of developmental delay in their children.

A variety of family situations mark the preschool period. Families of children who were identified in infancy as having medical or developmental problems may enter this period from a base of family stress, but also from a base of experience and support. Families receiving early intervention services will have had the opportunity for training in caregiving as well as child development services from the professional team. These families, however, face the daunting prospect of transition from family-centered early intervention services to child-centered preschool services. Other families enter the service delivery system at the preschool stage because the child's developmental delays are mild and were not evident earlier. For other families, the child's problems may have been extensive enough to warrant intervention services before this time, but appropriate referrals may not have been made or appropriate services may not have been available. Families confronting disability for the first time during the preschool period grieve and experience changes in family dynamics as they learn to provide for their child's needs and to participate in the service delivery system.

This chapter first discusses the impact on the family of the birth and diagnosis of a child with disabilities or medical problems. Then we consider educational opportunities for the young child as well as family involvement in early childhood intervention/education. Finally, forming and nurturing a partnership between families and professionals is addressed.

## BIRTH AND DIAGNOSIS

### ⊞ FOCUS 1

*What opportunities and risks exist for families as they respond to the birth and diagnosis of a child with disabilities or medical problems?*

### Learning the Diagnosis

When a child is born with a disability or medical problem, the medical-care system provides the infant and his or her family with their most basic opportunity, the opportunity to live. Babies who in the past would not have survived can now survive and thrive, often with no permanent disabilities (Kopp & Kaler, 1989). The risk for families comes with the task of learning to negotiate and function within the often confusing and complicated medical system, which for some families will be a lifelong task.

One of the most stressful events for parents is learning the child's diagnosis. More severe or medically evident disabilities (such as Down syndrome) are typically diagnosed shortly after birth, and in some cases before birth through prenatal testing, whereas learning disabilities may not be diagnosed until the preschool years or until school entry. The task of sharing diagnostic information with parents of infants and young children usually belongs to the physician, who may be joined by a social worker, psychologist, or other professional. These professionals may refer the family to an early intervention program where a team of professionals including occupational and physical therapists, early childhood educators, speech/language pathologists, nurses, and other professionals provide further diagnostic information.

Learning the diagnosis is a stressful event for parents as "disabilities are always unwanted and are usually unexpected" (Cooley, 1992, p. 91). However, receiving diagnostic information can be made less stressful by professionals who are sensitive to the impact of this news on the family. Suggestions for professionals include using accurate, nonstigmatizing language and showing acceptance of the child and optimism about his or her future (Parette, Hourcade, & Brimberry, 1990).

Leff and Walizer (1992) interviewed parents in order to better understand their feelings at the time of diagnosis. They offer additional guidelines for professionals conveying painful information. These guidelines are particularly salient because researchers (Quine & Rutter, 1994; Sloper & Turner, 1993) studying mothers of young children with disabilities found that the majority of the mothers were dissatisfied with the way they were first told about their child's problems. Leff and Walizer (1992, pp. 158–162) presented these parent-generated suggestions:

- When the initial diagnosis is given, make every effort to inform both parents together.
- Arrange for a quiet, comfortable setting. Privacy is crucial.
- Set aside time for the parents only. Avoid interruptions.
- Choose clear, direct, accurate statements. A simple sketch or drawing is often helpful to parents.
- Be sensitive to problems of conflicting information.
- Never be afraid to say, "I don't know."
- Follow-up is critical. Parents often need several meetings with the professionals involved in the diagnosis of their child.
- Give parents something to take away from the meeting. A written statement confirms the parent's understanding and can be shared with family members and friends.
- Hold out a hand of courage and hope. Support and empower parents with concrete aid.

Providing diagnostic information is stressful for professionals as well. One of the mothers interviewed by Leff and Walizer (1992) showed remarkable insight on this point when she said, "Bad news is bad news. Nothing can make the announcement of a serious problem light-hearted or painless; it is neither easy to hear nor easy to give such news" (p. 147). Certainly, the same feeling is reflected in the thoughts of Werner (1993) (see Window 7.1 on page 152).

### Families Respond

Gardner, Merenstein, and Costello (1993) remind us that "Loss is a fact of life, and not just of death. Every stage of development requires a loss of the privileges of the preceding stage and movement into the unknown of the next stage" (p. 531). For some parents, the loss of the pregnancy stage and the birth of their child is a traumatic event that has arrived too soon or is accompanied by ominous medical interventions. Some parents and infants start their lives together in neonatal intensive care units (NICU), a necessary setting of life support for the baby, but the place where a dream ends for parents. For other families, the diagnosis (and accompanying loss) comes later, but is still traumatic.

Loss is accompanied by a grief reaction, which in this case has three sources: "the loss of the 'perfect child,' the remaining child and his or her real difficulties, and the impact such a child's life has on the family" (Bruce et al., 1994, p. 38). These authors describe the psychological process of grieving as a coping strategy arising out of cognitive reappraisal. This reappraisal allows families to create new dreams and to set new goals. This is a more positive and functional orientation to the grief process than is sometimes presented, but the pain is real nevertheless. Furthermore, when the baby has problems at, or soon after birth, the parents are dealing with this loss at a time of increased physical and psychological vulnerability. The words of a new father reflect this vulnerability:

> Almost immediately after my daughter's birth, I was faced with a terrible choice. I could accompany my baby (who did not look at all like what I thought a newborn was supposed to look like) to the intensive care nursery or I could stay with my wife, who was in great physical and emotional distress, in the birthing room. We had always shared our decisions and responsibilities. Now, I was in the position of having to make a choice between my wife and our baby. I thought the baby was ugly. I thought we would all be better off if the baby died. I felt horrible for having these thoughts. But, I chose to go with the baby. Sharing the first six minutes of life with our baby was the most critical early intervention that could have happened for us. (Davis & May, 1991, p. 89)

For parents of children who are diagnosed with problems at birth, and even for parents of children whose problems are later resolved (many premature infants), this is the time of initial crisis. A review of the literature (Blacher, 1984) reflects parental responses of detachment, bereavement, and bewilderment at this time. Some of this bewilderment stems from the reality of caring for the child. This includes what they cannot do for the child (the medical-care system may dominate care for a period of time) and what they must do (such as learn to use feeding tubes, breathing monitors, and other technological supports). These parents are expected to both surrender control and develop mastery, which is enormously challenging. Fortunately, this crisis can also be the beginning of family-centered early intervention services that include both developmentally based educational programming for the child and supports for the family.

## EARLY CHILDHOOD EDUCATION

⊞   **FOCUS 2**

*What educational services are available for young children, and how are their families involved in these programs?*

### Early Intervention Programs

Some infants receive early intervention services in the NICU through the work of professionals such as nurses, occupational therapists, and developmental psychologists and through the guidance these professionals provide for families.

Then infants who meet the developmental criteria have the opportunity to transition from the NICU to an early intervention program, and professionals such as social workers are called on to facilitate the linkage of services between the NICU and the early intervention program. This transition requires careful coordination and has been targeted as an area of particular need for families (Cardinal & Shum, 1993). Other infants and toddlers and their families enter early intervention programs through referrals from a variety of health, education, and habilitation professionals and through self-referral. Some families are not served until later because appropriate referrals are not made or because the child's developmental delays do not meet the criteria to qualify for services.

Early intervention services, for infants and toddlers from birth to 36 months of age, are the result of amendments to the Individuals with Disabilities Education Act (IDEA), which provide federal incentives to states for provision of services for young children. These amendments were passed in 1986 and strengthened in 1991. These dates mark the implementation of more systematic and comprehensive services for infants and toddlers; however, federally funded model demonstration projects for early intervention have been in place since the late 1960s. Furthermore, a base of justification for these programs exists from federally funded early childhood programs such as Head Start and the Perry Preschool Project. These programs target young children considered at risk for delayed development because their families are economically disadvantaged. Research documenting outcomes of these programs indicate improved child and family functioning as well as cost effectiveness (Hymes, 1991; Zigler & Styfco, 1994).

Major components of early intervention services for infants and toddlers with developmental delay (P.L. 102-119, Part H of IDEA) were outlined by McDonnell (1995, pp. 109–111) and are presented here in a summarized form:

1. *Eligibility.* Participating states must provide services to infants and toddlers who have delayed development or who have a diagnosed physical or mental condition with a high probability of resulting developmental delay (e.g., cerebral palsy, Down syndrome). States determine the definition of developmental delay and may also serve infants and toddlers considered at risk.

2. *Individual family service plan (IFSP).* This is a required written document developed for every eligible child and his or her family. The IFSP reflects the goals, plan of action, services, and evaluation strategies that parents and multidisciplinary early intervention team members agree on as defining the individualized early intervention most important for that child and family.

3. *Service coordination.* A service coordinator is required as part of the IFSP to assist families in gaining access to identified early intervention services.

4. *Broadened range of services.* Early intervention programs include a broader range of services than special education programs for older children and ado-

lescents. For example, services such as family education and counseling, health-care services, and nutrition can be added to core instruction and therapy services.

5. *Interagency coordinating council.* Each participating state selects a lead agency and forms an interagency coordinating council. These councils include parents of infants and toddlers with developmental delays or disabilities, service providers, agency representatives, and representatives from higher education.

Enhancing the learning and development of the child while preventing secondary disabilities (such as behavior problems) and while maintaining or improving child health is a primary focus of early intervention, but this is done within a framework of family empowerment. McDonnell (1995) stated that "The empowerment of families is both an end goal and a means for reaching other goals" (p. 112).

## Family Involvement

In addition to empowerment, building on and increasing family strengths, addressing the needs of all family members, and supporting mutually enjoyable family relationships are stressed in early intervention programs and should occur within an atmosphere that advocates independence and inclusion for all family members (McDonnell, 1995). This is certainly challenging and not easily accomplished. Professionals who are used to being "child focused" may have difficulty becoming "family focused." Also, family focus may be interpreted as turning parents into teachers, which is appropriate if it is not overdone, if parent capabilities allow for this role, and if the parents' major role continues to be just that—their child's mother or father. This priority was advocated by Jody Lyon, Zak's mother (Window 7.2).

In some cases, teaching families to teach their children is unrealistic until other goals are met. These goals were delineated by Beckwith (1990) and include basic survival goals (nutrition, medical care, a safe environment); goals that focus on the parent–child relationship; goals involving family needs in areas such as social services or job training; and goals that focus on relationships within the family. Beckwith (1990) provided this reminder for professionals working with infants and their parents:

Parent-infant relationships are complex. The parent assumes multiple roles as protector, biological regulator, love object, teacher, and mediator of exploration in the environment. At the same time the parent must also deal with multiple competing and supporting relationships both within and outside the family. The task is demanding, and the responsibility is heavy; yet there are intuitive competencies within the parent and the infant that can be translated into success. The chances of success for risk groups are fostered when the community can provide adequate medical and child care as well as early intervention. (p. 70)

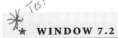

**WINDOW 7.2**

## *Zak's Mom*

ONCE AGAIN I FOUND MYSELF IN FRONT of yet another professional with my list of questions in hand. They tend to be under the categories of "What can I expect?" and "Is there anything I can do?"; the answers, more times than not, are along the lines of "We don't know" or "We can't be sure." This is a typical scene if your child has cerebral palsy. The one thing that professionals from all disciplines seem to agree on is that the best chance for balance, coordination, and quality of movement to develop is through a good program of therapy.

Zachary has had just that—numerous evaluations and frequent therapy sessions. I have had excellent home programs outlined for me, and I see a slow but continuous development of his strength and ability to control his movement. I have, however, spent a great deal of the last 22 months trying to think and behave as a therapist and feeling disappointed in myself if I don't. Because I am a single, working mother, my time with Zachary is limited. I feel driven to spend that time as therapist and patient, and feel it is selfish to want to be simply mother and son. Although I feel driven, I don't always choose to act on these impulses—thus the conflict.

I seem to hear my future self saying, "If I'd only worked fewer hours, if I'd let everything else go, I could have spent more time doing therapy." Intellectually, I know there will be no way to avoid those nagging thoughts. No matter how far Zachary advances, I'll wonder, "What if I'd done more? I could have. . . ." (But don't all mothers?)

I finally finished going through my two pages of questions. The doctor was extremely patient and informative. She smiled as I caught my breath and said something that eased the conflict I'd felt: "Don't worry too much about being a therapist. You're doing fine. It is equally important for Zachary to have a normal mother-son relationship." Those probably weren't her exact words, but I'd been given something I needed: permission to be a mom.

Since that consultation, I've come to terms with being "only human." If I could ensure that Zak could go through the day always moving in appropriate ways, flexing when he should flex, straightening when he should straighten, and play and learn and experience and appreciate . . . I would. But that is not possible. I do have a responsibility to help Zachary develop his motor skills, but I also have a responsibility to help him learn about life. So on those days when we have so much fun together or are so busy that bedtime comes before therapy time, I finally feel comfortable that I have given him something just as vital to his development—a real mom.

*Source:* From *Developmental Disabilities Special Interest Section Newsletter* by J. Lyon. Copyright © 1989 by the American Occupational Therapy Association, Inc. Reprinted with permission.

The structure of early intervention services includes families of infants and toddlers in the work of the team during the IFSP process. A visual representation of this process was presented by Olson and Kwiatkowski (1992) (Figure 7.1). As you can see, the family is involved in all phases of the IFSP process. Best outcomes for the children, families, and professionals involved in this process result when they follow this advice from Noonan and McCormick (1993): "It cannot be overemphasized that the IFSP and the process that generates the IFSP belongs to the family. Both family outcomes and child outcomes reflect the changes that family members want to see occur for their child and themselves" (p. 87).

Families involved in early intervention programs also play a role in determining where services are delivered. The parents might bring the child to a child development center to be seen by various professionals, or one or more professionals might go to the child's home. Many programs combine home-based and center-based services. Advantages to home-based services include being able to observe parent–child interaction in the setting in which parents and child spend most of their time. Also, being in the home allows professionals to get to know siblings and suggest ways to involve siblings in treatment programs or to give advice or make referrals to parents if siblings seem to be having problems related to adjustment to the attention needs of the infant (Blos & Davies, 1993).

Paying attention to the best match between programs and parents (Powell, 1993) and including families in service design and delivery is essential, but it should not be assumed that families will automatically welcome these services. For example, concerns of parents of babies with severe handicaps, as the babies entered early intervention programs, were addressed by Calhoun, Calhoun, and Rose (1989, pp. 148–150). Parental worries included the following:

- Accepting a place in an early intervention program underscored the seriousness and long-term nature of the child's handicap.
- The decision to enroll a child in an early intervention program may seem at odds with the family's recent decision to "care for the child ourselves" rather than seek institutionalization.
- Enrolling a baby in a structured educational and therapeutic program seems age inappropriate.
- Some parents expressed concerns about enrollment affecting the child's health and safety and disturbing the equilibrium of the family.

However, after participating in the early intervention program for periods ranging from 1 to 12 months, the parents articulated these benefits:

- Enrollment could lead to a more normal family life.
- Parents described a sense of relief because of shared responsibility for the child's care.

**FIGURE 7.1**    *The IFSP Process*

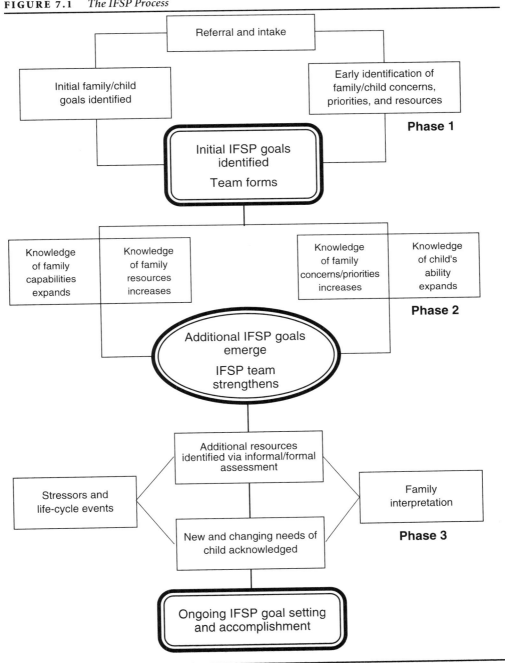

- Enrollment in a program leads parents to experience an enhanced sense of control by taking action, by doing something.
- Program enrollment is seen as producing developmental gains in children.

Even though parents were later able to identify program benefits, professionals should take these very legitimate initial concerns seriously as they should parental resources and family priorities.

## Preschool Education

Families of children who were identified and served as infants and toddlers face a major change at the time of the child's third birthday. The child must leave the early intervention program at this time. For some families, this intervention will have been sufficient and the child will no longer need services. Other children will now make the transition to school-based services. Others served in early intervention programs may still need services but not have disabilities severe enough to meet the criteria for inclusion in school services. Still others may be identified at this time and enter school services, although they were not served in early intervention programs.

Family stress is predictable at this transition point. For those transitioning from early intervention programs, it is difficult to leave the family-centered support of these programs, especially if the child is not eligible for school services. Professionals in early intervention programs must assist families with this transition by identifying and making referrals for the next services needed and by providing emotional support for the transition process. For example, an early intervention program can provide a transition reminiscing activity for the key professional and the parents. For this activity, the professional asks the parents to gather pictures and baby books. Together they talk about the changes that have occurred and the progress that has been made. This ritual of closure and mutual caring makes saying good-bye a little easier for the parents and for the professional.

Families whose children enter preschool special education programs experience many changes. One of the most significant is that the program at school becomes the educational focus, supplemented by home programs and home follow-up. McDonnell (1995, pp. 159–161) presented goals for preschool programs for children with disabilities that we summarize here:

1. Maximize the child's development in a variety of important developmental areas. Parents work with the IEP team to identify high-priority goals and create learning environments that facilitate learning and growth. For most preschool children this includes social, communication, motor, cognitive, preacademic, self-care, play, and personal management skills.

2. Develop the child's social interaction and classroom participation skills. This includes developing social skills and relationships with peers as well as learning to follow adult directions and classroom rules and routines and learning to complete activities without constant adult supervision or attention.

3. Prepare the child for inclusive school placements and provide support for the transition to kindergarten or elementary school. Maximizing skill development and practicing social skills with typical peers are important ways to prepare children. Transition planning involving the family, the preschool team, and the elementary team is also needed.

4. Increase community participation through support to family members and other caregivers. Developing social networks beyond the immediate family and the preschool is an important goal for the child. Also, preschool is a good time to support families in identifying and extending alternative caregivers so family members have more flexibility and more options to pursue their own interests.

### A Changing Role for Families

As noted in McDonnell's (1995) first point, parents will now be members of IEP teams (parent involvement in IDEA and IEP teams is discussed in more detail in Chapter 8). In addition to parents, these teams include a preschool special education teacher, an early education teacher, a school administrator, and other key professionals. Various therapists, child-care providers, and community health-care and social service providers are also important to the child's total program, but it may be difficult or impossible to gather all these individuals for one team meeting. The service coordinator from the early intervention program is no longer part of the team, so parents must now begin that role. This is a difficult job and a worrisome new role for parents. Barbara Ebenstein (1995), the mother of Risa, expressed these concerns: "How will we educate Risa? I worried about how I would communicate my daughter's special needs to our school district and how the district would respond. How could they possibly understand this beautiful child who loves without words?" (p. 62). Ebenstein used her parental concern and her professional ability as an attorney to develop these ten strategies for parents:

1. Keep "business" records. All communication should be in writing, and you should keep a copy of every document you submit.

2. Document all of your child's unaddressed needs.

3. Review your child's classification.

4. Cooperate with the school district's reasonable evaluation process.

5. Be sure the committee has accurate reports.

6. Build accountability into the child's IEP.

7. Work things out before the annual review.

8. Negotiate.

9. Consider all proposals for inclusion carefully.

10. Treat the annual review as your most important business meeting of the year. (pp. 62–63)

Professionals working with preschool children with disabilities could provide this list to parents and also link them with other parents and advocacy organizations as a means of helping them negotiate this new parental responsibility.

⊕   **FOCUS 3**

*How can the young child's needs for play and socialization experiences be addressed by the family and through early childhood education programs?*

### Play and Social Interaction

Play is the work of early childhood (Berger, 1994). It involves parents, siblings, toys, play equipment, and friends, and any or all of these may present challenges for a young child with disabilities. Professionals can help families incorporate play into therapy routines and encourage play for its own value. They can also recommend adapted toys and play equipment and promote sharing of parent-generated play ideas like this one suggested by Danny's parents:

> Our son, Danny, 5, does not like a traditional swing because his feet don't touch the ground when he is in it. He can't move the swing by himself, and feels uncomfortable when someone is pushing him and he can't stop the swing himself. So we hung a tire swing that he can lay across and propel with his feet still on the ground. He loves it! (Schopler, 1995, p. 70)

However, finding peers to play with may be more difficult. The child's disabilities or medical problems may limit casual play with neighborhood children or participation in child-care or church programs. School programs for preschool-age children, however, provide opportunities for social, motor, language, and cognitive development through play in a setting where the child's health and safety needs can be monitored.

Lack of opportunity for peer approval and peer interaction for preschool-age children with disabilities can result in a diminished sense of initiative and mastery in the child (Cook, 1988). Higher cognitive levels of play and increased verbal and social interactions have been documented when preschoolers with disabilities have play opportunities with peers with typical development (Goldstein & Kaczmarek, 1991; Guralnick & Groom, 1987). Preschool programs that integrate children with and without disabilities have received stronger endorsement for children with mild disabilities than for children with more severe disabilities (Cole et al., 1991). However, integration of children with more severe disabilities can also be successful if proper planning and preparation occurs (Demchak & Drinkwater, 1992; Drinkwater & Demchak, 1995).

Demchak and Drinkwater (1992) reviewed literature on the topic of preschool integration that revealed benefits for all involved. Benefits for the children with disabilities included more appropriate social interactions and increased self-initiations in social situations, more complex language/communication, more opportunities for skill generalization, and decreased inappropriate play. The children make as much progress as in segregated settings, and they are more likely to have friends without disabilities. There are also benefits for preschoolers without disabilities in integrated settings. These children tended to be more sensitive to and tolerant of individual differences, and they showed only positive gains in development and attitude change.

Parents of preschoolers generally have positive attitudes toward integration, and more positive attitudes are held by parents whose preschool children actually participate in such programs (Diamond & LeFurgy, 1994). Benefits perceived by parents include their children's preparation for dealing with the real world, more stimulating programs, increased communication skills with family members as well as with peers, and opportunities for families to get to know families with children with typical development (Demchak & Drinkwater, 1992). However, parents may be wary that their children will not receive needed services in these settings (Ebenstein, 1995). This may be the case if proper teacher preparation does not occur or if necessary supports are not in place.

## Staff Development

Participation in staff development programs, prior to working in integrated settings, can counter misinformation, fear, and negative attitudes while providing needed skill training, particularly in behavior management and in strategies to facilitate social interactions and communication exchanges. Ongoing consultation is another valuable support for teachers and other professionals because consultation can be directed toward strategies to enhance ongoing communication between general educators and special educators and between educators and parents (Demchak & Drinkwater, 1992).

Activities to prepare children and to promote interaction once programs are in place are also important strategies for teachers and are reassuring to parents. Using literature developed for preschool children to promote understanding and acceptance of differences can be effective (see Friedberg, Mullins, & Sukiennik,

1992, for an annotated bibliography). Also exciting are new programs such as the "child tested and teacher approved" buddy skills program (English et al., 1996, p. 62), which encourages preschool children to stay, play, and talk with a buddy (a child with a disability), or group friendship activities (Cooper & McEvoy, 1996), which use songs and games as expressions of friendship in integrated preschool classrooms.

## THE PARENT–PROFESSIONAL PARTNERSHIP

### ⊕   FOCUS 4

*What is involved in providing family-centered services?*

### Defining Family-Centered Services

Sussell, Carr, and Hartman (1996) remind professionals that "in intervention programs for children with disabilities, collaboration with families is a legal requirement, not just a nice thing to do" (p. 56). This legal requirement can be nice, if nice is defined as satisfying for parents and professionals and positive for children. However, these positive results do not just happen. They require both professional commitment to family-centered practices and hard work. Bailey et al. (1992c) have described family-centered services as "the provision of coordinated services based on a shared philosophy of how families are involved in every aspect of service delivery, whether it be assessment, child care, family support, therapeutic services, case management, team meetings, or consultation" (p. 9). A look back at the history of parent involvement begins with parents largely excluded from child assessment, program planning, and program implementation. These tasks were left to the professional experts. Later, there was a movement to involve parents as teachers of their children. Although positive in many ways, the teaching expectation can be an additional burden for parents, especially if resources are limited. Professionals are now moving to a practice that develops and sustains collaborative partnerships between professionals and parents. These partnerships focus on family priorities and include parents in every step of the service delivery process.

### The Challenge of Family-Centered Service Delivery

Research (Bailey, Palsha, & Simeonsson, 1991) documents that professionals find this family-centered collaborative role challenging, but it is seen as a priority, not just in the field of education, but in psychology (Roberts & Magrab, 1991), nursing (Krehbiel, Munsick-Bruno, & Lowe, 1991), and other fields. It is challenging because professionals must communicate and problem-solve effectively with one another, with a variety of agencies, and with families.

The best outcomes for young children and their families and the most satisfying experiences for professionals occur in situations of mutual respect and perspective taking. A key to accomplishing this goal is listening to one another. By listening to families, professionals can learn to respect parent knowledge of their child while remembering that each parent and each family system is unique and combines both strengths and needs. By listening to professionals, parents can gain knowledge about how to help their child and how to secure needed resources. Ann Oster (1985), a professional and parent, reminds us that "the only way to discover what any collection of human beings needs is by listening to each one" (p. 28). Also, possessing family-centered attitudes is necessary but not sufficient for developing family-centered services (McBride et al., 1993). Professionals must constantly monitor not only their intentions, but also the actual family focus of program implementation.

Professionals must also listen to and learn from one another and possess what Bricker and Cripe (1992, p. 65) termed "team player skills." Each family served by an early intervention program (child under age 3) has a service coordinator who assists families in all aspects of the early intervention program, and frequently one key professional is selected to be the person primarily involved with the child and the family. For preschoolers, the teacher usually provides this coordination of professionals and serves as the key professional. The selection of the key professional is typically based on the needs of the child and rapport established between professionals and parents during the assessment period. For example, a parent priority might be for the child to learn to sit independently. The occupational therapist might become the lead professional addressing this and other delays in motor development. Later, when the family wants to focus on improving the child's ability to communicate, the speech/language pathologist might work directly with the child and family or indirectly as a consultant to the occupational therapist.

When professionals are able to work in transdisciplinary teams (McGonigel, Woodruff, & Roszmann-Millican, 1994) and instruct one another (role release), it cuts down on the number of different relationships required of the young child and the family. McGonigel et al. (1994) provided suggestions for promoting role release for families and professionals involved in IFSP teams (see Table 7.1 on page 168).

Families are fortunate to have the range of expertise that multiple service providers direct toward the child's needs, but dealing with multiple providers can also be a source of stress for families (Beckman & Kohl, 1993). Professionals are challenged to maximize the positive benefits and minimize the stress. Despite these challenges, early intervention personnel report high levels of job satisfaction and job commitment (Kontos & File, 1992). Monitoring employee satisfaction

**TABLE 7.1** *Activities to Promote Role Release for Families and Professionals on Transdisciplinary Teams*

| Role Release Component | Activities |
| --- | --- |
| Role extension | • Read new articles and books within your discipline or about your child's condition.<br>• Attend conferences, seminars, and lectures.<br>• Join a professional organization in your field or a family-to-family network.<br>• Explore resources at libraries or media centers. |
| Role enrichment | • Listen to parents discuss their child's strengths and needs.<br>• Ask for explanations of unfamiliar technical language or jargon.<br>• Do an appraisal of what you wish you knew more about and what you could teach others. |
| Role expansion | • Watch someone from another discipline work with a child, and check your perception of what you observe.<br>• Attend a workshop in another field that includes some "hands-on" practicum experience.<br>• Rotate the role of transdisciplinary arena assessment facilitator among all service providers on the team. |
| Role exchange | • Allow yourself to be videotaped practicing a technique from another discipline; invite a team member from that discipline to review and critique the videotape with you.<br>• Work side by side in the center-based program, demonstrating interventions to families and staff.<br>• Suggest strategies for achieving an IFSP outcome outside your own discipline; check your accuracy with other team members. |
| Role release | • Do a self-appraisal—list new skills within your intervention repertoire that other team members have taught you.<br>• Monitor the performance of the service providers on your child's IFSP team.<br>• Present the "whole" child at a clinical conference.<br>• Accept responsibility for implementing, with the family, an entire IFSP. |
| Role support | • Ask for help when you feel "stuck."<br>• Offer help when you see a team member struggling with a complex intervention.<br>• Provide any intervention that only you can provide, but share the child's progress and any related interventions with the primary service provider and the family. |

*Source:* From *Meeting Early Intervention Challenges: Issues from Birth to Three* by L. Johnson et al. Copyright © 1994 Brookes Publishing Co., P.O. Box 10624, Baltimore, MD 21285-0624. Reprinted with permission.

and turnover (Palsha et al., 1990) and providing appropriate preservice and in-service training are vital components of effective family-centered services (Bailey, Palsha, & Simeonsson, 1991; Sexton et al., 1996).

---

⊕ **FOCUS 5**

*Identify three situations in which family–professional collaboration occurs in early intervention.*

### Involving Families in Assessment

Family-centered services begin with the assessment process. For parents, participation in this process is a new role that is being learned under stressful circumstances. Nor is it an easy role for professionals. How to conduct family-focused assessment was addressed by Davis and Gettinger (1995), who found a combination of self-report measures and structured interviews to be preferred by parents. Where to conduct the assessment was the focus of study for Rosenbaum and colleagues (1990), who compared the child's home and a children's treatment center. They found that both settings could be effective, but that home assessment enriched the information received through the opportunity for direct environmental observation. They suggested using the setting that the parents preferred.

The assessment process is family directed and includes developmental assessment of the child and assessment of the family. Providing family information (family strengths/needs, e.g., financial resources) is voluntary on the part of the family, and not all families feel comfortable providing this information. However, this information can be helpful to everyone involved because it allows families to inform professionals of family concerns, stressors, and needs as well as family strengths, resources, and supports. Family priorities for the child and the child's program—both current and long range—can also be ascertained through the process of family assessment (Beckman et al., 1993). Concrete suggestions on how to conduct child and family assessment, including sample forms, can be found in a variety of publications (e.g., McWilliam, 1992; Noonan & McCormick, 1993; Olson & Kwiatkowski, 1992).

Professionals depend on families to share their knowledge of the child and to help support the developing relationships between the professionals and the child. Parents depend on professionals to help them help their child develop optimal health, ability, and well-being. In all settings and circumstances, listening to parents is essential; assuming knowledge of family needs and priorities is ill advised. This was demonstrated in a study by Garshelis & McConnell (1993) that compared needs expressed by families of young children with family needs assessed by individual professionals and professional teams. The assessments of individual professionals matched those of mothers less than half the time, and teams were only slightly more adept at this task.

## Involving Families in Goal Setting

The assessment process leads to identification of parent priorities. These priorities can then be translated into IFSP goals for infants and toddlers and IEP goals for preschoolers. Developing family-focused goals can be challenging. In programs studied by researchers Bailey et al. (1990), most IFSP goals were child focused, rather than family focused. Additional research findings (Bailey et al., 1992b) indicated significant discrepancies between existing practices of family-centered services and ideal practices, as identified by professionals in early intervention programs. Campbell, Strickland, and La Forme (1992) advocated training for both professionals and parents as a means of increasing the family focus of IFSPs.

Vincent (1992) addressed the need for a better match between parent expectations and program goals and stressed that program participation may be jeopardized if this match is not made. Ethnic and cultural diversity can increase the risk of professional assumptions—rather than parental preferences—driving program planning and goal setting and can interfere with parent involvement if not taken into account (Sontag & Schacht, 1994; Vincent, 1992). However, attention to these issues can be major program strengths. Vincent (1992) provided this example: "Families particularly noted the importance of their relationship with a paraprofessional who spoke their language and came from their culture, especially when the professional staff did not" (p. 168).

Parent-generated priorities that lead to collaborative goals for child and family can be the starting point for mutually satisfying teaching and learning relationships among parents and professionals. Allowing parent priorities to shape goals can lead to increased parental involvement and increased trust in and respect for professionals.

## Involving Families in Program Implementation

Parents of children involved in early intervention and preschool programs combine the tasks of learning from professionals and teaching their children. The periods of infancy and early childhood are dynamic times of physical, cognitive, language, and social growth and development for children. Therefore, learning experiences for children must occur all the time, not just during a home visit by a professional or during the school day. Professionals can assist parents in learning to incorporate developmentally appropriate learning activities in the child's daily care and play routines.

In addition to working on developmental goals for the child, the team collaborates with parents to identify and utilize natural supports to accomplish goals that will benefit and empower the whole family (Noonan & McCormick, 1993). For example, the parents may need child care for their toddler while they work. The parents and the team can consider possible options. This might lead to an IFSP goal of enrolling the child in a child-care center serving children without developmental problems, which would meet the child-care need while giving the toddler cognitive, motor, and socialization experiences with toddlers with typical development. The team might then help the parents find an appropriate child-care center and provide support for the child within this community setting. This support could include staff training and consultation as well as modeling ways of working with the child for the child-care staff.

An important part of programming for young children is teaching parents how to incorporate IFSP/IEP goals into their daily care and play activities with their child. Learning to work with and enhance the development of their infants and preschoolers can be rewarding and empowering for parents. However, it can also be difficult for any parent at certain times and not possible for some parents some of the time (see Window 7.2 on page 159). For example, the work of Brinker, Seifer, and Sameroff (1994) suggested that some early intervention programs may demand too much of lower socioeconomic families. Professionals must be constantly vigilant concerning the impact of the programs they design. It is wise to heed the caution that although parent inclusion as equal team members is essential, flexible options that allow parents to determine, adjust, and readjust their levels of involvement are also necessary (Brotherson & Goldstein, 1992; Maple, 1987). Expecting too much of parents can be problematic, but expecting too little can be as well. This point was made by Vincent (1988), who warns professionals about attitude barriers in early intervention. She delineated the following inappropriate attitudes on the part of service providers as major barriers to effective communication and collaboration: (a) parents do not know what their children can do; (b) parents can't really identify appropriate goals for their children; (c) parents cannot teach their own children; and (d) parents need us to solve their problems for them (p. 3).

Professionals probably trained in the field of early childhood because they enjoy working with young children. Then they find that part of their job, in fact a very important part, is to teach adults—the parents of these young children. So they become adult educators with all the challenges this task can bring (Brookfield, 1992). Parents are as diverse as their children in terms of ability, motivation, and learning style. Professionals must learn to individualize for parents as they do for children. Motivation is critically important. Blum and Handleman (1992) remind professionals involved in teaching parents to teach their children that they "walk a fine line between being viewed as a task master and being appreciated for providing needed motivation" and of the importance of knowing "when to back off from pushing overloaded parents too hard, and when to persist and provide the needed steam" (p. 178).

Communication that involves affirmation can be a powerful component of parent–professional collaboration. Professionals can let parents know their positive feelings about the baby or young child and affirm positive parenting. This will be particularly appreciated by parents because praise from others may be limited. Parental praise is also appreciated by professionals. A teacher in a center-based early intervention program was deeply touched by a mother who came to pick up her infant and said, "I always know he has had a good day when he has been with you. I know you cuddle him because he smells like your perfume."

---

## ⊕  FOCUS 6

*How can professionals facilitate parental advocacy and coping responses?*

### Facilitating Parental Advocacy

In addition to wanting information about their child's condition, services for the child, and supports for the family, parents have expressed the need for information about the child's legal rights (Gowen, Christy, & Sparling, 1993). This is a relevant need because the early childhood period is the beginning of advocacy for parents (Pizzo, 1990). Advocacy has positive benefits in terms of both process and product. The process of advocating can support parental self-esteem and mastery (Patterson & Berry, 1997), and the product can be improved services for the child.

Service coordinators help parents of infants and toddlers secure needed services, but part of their role must be teaching parents how to advocate for their child, independent of this professional support. Parents can be taught skills such as how to acquire and file information about their child, including developmental milestones and medical history. They can also learn to use strategies such as keeping a communication notebook and telephone log of interactions with service providers (Beckman, Boyes, & Herres, 1993). The service coordinator is available to the family only during the brief period of eligibility for early intervention services, but the advocacy needs of the child may be lifelong. A continuum that moves the family from supported advocacy to independent parental advocacy to self-advocacy when the child becomes an adult is appropriate.

Professionals can also support parents in learning the communication skills that are necessary for advocacy. The family assessment can serve as a starting point. Professionals can ask for, listen to, and implement family priorities. This gives parents the message that what they think and feel is important, will be respected by the professional team, and will benefit their child. A relationship built on trust between the service coordinator and the parents can be the basis for productive relationships with the multiple microsystems awaiting this child and family. The service coordinator or another professional with a strong relationship with the parents can provide support for parents in team meetings and can go with parents to appointments with physicians or to visit school or child-care programs. These professionals can guide parents in not only asking questions and stating needs, but in understanding that they have the right to ask questions and receive needed information, advice, and support.

Even though their children are young and their parental role as advocates has just begun, some families have to advocate for their children at the exosystem level. Professionals can provide both direct and indirect support to families in this rather awesome task as they take on medical-care systems, school systems, welfare systems, and, as in the case of Jill Peterson, the mother of Kyle, the insurance industry (Window 7.3).

---

★ **WINDOW 7.3**

## *Journey down a Raging River*

KENT AND I WERE QUITE YOUNG when we took our two-week-old baby home from the hospital for the first time—accompanied by feeding tubes and heart monitors. We were completely naive to the journey we were facing. It is like taking a white water raft trip for the first time, only with no guide to tell you what to watch out for. So, you push your raft from the security of shore alone.

Your destination? To provide your child with every chance to be independent. You want equal opportunities for your child and all children with developmental disabilities. You load your raft with various books and resources. But most important, you have your family and love. The river looks challenging, but you face it with a positive attitude and determination. . . .

Ahead of you is your first sight of white water—and it's overwhelming. At only five months old, your child faces his first open-heart surgery. His heart defect is extremely rare. Only one surgeon qualifies to perform the operation. Unfortunately, this surgeon is not within your insurance plan. The doctor scheduled for the surgery has never performed a procedure even close to what your child needs.

You maneuver between the boulders blocking your course through the river. After numerous phone calls, letters, denial letters back, more phone calls, letters and meetings with insurance companies (and almost the entire chain of pediatric surgeons), you miraculously pull through the life-threatening rapids and your son is alive. You have convinced the right people that your son deserves a qualified surgeon. . . .

You realize that each day will be a fight. It is ironic that you continually assert yourself to give your child the same opportunities that many of us take for granted. Everyone deserves the right to proper medical care; to be fully integrated into the school systems; and to receive the necessary services to insure a quality education. The biggest challenge to you will be to teach society that everyone is human, with different abilities. So, climb back into your weathered raft and continue to meet the challenge of the river. But never lose focus of your destination.

*Source:* Reprinted with permission from PACER Center, (612) 827-2966.

## Facilitating Coping and Providing Support

An important coping response for all parents is experiencing a sense of control and competence in the parenting experience. Professionals can support family coping by addressing this need for control and looking for ways it can be achieved. For example, Lowenthal (1989) suggested that in the neonatal intensive care nursery it may be possible to give parents some choice and control over visiting times and feeding times, thereby instilling some sense of parental control in a setting in which their actual control is quite limited. Another suggestion for professionals is to help parents recognize that they still have control over some aspects of their life even when the care of their child is largely under the control of others. This story provides an example. The mother of a critically ill toddler had been at the hospital for 24 hours without a break. Her husband took over, and she went home to take a shower and a nap. She later related to the hospital social worker that when she got home, even though she felt tired and dirty, she could not rest or clean up until she spent time straightening her house. She found her behavior confusing until the social worker pointed out that she was seeking control. At the hospital, her son's life was in the control of the doctors and nurses and the hospital schedule. At home, she had the power to make her house neat and tidy. The social worker helped this mother look for other parts of her life over which she had control and worked with the medical staff to increase parental control over the child's care within the hospital.

Families, in order to cope effectively, also need tangible support. For families with newborns with medical and developmental problems, Julianne Beckett (1985), the mother of a young child with extensive medical needs, made these practical recommendations to professionals:

1. Secure funding to make sure that the child is coming home to a family whose biggest fear is not giving up every worldly possession to pay for home care.

2. Plan for some type of relief for the parents. They will never forget totally their responsibility for that child they brought home, but give them an opportunity to get away for a while to be who they are. (p. 13).

Families of young children whose problems are not as extensive or immediate also need support in order to cope with parenting demands. Valentine (1993) emphasized the importance of family assessment and planning. She described four typical family profiles: the well-supported family, the stressed family, the isolated family, and the overextended family, and suggested these profiles could be helpful to professionals for designing family supports. Sources of support designated by the families studied by Valentine included formal support from service providers, as well as natural supports including the extended maternal family, religious affiliation, and their places of employment.

Support needs frequently noted by families of young children include babysitting, respite care, more personal time, and someone to talk to (Bailey, Blasco, & Simeonsson, 1992a; Garshelis & McConnell, 1993). Keep in mind that these same needs might be articulated by families of a young child with typical development, but the needs of these families could likely be met through natural supports. Families with young children with developmental problems may need formal support in these areas as well as formal problem-solving support to help identify and utilize natural supports.

Professionals can work with parents to locate and train babysitters and respite-care providers. Help with child care also may help parents address the needs for personal time and for someone to talk to. Cooley (1992) addressed the support needs of families with infants with medical and developmental problems and stated that "families need support from familiar and trusted sources" (p. 103). Two-parent families can draw on their relationship for mutual support, and time away from child care can nurture this relationship. Also, having child care means that married or single parents can gain social support through social interaction with friends. Many parents further benefit by supplementing their existing friend networks with networks that include other parents of children with developmental problems.

Early intervention programs often provide parent support groups as part of the program. Attendance at support group meetings is voluntary, and mothers are more likely to attend than fathers. However, support groups specifically targeting fathers are endorsed by early intervention professionals and by the fathers themselves (Davis & May, 1991; May, 1992; Vadasy et al., 1986). The parent support groups typically meet weekly and are led by a social worker, nurse, or educator.

Krauss and colleagues (1993) studied the results of parent-group participation and found both beneficial and adverse outcomes. Parent-group attendance was associated with significant gains in perceived social support from peers but also with elevated personal strain and greater adverse impacts on social/familial relationships. These adverse impacts may, however, reflect awareness of the very real problems involved in rearing a child with disabilities. This awareness may be a healthy beginning to psychological growth and improved coping. However, the adverse impact could be due to the group structure that necessitates both sharing problems and listening to the problems of others. These findings point, once again, to the need to individualize services for families. Parent groups may be an important coping strategy for some parents and a source of stress for others or a source of support at one point, but not at another. Also, parent groups may serve to raise personal issues that need to be addressed one on one between the parent and a mental health professional as a follow-up to the group experience.

Parent support groups are but one means of parent-to-parent support, and other avenues, such as programs that link experienced parents with new parents (Smith, 1993), may be more appropriate for some families. Professionals can also provide support by simply helping parents meet and get acquainted with one another. This works best when parents are matched with parents of children with a similar disability and who have enough in common that they might have become friends even if they did not have children with similar developmental problems. In fact, parents of adults with disabilities report that their most enduring friendships are those in which their concern for their son or daughter with disabilities is but one aspect of many shared interests and values. Whether through formal parent support groups, structured pairings, or informal friendships, parents can help each other cope by finding meaning in their shared situation and by mutual empowerment.

During this first lifespan stage, parents must respond to their young child's ordinary needs for love and attention while addressing his or her extraordinary needs for medical care and developmental intervention. Today's parents are fortunate to have formal supports and professional assistance with these tasks. However, challenges to families remain. These challenges include accessing formal and natural supports and learning to be a team member and advocate while simultaneously learning the primary role of parent to a child with special needs. Professional intervention that helps parents learn these new roles and gather needed supports is crucial for parents both while their children are young and as they continue their lifespan journey.

## REVIEW

*FOCUS 1: What opportunities and risks exist for families as they respond to the birth and diagnosis of a child with disabilities or medical problems?*

- Parents may first interact with the medical-care system. Medical and other professionals have the task of sharing diagnostic information with parents. Accurate and complete information, sensitively conveyed, is greatly appreciated by parents.

- Parents of an infant or young child with medical or developmental problems must grieve the loss of the expected child while providing care that is often technically complicated and demanding.

*FOCUS 2: What educational services are available for young children, and how are their families involved in these programs?*

- Infants and toddlers with disabilities now have the opportunity to participate in early intervention programs that provide a wide range of home- and center-based, family-focused services.
- Family participation is an integral part of the IFSP process.
- Preschool-age children with disabilities participate in school-based services.
- Parents take on a new role as members of the IEP team.

*FOCUS 3: How can the young child's needs for play and socialization experiences be addressed by the family and through early childhood education?*

- Professionals can assist families in creating and adapting play equipment and activities for their young children.
- Social skills of young children with disabilities are enhanced when they participate in programs that include young children with typical development.

*FOCUS 4: What is involved in providing family-centered services?*

- Family-centered services include and involve families in every facet of service delivery.
- Delivering family-centered services is challenging because professionals must communicate and problem-solve effectively with each other, with a variety of agencies, and with families.

*FOCUS 5: Identify three situations in which family–professional collaboration occurs in early intervention.*

- The assessment process is family directed and includes developmental assessment of the child and assessment of family strengths, needs, and priorities.
- Family priorities are translated into IFSP goals for infants and toddlers and IEP goals for preschoolers.
- Professionals help parents incorporate developmentally based learning experiences within the child's daily care and play routines.

*FOCUS 6: How can professionals facilitate parental advocacy and coping responses?*

- The period of early childhood for children with developmental delay is the beginning of advocacy for parents. Professionals can support parents as they learn advocacy skills.
- Providing direct support, helping parents achieve control and mastery within the parenting experience, and helping parents access natural supports are all components of effective coping for parents.

# REFERENCES

Bailey, D. B., Blasco, P. M., & Simeonsson, R. J. (1992a). Needs expressed by mothers and fathers of young children with disabilities. *American Journal on Mental Retardation*, *97*, 1–10.

Bailey, D. B., Buysse, V., Edmondson, R., & Smith, T. (1992b). Creating family-centered services in early intervention: Perceptions of professionals in four states. *Exceptional Children*, *58*, 298–309.

Bailey, D. B., McWilliam, P. J., Winton, P. J., & Simeonsson, R. J. (1992c). *Implementing family-centered services in early intervention: A team-based model for change.* Cambridge: Brookline.

Bailey, D. B., Palsha, S. A., & Simeonsson, R. J. (1991). Professional skills, concerns, and perceived importance of work with families in early intervention. *Exceptional Children*, *58*, 156–165.

Bailey, D. B., Winton, P. J., Rouse, L., & Turnbull, A. P. (1990). Family goals in infant intervention: Analysis and issues. *Journal of Early Intervention*, *14*, 15–26.

Beckett, J. (1985). Comprehensive care for medically vulnerable infants and toddlers: A parent's perspective. In *Proceedings of Equals in this partnership: Parents of disabled and at-risk infants and toddlers speak to professionals* (pp. 7–14). Washington, DC: National Center for Clinical Infant Programs.

Beckman, P. J., Boyes, G. B., & Herres, A. (1993). Managing the information. In P. J. Beckman & G. B. Boyes (Eds.), *Deciphering the system: A guide for families of young children with disabilities* (pp. 39–48). Cambridge: Brookline.

Beckman, P. J., & Kohl, F. L. (1993). Working with multiple service providers. In P. J. Beckman & G. B. Boyes (Eds.), *Deciphering the system: A guide for families of young children with disabilities* (pp. 21–37). Cambridge: Brookline.

Beckman, P. J., Newcomb, S., Stroup, V., & Robinson, C. (1993). Gathering information about families. In P. J. Beckman and G. B. Boyes (Eds.), *Deciphering the system: A guide for families of young children with disabilities* (pp. 67–80). Cambridge: Brookline.

Beckwith, L. (1990). Adaptive and maladaptive parenting: Implications for intervention. In S. J. Meisels & J. P. Shonkoff (Eds.), *Handbook of early childhood intervention* (pp. 53–77). Cambridge: Cambridge University Press.

Berger, K. S. (1994). *The developing person through the life span* (3rd ed.). New York: Worth.

Blacher, J. (1984). Sequential stages of parental adjustment to the birth of a child with handicaps: Fact or artifact? *Mental Retardation*, *22*, 58–68.

Blos, P., & Davies, D. (1993). Extending the intervention process: A report of a distressed family with a damaged newborn and a vulnerable preschooler. In E. Fenichel & S. Provence (Eds.), *Development in jeopardy: Clinical responses to infants and families* (pp. 51–83). Madison: International Universities Press.

Blum, L. C., & Handleman, J. S. (1992). Consulting to families of a child with a developmental disability: Considerations for the home consultant. *Journal of Educational and Psychological Consultation*, *3*, 175–179.

Bricker, D., & Cripe, J. J. W. (1992). *An activity-based approach to early intervention*. Baltimore: Brookes.

Brinker, R. P., Seifer, R., & Sameroff, A. J. (1994). Relations among maternal stress, cognitive development, and early intervention in middle- and low-SES infants with developmental disabilities. *American Journal on Mental Retardation*, *98*, 463–480.

Brookfield, S. (1992, April). Why can't I get this right? Myths and realities in facilitating adult learning. *Adult Learning*, pp. 12–15.

Brotherson, M. J., & Goldstein, B. L. (1992). Time as a resource and constraint for parents of young children with disabilities: Implications for early intervention services. *Topics in Early Childhood Special Education, 12*, 508–527.

Bruce, E. J., Schultz, C. L., Smyrnios, K. X., & Schultz, N. C. (1994). Grieving related to development: A preliminary comparison of three age cohorts of parents of children with intellectual disability. *British Journal of Medical Psychology, 67*, 37–52.

Calhoun, M. L., Calhoun, L. G., & Rose, T. L. (1989). Parents of babies with severe handicaps: Concerns about early intervention. *Journal of Early Intervention, 13*, 146–152.

Campbell, P. H., Strickland, B., & La Forme, C. (1992). Enhancing parent participation in the individualized family service plan. *Topics in Early Childhood Special Education, 11*, 112–124.

Cardinal, D. N., & Shum, K. (1993). A descriptive analysis of family-related services in the neonatal intensive care unit. *Journal of Early Intervention, 17*, 270–282.

Cole, K. N., Mills, P. E., Dale, P. S., & Jenkins, J. R. (1991). Effects of preschool integration for children with disabilities. *Exceptional Children, 58*, 36–45.

Cook, S. S. (1988). The impact of the disabled child on the family. *Loss, Grief and Care, 2*, 45–52.

Cooley, W. C. (1992). Natural beginnings—unnatural encounters: Events at the outset for families of children with disabilities. In J. Nisbet (Ed.), *Natural supports in school, at work, and in the community for people with severe disabilities* (pp. 87–120). Baltimore: Brookes.

Cooper, C. S., & McEvoy, M. A. (1996). Group friendship activities. *Teaching Exceptional Children, 28*, 67–69.

Davis, P. B., & May, J. F. (1991). Involving fathers in early intervention and family support programs: Issues and strategies. *Children's Health Care, 20*, 87–92.

Davis, S. K., & Gettinger, M. (1995). Family-focused assessment for identifying family resources and concerns: Parent preferences, assessment information, and evaluation across three methods. *Journal of School Psychology, 33*, 99–121.

Demchak, M., & Drinkwater, S. (1992). Preschoolers with severe disabilities: The case against segregation. *Topics in Early Childhood Special Education, 11*, 70–83.

Diamond, K. E., & LeFurgy, W. G. (1994). Attitudes of parents of preschool children toward integration. *Early Education and Development, 5*, 69–77.

Drinkwater, S., & Demchak, M. (1995). The preschool checklist: Integration of children with severe disabilities. *Teaching Exceptional Children, 28*, 4–8.

Ebenstein, B. (1995, April). IEP strategies. *Exceptional Parent*, pp. 62–63.

English, K., Goldstein, H., Kaczmarek, L., & Shafer, K. (1996). "Buddy skills" for preschoolers. *Teaching Exceptional Children, 28*, 62–66.

Friedberg, J. B., Mullins, J. B., & Sukiennik, A. W. (1992). *Portraying persons with disability: An annotated bibliography of nonfiction for children and teenagers.* New Providence, NJ: Bowker.

Gardner, S. L., Merenstein, G. B., & Costello, A. J. (1993). Grief and perinatal loss. In G. B. Merenstein & S. L. Gardner (Eds.), *Handbook of neonatal intensive care* (3rd ed.) (pp. 530–563). St. Louis: Mosby.

Garshelis, J. A., & McConnell, S. R. (1993). Comparison of family needs assessed by mothers, individual professionals, and interdisciplinary teams. *Journal of Early Intervention, 17*, 36–49.

Goldstein, H., & Kaczmarek, L. (1991). Promoting communicative interaction among children in integrated intervention settings. In S. Warren & J. Reichle (Eds.), *Causes and effects in communication and language intervention* (pp. 81–111). Baltimore: Brookes.

Gowen, J. W., Christy, D. S., & Sparling, J. (1993). Informational needs of parents of young children with special needs. *Journal of Early Intervention, 17*, 194–210.

Guralnick, M. J., & Groom, J. M. (1987). The peer relations of mildly delayed and nonhandi-capped preschool children in mainstreamed playgroups. *Child Development, 58*, 1556–1572.

Hymes, J. L. (1991). *Early childhood education: Twenty years in review*. Washington, DC: National Association for the Education of Young Children.

Kontos, S., & File, N. (1992). Conditions of employment, job satisfaction, and job commitment among early intervention personnel. *Journal of Early Intervention, 16*, 155–165.

Kopp, C. B., & Kaler, S. R. (1989). Risk in infancy: Origins and implications. *American Psychologist, 44*, 224–230.

Krauss, M. W., Upshur, C. C., Shonkoff, J. P., & Hauser-Cram, P. (1993). The impact of parent groups on mothers of infants with disabilities. *Journal of Early Intervention, 16*, 8–20.

Krehbiel, R., Munsick-Bruno, G., & Lowe, J. R. (1991). NICU infants born at developmental risk and the individualized family service plan/process (IFSP). *Children's Health Care, 20*, 26–33.

Leff, P. T., & Walizer, E. H. (1992). The uncommon wisdom of parents at the moment of diagnosis. *Family Systems Medicine, 10*, 147–168.

Lowenthal, B. (1989). Alleviating stress in parents of high-risk premature infants. *Teaching Exceptional Children, 21*, 32–33.

Lyon, J. (1989). I want to be Zak's mom, not his therapist. *Developmental Disabilities Special Interest Section Newsletter*, The American Occupational Therapy Association, Inc., *12*, 4.

Maple, G. (1987). Early intervention: Some issues in co-operative teamwork. *Australian Occupational Therapy Journal, 34*, 145–151.

May, J. (1992, April/May). New horizons for fathers of children with disabilities. *Exceptional Parent*, pp. 40–43.

McBride, S. L., Brotherson, M. J., Joanning, H., Whiddon, D., & Demmitt, A. (1993). Implementation of family-centered services: Perceptions of families and professionals. *Journal of Early Intervention, 17*, 414–430.

McDonnell, A. P. (1995). Early intervention programs for infants and toddlers with disabilities and their families. In J. J. McDonnell, M. L. Hardman, A. P. McDonnell, & R. Kiefer-O'-Donnell (Eds.), *An introduction to persons with severe disabilities* (pp. 100–139). Boston: Allyn & Bacon.

McGonigel, M. J., Woodruff, G., & Roszmann-Millican, M. (1994). The transdisciplinary team: A model for family-centered early intervention. In L. J. Johnson, R. J. Gallagher, M. J. LaMontagne, J. B. Jordan, J. J. Gallagher, P. L. Huntinger, & M. B. Karnes (Eds.), *Meeting early intervention challenges: Issues from birth to three*. Baltimore: Brookes.

McWilliam, R. A. (1992). *Family-centered intervention planning: A routines-based approach*. Tucson: Communication Skill Builders.

Noonan, M. J., & McCormick, L. (1993). *Early intervention in natural environments: Methods and procedures*. Pacific Grove, CA: Brooks/Cole.

Olson, J., & Kwiatkowski, K. (1992). *Planning family goals: A systems approach to the IFSP*. Tucson: Communication Skill Builders.

Oster, A. (1985). Keynote address. In *Proceedings of Equals in this partnership: Parents of disabled and at-risk infants and toddlers speak to professionals* (pp. 27–33). Washington, DC: National Center for Clinical Infant Programs.

Palsha, S. A., Bailey, D. B., Vandiviere, P., & Munn, D. (1990). A study of employee stability and turnover in home-based early intervention. *Journal of Early Intervention, 14,* 342–351.

Parette, H. P., Hourcade, J. J., & Brimberry, R. K. (1990). The family physician's role with parents of young children with developmental disabilities. *Journal of Family Practice, 31,* 288–296.

Patterson, L., & Berry, J. O. (1997). *Parental advocacy and child disability: Personal and social characteristics of an advocate.* Poster session presented at the annual conference of the Council for Exceptional Children, Salt Lake City, UT.

Peterson, J. (1995, September). Each day becomes a journey down a raging river. *The Pacesetter,* p. 10.

Pizzo, P. (1990). Parent advocacy: A resource for early intervention. In S. J. Meisels & J. P. Shonkoff (Eds.), *Handbook of early childhood intervention* (pp. 668–678). Cambridge: Cambridge University Press.

Powell, D. R. (1993). Emerging directions in parent-child early intervention. In D. R. Powell (Ed.), *Parent education as early childhood intervention: Emerging directions in theory, research, and practice* (pp. 1–22). Norwood, NJ: Ablex.

Quine, L., & Rutter, D. R. (1994). First diagnosis of severe mental and physical disability: A study of doctor-parent communication. *Journal of Child Psychology and Psychiatry, 35,* 1273–1287.

Roberts, R. N., & Magrab, P. R. (1991). Psychologists' role in a family-centered approach to practice, training, and research with young children. *American Psychologist, 46,* 144–148.

Rosenbaum, P., King, S., Toal, C., Puttaswamaiah, S., & Durrell, K. (1990). Home or children's treatment centre: Where should initial therapy assessments or children with disabilities be done? *Developmental Medicine and Child Neurology, 32,* 888–894.

Schopler, E. (1995). *Parent survival manual: A guide to crisis resolution in autism and related developmental disorders.* New York: Plenum.

Sexton, D., Snyder, P., Wolfe, B., Lobman, M., Stricklin, S., & Akers, P. (1996). Early intervention inservice training strategies: Perceptions and suggestions from the field. *Exceptional Children, 62,* 485–495.

Sloper, P., & Turner, S. (1993). Determinants of parental satisfaction with disclosure of disability. *Developmental Medicine and Child Neurology, 35,* 816–825.

Smith, P. M. (1993). Opening many, many doors: Parent-to-parent support. In P. J. Beckman & G. B. Boyes (Eds.), *Deciphering the system: A guide for families of young children with disabilities* (pp. 129–141). Cambridge: Brookline.

Sontag, J. C., & Schacht, R. (1994). An ethnic comparison of parent participation and information needs in early intervention. *Exceptional Children, 60,* 422–433.

Sussell, A., Carr, S., & Hartman, A. (1996). Families R Us: Building a parent/school partnership. *Teaching Exceptional Children, 28,* 53–57.

Vadasy, P. F., Fewell, R. R., Greenberg, M. T., Dermond, N. L., & Meyer, D. J. (1986). Follow-up evaluation of the effects of involvement in the fathers program. *Topics in Early Childhood Special Education, 6,* 16–31.

Valentine, D. P. (1993). Children with special needs: Sources of support and stress for families. *Journal of Social Work and Human Sexuality, 8,* 107–121.

Vincent, L. J. (1988). What we have learned from families. *OSERS News in Print, 1,* 3.

Vincent, L. J. (1992). Families and early intervention: Diversity and competence. *Journal of Early Intervention, 16,* 166–172.

Werner, S. (1993). Through the door. In J. A. Spiegle & R. A. van den Pol (Eds.), *Making changes: Family voices on living with disabilities* (pp. 125–126). Cambridge: Brookline.

Zigler, E., & Styfco, S. J. (1994). Is the Perry Preschool better than Head Start? Yes and no. *Early Childhood Research Quarterly, 9,* 269–287.

# CHAPTER EIGHT

# Families and Schools[1]

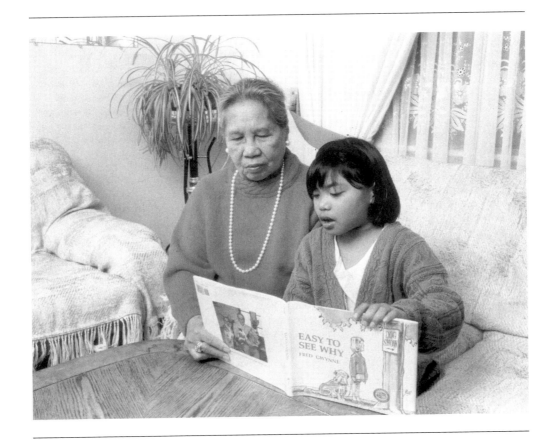

---

[1]This chapter was coauthored by Monica Ferguson, Fairbanks North Star Borough School District, Fairbanks, Alaska.

✦ **WINDOW 8.1**

## Ricardo

RICARDO GALLEGHOS, A THIRD GRADER AT Bloomington Hill Elementary School, has recently been referred by his teacher, Ms. Thompson, to the school's special services committee for an evaluation. During the first four months of school, Ricardo has continued to fall further behind in reading and language. He entered third grade with some skills in letter and sound recognition, but had difficulty reading and comprehending material beyond a first grade level. It was clear to Ms. Thompson that Ricardo's language development was delayed as well. He had a very limited expressive vocabulary and had some difficulty following directions if more than one or two steps were involved.

Ms. Thompson contacted Ricardo's mother, Maria Galleghos (a single parent), saying she would like to refer Ricardo for an in-depth evaluation of his reading and language skills. A representative from the school would be calling Ms. Galleghos to explain what the evaluation meant and get her approval for the necessary testing. The school psychologist, Jean Andreas, made the call. During the phone conversation Ms. Galleghos reminded the school psychologist that the primary language spoken in the home was Spanish even though Ricardo, his mother, and siblings spoke English as well. Ms. Andreas indicated that the assessment would be conducted in both Spanish and English in order to determine if Ricardo's problems were related to a disability in reading or problems with English as a second language.

Following written approval from Ricardo's mother, the school special services team conducted an evaluation of Ricardo's academic performance. The formal evaluation included achievement tests, classroom performance tests, samples of Ricardo's work, behavioral observations, and anecdotal notes from Ms. Thompson. An interview with Ms. Galleghos was conducted as part of the process to gain her perceptions of Ricardo's strengths and problem areas and to give her the opportunity to relate pertinent family history.

The evaluation confirmed his teacher's concerns. Ricardo was more than two years below what was expected for a child his age in both reading and language development. Ricardo's difficulties in these areas did not seem to be primarily related to the fact that he was bilingual, but the issue of English as a second language would need to be taken into consideration in developing an appropriate learning experience.

The team determined that Ricardo qualified for special education services as a student with a specific learning disability. Once again, Ms. Andreas contacted Ms. Galleghos with the results, indicating that Ricardo qualified for special education services in reading and language. Ms. Andreas pointed out to Ms. Galleghos that as a parent of a student with an identified disability, she had some specific legal rights which would be further explained to her both in writing and orally.

One of those rights is to participate as a partner in the development of Ricardo's individualized education program (IEP). Ms. Andreas further explained that a meeting would be set up at a mutually convenient time to develop a plan to assist Ricardo over the next year. Prior to that formal meeting, however, Ms. Andreas asked Ms. Galleghos to meet with her and the special education teacher, Mr. Lomas, to talk about how IEP teams work and what everyone needed to do in order to be prepared and work together to help Ricardo. Ms. Galleghos was asked to think about the long-range goals she has for Ricardo. What does she see as important for Ricardo to learn in school? What are her experiences at home that would help the team better understand Ricardo's needs and interests, particularly in the areas of reading and language development?

For most children, basic patterns of learning and development are established within the first five years of life under the watchful guidance of parents
and other family members. Through interaction within the family, the child en-
gages in many early learning experiences, such as a trip to the grocery store, a walk
outside to watch the cat chase a butterfly, or sitting on a parent's lap listening to
a bedtime story. As children grow older, their experiences outside the home
broaden. Expanding on the foundation laid by the family, preschool programs
provide further opportunities for learning. Through preschool, children use the
early concrete experiences provided by the family as a base on which to build further understanding of the world around them.

At about age 5 or 6, both the child and the family face a major life passage: the
transition to elementary school. As was true with preschool, the child's time away
from home continues to increase. Although parents still play a critical role in
shaping the child's development, the school becomes an additional influence on
learning and behavior as the child spends about six hours a day outside the family sphere. For families with a child who has been identified as disabled prior to
age 5, expectations for elementary school are well grounded in their experiences
with early intervention and preschool programs. For families with a child who has
*not* been identified as disabled before age 5, the initial recognition that their child
has a disability will come through interactions with educators. Such is the case for
Ricardo from Window 8.1. Ricardo's mother learned of his disability through an
evaluation process that took place when he was in third grade and had fallen significantly behind his peers in reading and language development.

In this chapter, we address the relationship between families that have a child
with a disability and the schools that serve them. We begin with a discussion of
the legal basis for parents' participation in the education of children with disabilities as mandated in the Individuals with Disabilities Education Act (IDEA).
Using the basic tenets of IDEA, we then examine ways to build effective home-
school partnerships.

## THE INDIVIDUALS WITH DISABILITIES
## EDUCATION ACT (IDEA)

For the better part of the twentieth century, families faced a school system that was
at best apathetic to the needs of children with disabilities, and at worst discriminatory. For many parents, their only option was to take whatever the school was
willing to give in providing an education to their child. The school did not have to
adapt to the individual needs of the child; the child had to adapt to what the school
could provide, or face exclusion from public education. For many children with
disabilities and their families, exclusion became the norm. This standard changed
with the educational reforms of the 1960s and 1970s, eventually culminating in the
U.S. Congress passing Public Law 94-142, the Education for All Handicapped
Children's Act of 1975 (renamed the Individuals with Disabilities Education Act

[IDEA] in 1990). IDEA brought a new era of *rights-based education* that, among other important requirements, mandated parental involvement in the education of the child with disabilities.

## ⊕  FOCUS 1

*Identify the four major requirements of IDEA.*

IDEA was originally passed by the U.S. Congress in 1975 to ensure that all children with disabilities would have access to a free and appropriate public education designed to meet their unique needs. Every eligible child with a disability is to receive specialized instruction that is designed and reasonably calculated to provide educational benefit. Today, more than 5.2 million eligible students with disabilities receive special education and related services through the provisions of IDEA (U.S. Department of Education, 1996). Under current law, appropriate education includes access to special education in all settings, including the workplace and training centers. IDEA also stipulates that students with disabilities are to receive the related services necessary to ensure that they directly benefit from their educational experience. Related services include special transportation and other support services, such as speech pathology, psychological services, physical and occupational therapy, recreation, rehabilitation counseling, social work, and medical services. The act describes eligible students by disability condition and includes those with specific learning disabilities, mental retardation, serious emotional disturbance, speech or language disabilities, vision loss (including blindness), hearing loss, orthopedic impairments, other health impairments, deaf-blindness, multiple disabilities, autism, and traumatic brain injury. To ensure that each of these students receives a free and appropriate public education IDEA provides for the following:

• nondiscriminatory and multidisciplinary assessment of educational needs
• an individualized education program (IEP)
• education in the least restrictive environment (LRE)
• parent involvement in the education of their child with disabilities.

Nondiscriminatory and multidisciplinary assessment means (1) testing students in their native or primary language, (2) using evaluation procedures selected and administered to prevent cultural or racial discrimination, (3) using assessment tools validated for the purpose for which they are being used, and (4) conducting assessment through a multidisciplinary team that employs several pieces of information in order to formulate an individualized education program and determine educational placement in the least restrictive environment. Using the assessment information gathered on each child, the multidisciplinary team formulates an individualized education program (IEP). The basic requirements of the IEP include identifying each student's (a) present level of educational performance, (b) annual goals and short-term objectives, (c) related services, (d) beginning and ending dates for special education services, (e) appropriate percentage of time in a general education classroom, and (f) annual performance on the established goals and objectives. Once the IEP has been written and agreed upon by the multidisciplinary team, which includes the parents, a decision is made regarding where the student will receive their educational program. IDEA mandates that students with disabilities are to be educated in the least restrictive environment (LRE). LRE is defined in law as educating student with disabilities with their nondisabled peers to the maximum extent appropriate. "Appropriate" placement is determined by the needs of the student as designated in the goals and objectives of the IEP. In order to meet the basic requirements of the LRE provision, schools are required to offer a continuum of placements that range from placing the student in a general education classroom with support services to homebound and hospital programs.

Parents play a vital role in each stage of the process just described. IDEA requires that parents and professionals become partners in the education of the child with disabilities. This partnership designates specific rights for parents as members of the multidisciplinary team.

## PARENT INVOLVEMENT AS MANDATED IN IDEA

### ⊞ FOCUS 2

*Identify the ways that parents of children with disabilities are required by law to be directly involved in the planning and evaluation of their child's educational program.*

Parents' participation in the education of their child with a disability is clearly stipulated in IDEA. Legally, the law requires that parents be afforded the opportunity to participate as a member of the educational team in the planning and evaluation of their child's IEP. Practically, the law provides the framework for building a collaborative partnership between parents and educators to provide an appropriate education for the child with a disability.

IDEA outlines several ways in which parents have the opportunity to be directly involved:

- Consent in writing before the child is initially evaluated.
- Consent in writing before the child is initially placed in a special education program.

- Request an independent education evaluation if they feel the school's evaluation is inappropriate.

- Request an evaluation at public expense if a due process hearing finds that the public agency's evaluation was inappropriate.

- Inspect and review educational records and challenge information believed to be inaccurate, misleading, or in violation of the privacy or other rights of the child.

- Request a copy of information from the child's educational record.

- Request a meeting with the multidisciplinary team at any time to review their child's progress and/or appropriateness of the goals and objectives.

- Request a hearing concerning the school's proposal or refusal to initiate or change the identification, evaluation, or placement of the child or the provision of a free, appropriate public education.

- Participate on the individualized education program (IEP) committee that considers the evaluation, placement, and programming of the child.

### Parents and the IEP Process

**FOCUS 3**

*Identify each of the phases leading to a completed IEP. What are the roles of parents in each phase?*

The fundamental purpose of the IEP is to ensure that students with disabilities have access to an appropriate education based on individual need. The phases leading to a completed IEP involve referral for special education services, assessment of the student's educational need and eligibility, and development of the IEP concluding with placement in the least restrictive environment.

*Referral.* Referral for special education services occurs at different times for different children depending on individual functioning and need. For children with more severe disabilities, referral usually occurs very early in their educational life, often during preschool. For children with more mild to moderate disabilities, referral is initiated as they fall behind in their academic or social learning and become at risk for educational failure. This can occur at any time during the elementary or secondary school years, and referral is most often initiated by the general education teacher. Such was the case for Ricardo. His teacher observed him falling further and further behind in his learning. A request was made to the school's child-study team or special services committee for an assessment to determine qualification for additional support services through special education.

At a minimum, this team should consist of the school principal, school psychologist, and a special education teacher. It may also include a general education teacher, speech and language specialist, school nurse, occupational therapist, or other support personnel as determined by the child's needs.

A special services team may choose one of two paths following an initial referral: (1) develop and implement adaptive instruction in the general education classroom, or (2) conduct formal assessment for special education services. The purpose of adaptive instruction is to provide additional support services to children who are at risk of educational failure in an attempt to meet their needs and prevent an inappropriate labeling of the student for special education. In the process of developing an adaptive program, parents are notified that the child is having difficulty and are asked to meet with the school's child-study team. The team and the parents discuss the student's needs and make recommendations for instructional adaptions within the general education classroom. Instructional adaptations vary depending on individual need, but most often involve modifying a curriculum, changing the seating arrangement, changing the length and difficulty of homework or classroom assignments, using peer tutors or volunteer parents to assist with instructional programs, or implementing a behavior management program (see Figure 8.1 on page 190). The general education teacher implements the necessary adaptions and documents student progress over a predetermined period of time. If the modifications are successful, the referral for special education is terminated. The teacher has successfully implemented alternative strategies that eliminate the need for special education. However, if the team determines that the child's educational progress is not satisfactory, the referral process for special education services continues.

Once the formal referral process is initiated, the child-study team (referred to in IDEA as the multidisciplinary team) reviews the information documented by the classroom teacher or other education professional describing the child's difficulties. Documentation may include results from achievement tests, classroom performance tests, samples of student work, behavioral observations, or anecdotal notes (such as teacher journal entries). The team decides whether any additional assessment information is needed in order to determine eligibility for special education. At this time, "a written notice must be provided to parents regarding their child's educational performance indicating that the school proposes to initiate or change the identification, evaluation, or educational placement of the child" (Federal Register, 1977, p. 42495). The content of the notice must include the following:

- a full explanation of the procedural safeguards available to the parents;
- a description of the action proposed or refused by the agency, why the agency proposes or refuses to take the action, and a description of any options the agency considered and the reasons why those options were rejected;

**FIGURE 8.1**   *Classroom Adaptations*

MATERIALS/CURRICULUM
_____ Individualize reading program
_____ Provide taped novels when possible
_____ Provide large print materials
_____ Read material to student when possible
_____ Modify vocabulary in written directions
_____ Modify curriculum in content area(s)
_____ Complete spelling activities in resource
_____ Modify the level of weekly spelling words
_____ Modify the number of weekly spelling words
_____ Individualize math program
_____ Permit use of multiplication chart
_____ Provide graph paper for math problems
_____ Provide reference chart-numbers
_____ Reduce number of math problems per page
_____ Provide raised line paper for writing
_____ Provide reference chart-letters
_____ Use hands on materials when possible
_____ Use audiovisual materials to supplement
_____ Use pictures/diagrams to demonstrate
_____ Other:

TEACHING TECHNIQUES/STYLES
_____ Provide one-on-one help when possible
_____ Provide adult tutor when possible
_____ Provide immediate feedback when possible
_____ Provide more repetition than expected
_____ Use multisensory approaches
_____ Emphasize visual in teaching reading
_____ Emphasize auditory in teaching reading
_____ Use language experience method
_____ Use sequential, step-by-step approach
_____ Teach use of mnemonic devices
_____ Use cooperative learning situations
_____ Use partner writing
_____ Provide way for student to express needs
_____ Other:

CLASSROOM ENVIRONMENT
_____ Provide predictable routine
_____ Special seating to reduce distractions
_____ Special seating due to poor vision
_____ Provide isolated work space
_____ Other:

TESTS
_____ Read tests orally to student
_____ Change format of tests
_____ Permit open book tests
_____ Longer time to complete tests
_____ Permit oral or taped responses
_____ Reduce number of items
_____ Require fewer correct responses

STUDY/WORK AIDS
_____ Use colored overlays when reading
_____ Provide paper with lines for assignments
_____ Permit student to print or type assignments
_____ Help student organize materials
_____ Provide assignment notebook
_____ Provide peer tutor to help study
_____ Provide study skills assistance
_____ Highlight key words/directions on worksheets
_____ Show student how to highlight content materials
_____ Provide study guides
_____ Provide visual cues for margins/boundaries
_____ Permit student to make oral reports
_____ Break assignments into small segments
_____ Other:

EQUIPMENT
_____ Provide calculator
_____ Provide computer when possible for assignments
_____ Provide tape recorder
_____ Uses a hearing aid
_____ Needs adaptive P.E. equipment
_____ Other:

STANDARDS/EXPECTATIONS
_____ Provide extra time to complete assignments
_____ Adjust length of assignments
_____ Base grade on number of problems completed
_____ Cut pages in half
_____ Specify level of success expected
_____ Specify time expectations
_____ Specify how to get help
_____ Provide extra instruction
_____ Have student restate/repeat directions
_____ Clearly state contingencies for incomplete work
_____ Work in small heterogeneous groups
_____ Work in small homogeneous groups
_____ Increased level of parent contacts
_____ Consider medical factors such as A.D.D.
_____ Remind student frequently to stay on task
_____ Consider disabilities when grading
_____ Other:

BEHAVIOR
_____ Needs behavior management plan

[1]Special thanks to Char Bailey, Pearl Creek Elementary School, Fairbanks Northstar Borough School District, who developed the original list of instructional modifications from which this figure is drawn.

- a description of each evaluation procedure, test, record, or report the agency used as a basis for the proposal or refusal; and

- a description of any other factors which are relevant to the agency's proposal or refusal. (Federal Register, 1977, p. 42495)

Following a written notice the school must *seek* <u>*consent*</u> *in writing from the parents in order to move ahead with the evaluation process.* Informed consent means that parents:

- have been fully informed of all information relevant to the activity for which consent is sought, in their native language or other mode of communication;

- understands and agrees in writing to the carrying out of the activity for which their consent is sought, and the consent describes that activity and lists the record (if any) which will be released and to whom; and

- understands that the granting of consent is voluntary . . . and may be revoked at any time. (Federal Register, 1977, p. 42494)

***Assessment of Student Functioning Level and Eligibility.*** Once written consent has been obtained from parents, the multidisciplinary team may move ahead to assess the child's educational performance. The purpose of this assessment is to evaluate the overall functioning level of the child and determine whether the child meets eligibility requirements under one of the disability categories within the law. The assessment should include the child's performance in both school and home environments. Information regarding how the child functions at home may be collected through parent/family interviews or direct observation by an education professional. Sattler (1988) suggests that parent interviews include information on (a) concerns regarding the child's educational program, (b) perceptions of the child's strengths as well as problem areas, and (c) a family history.

Once the assessment process has been completed, a decision is made regarding the child's eligibility for special education. If the child is not eligible for special education, he or she remains in the general education setting and may receive additional help but not as a child with a disability. If the child is eligible, the next step in the process is to develop the IEP.

***Developing the IEP and Placing the Child in the Least Restrictive Environment.*** The multidisciplinary team, including the child's parents, analyzes the assessment information, describes student functioning, and develops annual goals and short-term objectives. The first step in the development of a student's IEP is to determine who are the appropriate education professionals to be involved in the process and appoint someone (such as the special education teacher, school psychologist, or school principal) as the team coordinator. Among other responsibilities, the team coordinator serves as liaison between the school and the family. As such, it is the coordinator's charge to (a) inform parents regarding the process of IEP development, (b) work directly with parents in ascertaining their concerns regarding the IEP process, (c) assist parents in developing specific goals they would like to see their child achieve, (d) schedule IEP meetings that are mutually convenient for both team members and parents, and (e) lead the IEP meetings (see Window 8.2).

Prior to conducting the IEP meeting, parents should be provided written copies of all assessment information on their child. Individual conferences with members of the multidisciplinary team or a full team meeting may be necessary prior to the development of the IEP in order to assist parents in understanding and interpreting assessment results. Analysis of the assessment information should include a summary of the child's strengths as well as areas in which the child may require specialized instruction beyond his or her current program.

Once there is mutual agreement between educators and parents on the interpretation of the assessment results and the child's specific disability area, the team coordinator should organize and lead the development of the student's IEP. The purpose of the IEP meeting is for the multidisciplinary team to (a) agree on the annual goals and objectives for the student, (b) determine necessary related services, if any, the student requires, (c) establish beginning and ending dates for special education services, and (d) decide the least restrictive environment in which the student should receive specialized instruction. The student's educational placement is determined only after educators and parents have agreed on annual goals and short-term objectives. The decision regarding placement rests on two factors. First, what is the most appropriate placement for the student given his or her annual goals? Second, which of the placement alternatives under consideration is consistent with the principle of the least restrictive environment? *The student is to be educated with nondisabled peers to the maximum extent appropriate.*

The IEP process is most successful when parents are viewed as valued and equal members of the multidisciplinary team. Educators should encourage parents to not only share their expectations for the child, but to express approval for or concerns about the goals and objectives that are being proposed by educators on the team. It is most important that the student's IEP is the result of a collaborative process that reflects the views of both the school and the family.

If parents and professionals cannot come to agreement on what constitutes an appropriate education for the child, there is a right of appeal. Parents have the right to make a formal complaint and seek a due process hearing as a means to resolve the disagreement. Parental appeal rights include access to legal counsel, the right to an independent evaluation of the child, and an opportunity to present

---

☆ **WINDOW 8.2**

---

## *Developing Ricardo's IEP: A Parent–Professional Partnership*

### *Before the IEP Meeting*

- Ms. Galleghos (Ricardo's mother) was invited by Jean Andreas (the school psychologist) to Ricardo's third-grade classroom to observe what was being taught and how he was doing both academically and socially.

- Ms. Galleghos was sent a written invitation to the IEP meeting, indicating time, location, and date the meeting would take place. She was also provided with the names and titles of everyone who would be participating. Ms. Galleghos's due process rights (written in Spanish as per her request) were attached to the note. The invitation was sent to Ms. Galleghos with ample notice to allow her time to make arrangements to attend. The professionals on the team, including Ricardos's third grade teacher (Ms. Thompson), were also given ample notice regarding the date and time for the meeting.

- One week prior to the meeting, Ms. Galleghos was called by Jean Andreas to see if she had any questions and to ensure her understanding of the meeting's purpose. During the call, Ms. Andreas assured Ms. Galleghos that the team welcomed her full participation in developing Ricardo's IEP. She listened carefully to issues and concerns raised by Ms. Galleghos relative to Ricardo's educational program. She wrote down Ms. Galleghos's comments so they could be further discussed by all the team members during the meeting. Ms. Galleghos was also encouraged to write down her goals, suggestions, and concerns and bring them to the meeting.

- Documentation (work samples, charting, assessments, notations on classroom observations, grades) of student progress was collected and organized so that it could be reported on during the meeting.

### *During the IEP Meeting*

- Ms. Andreas introduced all participants and explained the reason for the meeting and suggested that she serve as a facilitator to help keep the discussion focused. In addition to Ms. Andreas (who served as team leader and school district representative), the meeting participants included Ms. Galleghos, Mr. Lomas (special education teacher in learning disabilities), and Ms. Thompson.

- Mr. Lomas and Ms. Andreas reviewed the team's evaluation of Ricardo's academic performance. Ms. Thompson discussed what strategies had worked with Ricardo in her classroom, as well as the approaches that seemed to be less productive.

- Ms. Galleghos was asked to talk about Ricardo's life outside of school. She discussed what she saw as his major strengths, his role within the family, personal interests, and so on.

- Ms. Andreas led the discussion on Ricardo's general areas of need as identified in the evaluation and by his mother. Possible strategies to assist Ricardo with his reading and language were suggested by various team members.

*continued*

★ **WINDOW 8.2** *(continued)*

- The parent/professional team addressed what would be realistic goals for Ricardo during the year that would build on his strengths and help him develop his reading and language skills more effectively. Possible curriculum modifications, adaptations, and accommodations were discussed. Specific goals and objectives were written down and the team identified ways to evaluate progress in a meaningful way.

- The team agreed on Ricardo's annual goals, short-term objectives, methods, materials, and procedures to be used, the personnel responsible, and time lines for implementing the IEP.

- Finally, the team addressed the issue of what constituted the least restrictive environment to implement Ricardo's IEP. The team agreed that Ricardo should only be removed from the general education classroom for times when such a placement could not meet his needs. It was agreed that based on the IEP, it would be most appropriate for Ricardo to spend the majority of his day in the general education classroom, with Mr. Lomas consulting directly with Ms. Thompson on the necessary specialized instruction in the areas of reading and language. Mr. Lomas would work directly with Ricardo for two hours a day providing further instruction and support in the identified instructional content areas.

- At the close of the meeting, Ms. Andreas checked directly with Ms. Galleghos and other team members to find out if there were any further issues or questions. Ms. Galleghos was interested in parent organizations in the area of learning disabilities. She was referred to a local learning disabilities organization.

- Ms. Galleghos was provided a copy of Ricardo's IEP, and was invited to visit and/or volunteer in Ricardo's classroom at her convenience.

*Follow-Up on the IEP Meeting*

- In order to be responsive to parent concerns, Ms. Galleghos was contacted at least weekly to review Ricardo's progress with Mr. Lomas and Ms. Thompson. The discussion included suggested home activities that could reinforce the learning taking place in school.

- Periodic face-to-face meetings with Mr. Lomas and Ms. Thompson were set up to provide the opportunity for a more in-depth analysis of progress.

witnesses and written evidence. In many states, there is an initial attempt to resolve disputes between parents and school districts through a process known as mediation. Mediation involves a third-party arbitrator who works with both parents and educators to reach a mutually agreeable solution. If a compromise is not possible, parents may then move forward with their formal complaint, which may be taken beyond the district and into civil court if necessary.

## *Differing Perspectives on Parent Involvement in the IEP Process*

⊞   **FOCUS 4**

*Identify possible barriers to active parental participation in the IEP process.*

The IEP process is the bedrock of parent involvement in the education of students with disabilities. Although the legal mandate to involve parents is clear, there is great variability in actual practice. The Robert Wood Johnson Foundation conducted a longitudinal study of children with disabilities in five large metropolitan school districts (*Serving Handicapped Children*, 1988). The researchers found that although parents were generally satisfied with special education services, many were not attending IEP meetings. In fact, less than half of the parents surveyed had ever attended their child's IEP meeting. This research corroborated an earlier study by Goldstein and colleagues (1980).

A report from the National Council on Disability (NCD) (1995) also found mixed results relative to parental satisfaction and involvement in the IEP process. Again, although some parents indicated the process is effective and they are engaged as an active member in decision making, others expressed considerable concern regarding barriers to parental participation (see Point of Interest 8.1 on page 196).

Powell and Graham (1996) summarized some of these concerns:

> IDEA's provisions for a parent–professional partnership are far from a reality for many families. True parent–professional partnerships seem to be atypical. In too many cases schools remain impregnable, mysterious places into which parents are allowed to venture for prescribed activities and sometimes only because of existing federal and state mandates. In many schools parents are still viewed as uninvited guests whose participation is required, not welcomed. (p. 607)

The available evidence suggests several barriers to parent participation, including low parental attendance at IEP meetings, scheduling meetings at times that are inconvenient to parents, use of educational jargon, a lack of adequate skills and available information for parents, an overall devaluing of parent input into the decision-making process, inadequate preparation of professionals to work with families, and time constraints (NCD, 1995; Powell & Graham, 1996). In regard to time constraints, the NCD reported that it is very difficult to accomplish the various IEP tasks in the time available. Silverstein, Springer, and Russo (1988) found that the average IEP meeting lasts about one hour. For many parents there is the concern that they will not be able to process the amount of information presented and make the appropriate decisions within this limited time frame.

---

◆ **POINT OF INTEREST 8.1**

---

*Parent Perspectives on the IEP Process*

A KEY TO MICHAEL'S SUCCESS has been the teamwork of all the educational professionals involved in Michael's program. The IEP process has allowed us to carefully plan
and individually tailor Michael's educational goals and objectives.

*Susan Tachau, Philadelphia, PA*

In regard to the IEP process itself, I wish it stood for "Individual Encouragement to Parents." If we could change it, I would change it. In many ways this public law has become
our enemy. Educators are being consumed by accountability and the IEP process itself.
This process is not a true process at all sometimes until due process . . . the reason being
minimal parent involvement until it's too late. The IEP process is so labor intensive that
it actually drives us away from the child instead of closer to the child. It has become a
burden to our professionals. You may have five to eight professionals on a team and not
one of those really possesses a true trusting relationship with parents. Not one sees the
big picture of this child's life, because they are caught up in the accountability, they are
caught up in time, which also becomes their enemy.

*Kathy Davis, Des Moines, Iowa*

*Source:* National Council on Disability (1995, May 9). Improving the implementation of the Individuals with Disabilities Education Act: Making schools work for all of America's children. Washington, D.C.: Author. pp. 56–57.

---

The NCD report also suggested that the use of educational jargon and highly
technical language by various education professionals was a barrier to full participation at IEP meetings. Ysseldyke, Algozzine, and Mitchell (1982) reported that
parents only comprehend about 27 percent of the language used by professionals
in the IEP process. Language issues may become even more complex for parents
from ethnic minority backgrounds. Research suggests that appropriate oral and
written communication is critical to active involvement of minority parents in
the education of students with disabilities (Harry, 1992; Harry, Allen, & McLaughlin, 1995). Although federal law requires written communication to be in the parents' native language, this is often not the case. Harry reports that important
documents are sent home to parents in English, contain unfamiliar words, and
are presented to parents with little or no feedback regarding their understanding
of what has been written.

Although the law mandates that parents and educators share the responsibility of making decisions for the child's educational program, it does not define the
type and quality of parent participation. Beyond the legal requirements imposed
on schools for parent involvement in the education of students with disabilities,

there are some very compelling philosophical, conceptual, and practical reasons for developing strong home–school partnerships.

## BEYOND IDEA: BUILDING POSITIVE HOME–SCHOOL PARTNERSHIPS

### *Laying the Foundation*

> Parents take their child home after professionals complete their services and parents continue providing the care for the larger portion of the child's waking hours. . . . No matter how skilled professionals are, or how loving parents are, each cannot achieve alone what the two parties, working hand-in-hand, can accomplish together. (Peterson & Cooper, 1989, pp. 208, 229)

What we know about schools is that they are most successful when they establish positive relationships with the family (Hardman, Drew, & Egan, 1996; Newton & Tarrant, 1992). This is true for all children, but takes on even more meaning when we are addressing the challenges facing students with disabilities and their families. A fundamental component of a strong home–school relationship is a clear understanding of each other's philosophical and practical approaches to meeting the needs of the child with a disability. Without this understanding, it is not possible to develop the collaborative ethic necessary to establish a consistent and meaningful program for the child that promotes growth in both school and home environments.

Children are first and foremost members of a family unit. As they grow older, their learning experiences extend beyond the family into the school and finally into the vast environment we call community. As children mature, they are nurtured across a variety of environments in which one context (home, school, or community) influences and interrelates with the others. For example, an infant and toddler's early experiences at home, or in preschool, play a significant role in how prepared a child is for learning and interacting in the academic and social environment of kindergarten and beyond.

The significant role played by parents during the early intervention and preschool years must continue and be supported as the child with a disability moves on to elementary school. Although parents are often described as the child's first teacher and mentor during the early years of life, this does not mean that their role diminishes as the child moves on to formal schooling. The reality is that during the school years the majority of the child's waking hours are spent under the supervision and with the interaction of the family. Thus the family must be viewed as a critical partner in the education of the child with a disability.

*Components of a Home–School Partnership*

**⊕     FOCUS 5**

*What are the two components of an effective home–school partnership?*

A home–school partnership is a critical building block in providing an appropriate and successful educational experience for the elementary school-age child with disabilities. Fostering this partnership is a challenge that goes far beyond giving lip service to the importance of parent involvement. There are two basic components to establishing and maintaining an effective home–school partnership. First, both professionals and parents must strive to understand and respect each other's needs, differences, and constraints. Second, communication between school and home must occur often, and in an atmosphere of openness and mutual trust (see Chapter 6).

Although educators spend a significant amount of time discussing the importance of educating students with and without disabilities side by side to the maximum extent appropriate, they often do not give equal time to the value of parents and educators working together in a similar fashion. In a survey on home–school communication, Epstein (1986) reported that more than nine out of every ten teachers say they have direct communication with parents on an ongoing basis. Yet, one out of every three parents reports they had no conference with their child's teacher during the year; two out of three never talk to the teacher over the telephone.

By getting to know the family and taking the time to learn about their attitudes and beliefs, the school sends a message of respect. Collaboration is most successful when parents and educators:

- acknowledge and respect each other's differences in values and culture
- listen openly and attentively to the other's concerns
- value varying opinions and ideas
- discuss issues openly and in an atmosphere of trust
- share in the responsibility and consequences for making a decision.

There are many ways that educators can communicate how much they value parent involvement long before the special education referral process even begins. These strategies range from a more personalized approach to the individual needs of the child and family to more general forms of communication that attempt to involve parents in the activities of the school.

### Benefits of a Home–School Partnership

⊞ **FOCUS 6**

*Discuss the ways in which all members of the educational team benefit from parent participation in the child's educational program.*

All members of the school team, including the child, parents, educators, and other involved professionals, may benefit significantly from a home–school alliance. *Children* benefit because their learning can be taught and applied across both school and home environments. As communication between parents and educators increases, student progress can be more readily evaluated and reinforced. Additionally, opportunities to solve difficult learning or social problems often occur early enough in the situation that a positive solution may be possible. As participating members of the collaborative team, *parents* acquire the attitudes and skills necessary to work effectively with their child in areas such as communication, behavior, and academics. Parents feel valued as equal members of the team, and in turn a positive attitude toward the school is developed and fostered. *Educators* also profit from working closely with parents. Through interacting with parents, teachers gain access to critical information about the needs and functioning level of the child beyond the school setting and into the broader context of home and community. The school's sensitivity to family values and daily stress is dramatically increased, allowing the school to genuinely address the needs of each student with a disability (Dettmer, Thurston, & Dyck, 1993; see Point of Interest 8.2).

---

◆ **POINT OF INTEREST 8.2**

## Ten Reasons Why Schools Should Have a Collaborative Partnership with Families

1. Recognizes that the child is a member of a home and a school community. Each influences the other.
2. Enables family and school to work together toward a common outcome.
3. Increases opportunities for students to succeed.
4. Includes the parents, who play a primary role in the child's development throughout the school years and have an important influence on the child's learning.
5. Creates a positive relationship between home and school.
6. Helps teachers learn more about the family, which increases effectiveness with the student.
7. Addresses concerns about the student as they arise.
8. Allows for mutual problem solving.
9. Encourages collaborative decision making.
10. Fosters shared responsibility for implementation of school program and home activities.

## Moving from Involvement to Collaboration

**✛   FOCUS 7**

*Distinguish between involvement and collaboration in the educational process.*

*Involving* parents in their child's education does not mean they have become a *collaborative* member of the child's educational team. In order to understand how parents become active participants in shared educational decision making, we must distinguish between the terms involvement and collaboration. *Involvement* can be described as a "one-way communication process" in which the school imparts information to parents in much the same manner that parents give information to their child when they are using a didactic approach to teaching (Dettmer et al., 1993). As such, parent involvement may be passive in that information flows one way: school to home. Parent concerns and interests may not be heard or addressed. Thus decisions regarding the child's education are solely in the hands of education professionals. Parent *involvement* activities may include student progress conferences; parent information and training meetings; school or class newsletters; parent support in the classroom: follow-up on homework assignments, tutoring students, or preparing materials. In each of these activities the school is offering a system of one-way communication that is missing a key ingredient for a successful partnership: mutual problem solving and shared decision making (Dettmer et al., 1993).

   *Collaboration*, in contrast, suggests a two-way communication process in which there is an established partnership between the home and school and decisions are made jointly. The process involves two or more parties who share information, consider each other's input in the problem-solving process, and reach a joint resolution. Implied within the collaborative ethic is that a mutual respect exists between the two parties and each views the other as a competent member of the team (Dettmer et al., 1993). Table 8.1 describes some of the many characteristics of successful home–school partnerships.

## Communication Strategies

**✛   FOCUS 8**

*Identify three forms of communication commonly used by schools.*

The specific strategies used by educators to communicate with parents positively correlates with how successful they are in establishing the bond between home and school. Essentially schools use three forms of communication: (1) in-person contact, (2) phone calls, and (3) written information. Every form of communication is important, and each serves a different purpose.

**TABLE 8.1**    *Components of Effective Home–School Partnerships*

*Successful programs*

1. Are designed with the expectation that parents will be collaborators.
2. Tailor activities to meet the needs of the particular parents involved.
3. Include a variety of types of parental involvement.
4. Utilize creative and flexible program activities.
5. Communicate expectations, roles, and responsibilities.
6. Consider staff skills and available resources.
7. Recognize variations in parents' skills.
8. Are characterized by a balance of power so that parents are involved in decision making and administrative decisions are explained.
9. Provide increased opportunities for interaction.
10. Expect problems but emphasize solutions.
11. Empower parents and school personnel.
12. Are minimally intrusive.
13. Are clear and specific.
14. Are designed with obtainable goals and objectives.
15. Have an acceptable cost-return ratio.
16. Assess parents' and school personnel's perceptions of the program.

*Source:* Welch & Sheridan (1995).

***In-Person Contact.*** Face-to-face communication between educators and parents can occur in a variety of situations, including regularly scheduled parent–teacher conferences (group or individual), informal school meetings, home visits, or parent information/training seminars. Regardless of the situation, the general rule is the more direct the contact, the greater the impact. However, some in-person contact (such as regularly scheduled parent–teacher conferences) may be perfunctory rituals that are viewed as necessary evils occurring once or twice per year (Epstein, 1986). Unfortunately, in many schools the *group* parent–teacher conference may be the primary or only form of direct communication between home and school. Group conferences are the traditional "back-to-school" nights or schoolwide meetings in which parents may have no more than five minutes with an individual teacher. Welch and Sheridan (1995) suggest that these conferences are primarily used to "discuss with groups of parents the programs, policies and issues of importance to large numbers of parents and students" (p. 334). Whereas the group conference is more general in scope, the *individual* conference is a more personalized school meeting that is "child and family-centered." These meetings are usually held to give teachers a chance to let parents know how well the child is doing in school and/or deal with specific areas of academic or social concern. They may be set up by appointment or handled on a drop-in basis if the parents arrive unannounced either before or after school.

Another form of in-person contact is the home visit. Home visits may occur for several reasons. Parents may lack transportation or are unable (perhaps unwilling) to come to the school. One positive aspect of home visits is that they communicate the professional's willingness to meet in surroundings that are comfortable and familiar to parents. Home visits also give the professional the opportunity to interact within the family culture and to observe the child in a natural setting. Prior to setting up a home visit, professionals must take the time to ensure that the parents are comfortable in opening up their home and do not see the visit as an unwanted intrusion into their private lives.

Parent information/training seminars are also an important form of in-person contact (see Point of Interest 8.3). Parents approach the school setting with varying levels of information, experience, and degrees of comfort in working with school personnel. It is the school's responsibility to identify the parents' knowledge base and individual needs/preferences as a basis for providing useful infor-

---

♦ **POINT OF INTEREST 8.3**

*Parent Training and Information Centers (PTICs)*

IN 1983, THE U.S. CONGRESS AUTHORIZED a national program to provide information and training to parents of students with disabilities to assist them in the following:

- better understanding the nature and needs of their children's disabling condition
- locating follow-up support for their child's special education program
- communicating more effectively with special and general educators, administrators, related services personnel, and other relevant professionals
- participating fully in educational decision making, including the development of their child's IEP
- obtaining information about the range of options, programs, services, and resources available at the national, state, and local levels for students with disabilities and their families
- understanding the provisions of the Individuals with Disabilities Education Act.

Administered through the U.S. Department of Education, PTICs are parent directed and now located in every state. Congress recently authorized new centers to serve parents of minority children with disabilities. For information on parent training and information in any given state, contact the state PTIC, the state Office of Education, or the U.S. Department of Education (Office of Special Education Programs).

mation and training as necessary. Parent training seminars may include information on community resources for families, general topics such as the benefits of parents and teachers working in collaboration, or special topics related to identified parent needs such as behavior management programs in the home.

***Phone Calls.*** Although not as direct or effective as in-person contact, a phone call can be an efficient way to (a) give and receive information quickly, (b) follow up after face-to-face conferences, (c) provide parents with regular (such as weekly or monthly) reports on student progress, or (d) deal with an immediate crisis. A primary advantage to a phone call is that it does not require travel. Parents can communicate with teachers in the comfort of their home or at work; teachers can make a phone call that is convenient to their busy daily schedule or choose to talk with a parent during the evening or weekend. A disadvantage of a phone call is that the communication is limited to auditory input. Nonverbal communication, such as body language or gesturing, cannot be taken into account during the interaction.

***Written Information.*** The least personal of the three forms of communication is written information. As is true with in-person contact, written information can be both general in nature or specific to the individual child. Examples of general written information include class newsletters or flyers that highlight upcoming school or class events. Written information that focuses on an individual child includes (a) progress reports (ranging from daily school–home notes to term report cards), (b) daily interactive journals between parents and teachers, or (c) notification of a forthcoming parent–teacher conference. Written information shared between school and home is both time efficient and cost effective. Ongoing two-way communication can be established without the difficulties inherent in attempting to set up formal meetings or catch someone with a phone call. For example, in the case of brief daily progress reports (also known as school–home notes), there is little investment of teacher time with a good potential for positive return. Welch and Sheridan (1995) suggest school–home notes can take many forms, including "a brief half-page document on which teachers can tally occurrences of target behaviors (such as work completed or on-task behaviors) or lengthier, open-ended forms on which teachers and parents can write comments to each other" (p. 332) (see Figure 8.2 on page 204).

The drawbacks to written information are obvious. It is not helpful when dealing with an immediate crisis or with issues that require in-person contact and a team effort. Additionally, given that the child may be the emissary of written information, there has to be some system to ensure that school–home notes reach their intended destination. This problem can be resolved if both the school and home can access e-mail on their respective computers.

**FIGURE 8.2**    *Daily School–Home Note*

*Weekly School–Home Note*

*week of* _____

_____ follows rules

_____ helpful to classmates and teacher

_____ knows sight words

_____ understands math for the week

_____ comprehending new reading material

_____ finishes assignments on time

Comments:

Parent Signature: _____.

*Source:* Sue McIntosh, Fairbanks North Star Borough School District, Badger Road Elementary School, first grade.

### Encouraging Parents to Participate in School Governance and Volunteer Activities

**⊞   FOCUS 9**

*What strategies can be used to increase parent participation in school governance and volunteer activities?*

Many parents of children with disabilities may feel disenfranchised from the school because their child is identified as different. They perceive themselves labeled in the same way as their child. As such, schools have to make an extra effort to encourage and support parents of students with disabilities to participate in school decision making. A typical approach, such as sending home written information encouraging involvement in school governance, may not be effective. One strategy to encourage participation involves the teacher or school principal taking the time to make an in-person contact with parents of students with disabilities as a means of personally seeking their participation in the school planning council or parent–teacher association.

A variety of volunteer opportunities can be made available to parents or other family members. Volunteer opportunities run the gamut from assisting with out-of-school activities (such as field trips, sporting events, back-to-school nights) to working in the computer lab or serving as an in-class tutor.

Regarding out-of-school activities, a personal contact may once again be necessary to let parents know the school values and encourages their child's participation in clubs, sports, or other extracurricular activities. As the child feels more welcome and comfortable in these activities, the parents may also be more willing to help out.

A stronger commitment is required from parents who are willing to volunteer as computer lab/library assistants or tutors in the classroom. Parents may have to commit as little aş an hour each day or as much as twenty hours a week to serve as an in-class volunteer. It is important for parents to meet their volunteer commitment consistently because the school is relying on them to work directly with children in a class or lab setting. The school must also commit to providing parents with adequate training and support so their tutoring responsibilities can be carried out successfully. Despite the fact that in-class volunteering requires considerable time and effort, it can have some significant benefits for both parents and teachers. Parents feel valued and are more connected to the life of the school. As volunteers, they learn about the nature and scope of instruction programs, how the school functions, and the daily pressures faced by teachers. Teachers benefit through the development of a sustained and collaborative relationship with parents that creates a closer bond between home and school. Teachers also profit from the additional expertise and assistance that parent volunteering brings to their classroom.

## Some Final Thoughts on the Role of Parents in the Learning Process

 **FOCUS 10**

*Distinguish between parents in the role of trainers versus parents in the role of facilitators of child-initiated learning.*

Parental roles in a child's learning are often viewed from two somewhat different perspectives: (1) the parent as a trainer imparting information to the child (the didactic model), or (2) the parent in the role of a facilitator for learning as the child interacts in the natural setting of the family (the environmental model). In the didactic model, parents become trainers, and the child is the recipient of the parent's knowledge and skills. The effectiveness of parents as trainers has been called into question by some professionals because (a) the model is disruptive to the typical everyday functioning of the family unit, and (b) intervention techniques are not used appropriately or consistently over time (Rainforth, York, & Macdonald, 1992). Additionally, many parents are not willing to be trainers because of the inordinate demands of being both a parent and a teacher (Bailey & Wolery, 1992; Benson & Turnbull, 1986; McDonnell et al., 1995).

In contrast to the didactic approach, an environmentally based model promotes child-initiated learning within the context of "typical family interactions." The model creates an opportunity for parents to facilitate learning by assisting the child as specific skills are developed and applied in the home. The environmental model removes the parent from the role of trainer in order to capitalize on activities that are interesting to the child, thus increasing a motivation to learn (Rainforth et al., 1992). Although the positive aspects of the environmental model are in its orientation to child-initiated learning, there may be times when parent-directed instruction is necessary in order for the child to develop skills in an efficient and effective manner (such as learning to tie one's shoe, solving difficult math or reading homework assignments, or using public transportation). The reality is that *both* parent roles may be necessary depending on family dynamics and the needs of the child. How each of these roles is played out during the elementary school years often depends on the nature of the relationship between the parents and educators.

## REVIEW

*FOCUS 1: Identify the four major requirements of the Individuals with Disabilities Education Act.*

- Nondiscriminatory and multidisciplinary assessment of educational needs.
- An individualized education program (IEP).
- Education in the least restrictive environment (LRE).
- Parent involvement in the education of their child with disabilities.

*FOCUS 2: Identify the ways that parents of children with disabilities are required by law to be directly involved in the planning and evaluation of their child's educational program.*

- Consent in writing before the child is initially evaluated.
- Consent in writing before the child is initially placed in a special education program.
- Request an independent education evaluation if they feel the school's evaluation is inappropriate.
- Request an evaluation at public expense if a due process hearing finds that the public agency's evaluation was inappropriate.
- Inspect and review educational records and challenge information believed to be inaccurate, misleading, or in violation of the privacy or other rights of the child.

- Request a copy of information from the child's educational record.
- Request a meeting with the multidisciplinary team at any time to review their child's progress and/or appropriateness of the goals and objectives.
- Request a hearing concerning the school's proposal or refusal to initiate or change the identification, evaluation, or placement of the child or the provision of a free, appropriate public education.
- Participate on the individualized education program (IEP) committee that considers the evaluation, placement, and programming of the child.

*FOCUS 3: Identify each of the phases leading to a completed IEP. What are the roles of parents in each phase?*

- Referral for special education services: Parents are notified their child is having difficulty and are asked to meet with the school's child-study team. Parents and team members discuss possible instructional adaptations as part of the prereferral process. If instructional adaptions are inadequate, a formal referral is initiated. At this time a written notice must be provided to parents regarding their child's educational performance indicating that the school proposes to initiate or change the identification, evaluation, or educational placement of the child. Following the written notice, parents must consent in writing in order for the school to continue with the evaluation process.
- Assessment of the student's educational need and eligibility: The assessment should include the child's performance in both school and home environments.
- Development of the IEP concluding with placement in the least restrictive environment: The parents and the school team analyze the assessment information, describe student functioning, and develop annual goals and short-term objectives. The team coordinator is charged to work directly with, and assist, parents as a means to facilitate their participation in the IEP process. The team members, including the parents, must also agree on what constitutes the least restrictive environment for the child given his or her annual goals.

*FOCUS 4: Identify possible barriers to active parental participation in the IEP process.*

- Low parental attendance at IEP meetings.
- Scheduling meetings at inconvenient times for parents.
- Professionals' use of educational jargon.
- Devaluing of parent input.

- Lack of adequate skills and available information for parents.
- Inadequate preparation of professionals to work with parents.
- Lack of time.

*FOCUS 5: What are the two components of an effective home–school partnership?*

- Professionals and parents must strive to understand and respect each other's needs, differences, and constraints.
- Communication between school and home must occur often and in an atmosphere of openness and mutual trust.

*FOCUS 6: Discuss the ways in which all members of the educational team benefit from parent participation in the child's educational program.*

- *Children* benefit because their learning can be taught and applied across both school and home environments. Student progress can be more readily evaluated and reinforced. Additionally, opportunities to solve difficult learning or social problems often occur early enough in the situation that a positive solution may be possible.
- *Parents* acquire the attitudes and skills necessary to work effectively with their child in areas such as communication, behavior, and academics. Parents feel valued as equal members of the team, and in turn a positive attitude toward the school is developed and fostered.
- *Educators* gain access to critical information about the needs and functioning level of the child beyond the school setting and into the broader context of home and community. The school's sensitivity to family values and daily stress is dramatically increased, allowing the school to genuinely address the needs of each student with a disability.

*FOCUS 7: Distinguish between involvement and collaboration in the educational process.*

- *Involvement* is a "one-way communication process" in which the school imparts information to parents. Parent concerns and interests may not be heard or addressed.
- *Collaboration* suggests a two-way communication process, an established partnership between the home and school in which decisions are made jointly. The process involves two or more parties who share information, consider each other's input in the problem-solving process, and reach a joint resolution.

*FOCUS 8: Identify three forms of communication commonly used by schools.*

- In-person contact involves regularly scheduled parent–teacher conferences, informal school meetings, home visits, or parent information/training seminars. Parent–teacher conferences may be in a group or with individual parents. Group conferences include "back-to-school" nights or schoolwide meetings. The *individual* conference or more *informal* school meeting is "child and family-centered." These meetings are usually held to reinforce an individual child's progress or deal with specific areas of academic or social concern. Home visits may be necessary when parents lack transportation or are unable (perhaps unwilling) to come to the school. Parent training seminars may include information on community resources for families, general topics such as the benefits of parents and teachers working in collaboration, or special topics related to identified parent needs.

- Phone calls may be an efficient way to (1) give and receive information quickly, (2) follow up after face-to-face conferences, (3) provide parents with regular (such as weekly or monthly) reports on student progress, or (4) deal with an immediate crisis.

- Written information includes class newsletters or flyers that highlight upcoming school or class events. Written information that focuses on an individual child includes (1) progress reports (ranging from daily school–home notes to term report cards), (2) daily interactive journals between parents and teachers, or (3) notification of a forthcoming parent–teacher conference.

*FOCUS 9: What strategies can be used to increase parent participation in school governance and volunteer activities?*

- Encourage participation by having the school principal or classroom teacher take the time to make an in-person contact with parents of students with disabilities as a means of personally seeking their involvement in the school planning council or parent–teacher association.

- A personal contact may also be necessary to let parents know the school values and encourages their child's participation in clubs, sports, or other extracurricular activities. For volunteer activities, the school must commit to providing parents adequate training and support so their tutoring responsibilities can be carried out in an informed manner.

*FOCUS 10: Distinguish between parents in the role of trainers versus parents in the role of facilitators of child-initiated learning*

- The parent as a trainer imparts information to the child, and the child is the recipient of parent knowledge and skills.

- In the role of facilitator, learning is child directed. The parent assists the child in developing and applying specific skills in the home.

## REFERENCES

Bailey, D. B., & Wolery, M. (1992). *Teaching infants and preschooler with disabilities* (2nd ed.). New York: Merrill.

Benson, H. A., & Turnbull, A. P. (1986). Approaching families from an individualized perspective. In R. H. Horner, L. H. Meyer, & H. D. Fredericks (Eds.), *Education of learners with severe handicaps: Exemplary service strategies* (pp. 127–157). Baltimore: Brookes.

Dettmer, P., Thurston, L. P., & Dyck, N. (1993). *Consultation, collaboration, and teamwork: For students with special needs* (pp. 323–326). Boston: Allyn & Bacon.

Epstein, J. L. (1986). Parents' reactions to teacher practices of parent involvement. *Elementary School Journal, 86,* 277–294.

Goldstein, S., Strickland, B., Turnbull, A. P., & Curry, L. (1980). An observational analysis of the IEP conference. *Exceptional Children, 46*(4), 278–286.

Hardman, M. L., Drew, C. J., & Egan, M. W. (1996). *Human exceptionality* (5th ed.). Boston: Allyn & Bacon.

Harry, B. (1992). *Cultural diversity, families, and the special education system: Communication and empowerment.* New York: Teachers College Press.

Harry, B., Allen, N., & McLaughlin, M. (1995). Communication versus compliance: African-American parents' involvement in special education. *Exceptional Children, 61*(4), 364–377.

McDonnell, J., Hardman, M., McDonnell, A. P., & Kiefer-O'Donnell, R. (1995). *Introduction to persons with severe disabilities.* Boston: Allyn & Bacon.

National Council on Disability. (1995, May 9). *Improving the implementation of the Individuals with Disabilities Education Act: Making schools work for all of America's children.* Washington, DC: Author.

Newton, C., & Tarrant, T. (1992). *Managing change in America's schools.* London: Routledge.

Peterson, N. L., & Cooper, C. S. (1989). Parent education and involvement in early intervention programs for handicapped children: A different perspective on parent needs and parent-professional relationships. In M. J. Fine (Ed.), *The second handbook on parent education* (pp. 197–234). New York: Academic.

Powell, T. H., & Graham, P. L. (1996). Parent-professional participation. In National Council on Disability, *Improving the implementation of the Individuals with Disabilities Education Act: Making schools work for all of America's children* (supplement) (pp. 603–633). Washington, DC: Author.

Rainforth, B., York, J., & Macdonald, C. (1992). *Collaborative teams for students with severe disabilities: Integrating therapy and educational services* (pp. 46–47). Baltimore: Brookes.

Sattler, J. M. (1988). *Assessment of children.* San Diego: Sattler.

*Serving handicapped children: A special report.* (1988). Princeton, NJ: The Robert Wood Johnson Foundation.

Silverstein, J., Springer, J., & Russo, N. (1988). Involving parents in the special education process. In S. L. Christensen & J. C. Conoley (Eds.), *Home-school collaboration: Enhancing children's academic and social competence.* Silver Spring, MD: National Association of School Psychologists.

U.S. Department of Education. (1995). *Seventeenth Annual Report to Congress on the Implementation of the Individuals with Disabilities Education Act.* Washington, DC: Author.

Welch, M., & Sheridan, S. M. (1995). *Educational partnerships: Serving students at risk.* Fort Worth: Harcourt Brace.

Ysseldyke, J. E., Algozzine, B., & Mitchell, J. (1982). Special education team decision making: An analysis of current practice. *Personnel and Guidance Journal, 60*(5), 308–313.

# Families and the Transition from School to Adult Life[1]

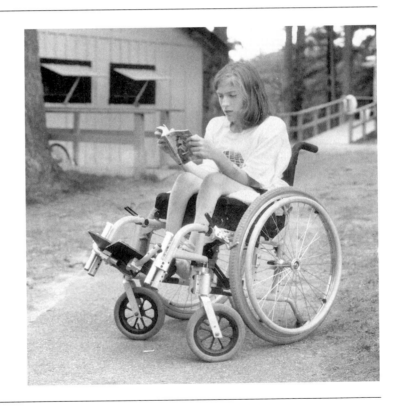

---

[1]This chapter was coauthored by Loxi Calmes, Department of Special Education, University of Utah.

★ WINDOW 9.1

## Lisa

O N A COOL SPRING MORNING IN MARCH, seven professionals from a variety of different backgrounds are gathered in a conference room at Eastridge High School with Lisa O'Neil and her parents. They are meeting to initiate plans for Lisa's transition from school into adult life. Lisa, labeled as emotionally disturbed throughout elementary school and junior high, is now 17 years old and within two years of exiting high school. Along with Lisa and her parents (Sarah and Gene O'Neil), this initial planning meeting includes the high school principal (Sally Monroe), a special education teacher with background in transition planning (Dennis Cochran), and the school psychologist (George Rivera).

Lisa, her parents, and Dennis Cochran have talked for about an hour prior to the meeting, reviewing Lisa's educational progress and outlining some of their thoughts about what lies ahead after school is over. After some greetings and formal introductions, Sally Monroe reviews the purpose and agenda for the meeting. In addition to developing Lisa's individual education program (IEP) and a formal transition plan, the team must also review evaluation data to determine whether she is still eligible for special education services next year.

To a large degree, today's meeting represents a celebration and encouragement for a young woman who has begun making a dramatic turnaround in her attitude and performance in school over the last seven months. After a very difficult freshman year of cutting classes, Lisa appears back on track toward graduation. With the support of her friends, family, and teachers, she is attending and passing most of her courses.

Following a somewhat lengthy and detailed report of the evaluation information to determine Lisa's continuing eligibility for special education, the team establishes that Lisa is eligible next year. During the report, Mr. and Mrs. O'Neil indicate both their agreement with the evaluation information as well as areas of concern regarding the results. They ask questions and provide additional information for clarification. With some prompting from Dennis Cochran and George Rivera, Lisa also answers questions from the team and shares some of the ways she is learning to be successful in school.

After an hour of outlining the testing information and Lisa's current level of performance, Sally Monroe focuses the team's attention on writing an IEP for Lisa that will include a transition planning component. Mr. and Mrs. O'Neil speak out indicating that Lisa has strong interest in becoming a fish and game warden. Lisa confirms the comments from her parents, reiterating that "she really likes the outdoors and would enjoy working in a national forest." The discussion then centers on the opportunities and support Lisa would need to achieve this goal. Sally Monroe emphasizes the need for Lisa to pass her academic classes successfully and receive her high school diploma. "Without a high school diploma, she may not be eligible to work for agencies such as the Forest Service or the State Fish and Game." The team develops goals and short-term objectives to support Lisa's effort to meet high school graduation requirements, along with who will be responsible for providing the necessary assistance and the time lines for completion.

*continued*

Attention is then directed to the supports necessary for Lisa to transition out of school successfully and into a job that is consistent with her preferences and ability. Lisa, her parents, and other team members identify various activities for Lisa that are to be completed over the next year, including learning organizational skills, opportunities for work experience in an outdoor setting that will involve job shadowing, and developing independent living skills. Each area of support is then written into Lisa's IEP as an annual transition goal with short-term objectives. The plan also includes opportunities for Lisa and her parents to receive training on how they can be actively involved in the process of transition planning during the next two years. Mr. Cochran informs Lisa and her parents that they will be receiving more information on the types of support that may be made available after Lisa exits school, including vocational rehabilitation, job service, and community mental health.

Once the goals, short-term objectives, responsible persons, and time lines are completed, the team discusses the need for other professionals to be involved in planning for Lisa's transition out of school. Sally Monroe suggests that the team be expanded to include a vocational rehabilitation counselor and someone from the local job services agency. Team members agree and Dennis Cochran is given the responsibility of contacting the appropriate individuals.

The meeting is concluded a full two hours after it began. Mr. Cochran lets Lisa and her parents know that they are welcome to contact him if they have any further suggestions, questions, or concerns regarding the individualized education program or formal transition plan. Copies of the paperwork are then given to Lisa and her parents. Mr. and Mrs. Neil return to their jobs, Lisa to class, and team members begin thinking about their next transition planning meeting.

In reflecting on the meeting, Lisa commented to Mr. Cochran that this was the first time one of these meetings meant anything to her. Lisa told Mr. Cochran that the meeting gave her an opportunity to hear how she was doing and what she needed to do if she was to graduate from high school and get a job. She was pleased that her parents were there because that way they'd know she was "telling the truth" about how school was going. Most of all, she liked hearing what the principal had to say, and enjoyed getting the chance to talk with her.

For Mr. and Mrs. O'Neil, the meeting was a way to become more informed about their daughter's educational experiences and to begin thinking about what life was going to be like when she was no longer in high school. Over the years, they had dreaded attending special education meetings because they were so negative. The teachers always complained about Lisa's "bad" attitude and lack of motivation. This meeting was different. For the first time, Mr. and Mrs. O'Neil felt that Lisa really had a chance to graduate and move on to some level of independence as an adult.

A DOLESCENCE IS A TIME OF CHANGE AND STRESS for both the teenager and the family. The very term *adolescence* may conjure up such images as "turbulent teens," "nightmare years," "storm and stress," and "generation gap." The challenges faced by adolescents making the transition to adult life are both numerous and complex. For Lisa in Window 9.1, her elementary school years and early adolescence were marked by a period of unrest and open rebellion. Described by her teachers as having a bad attitude and lacking motivation, she regularly cut classes at school. As she entered high school, Lisa was at serious risk of dropping out. At 17, with the support of friends, family, and school personnel, Lisa seems to be moving in a different direction toward adult life. Along with her family and school support personnel, Lisa is planning for the future. The time for transition planning is short, and within the next year or two Lisa must be able to (a) understand personal significance and build self-esteem; (b) establish philosophy and values; (c) make adjustments toward independence; (d) develop relationships with adults and authority figures; (e) cultivate relationships with peers and the opposite sex; and (f) engage in occupational roles (Hendry et al., 1993). For Lisa and other adolescents with disabilities, meeting these challenges can take on added significance as they try to weather the storm of adolescence, cope with the realities of a disability, and move on to adult responsibilities.

A strong alliance between the family and the school is an important element in a successful transition from adolescence into adult life. Successful transition necessitates that both formal (government-sponsored) and natural family supports are in place (McDonnell, Wilcox, & Hardman, 1991; Morningstar, Turnbull, & Turnbull, 1996; Szymanski, 1994). Historically, much of the emphasis has been on providing formal supports (such as health care, employment preparation, and supported living), and society is only beginning to realize the importance of the family and other natural support networks in preparing the adolescent with disabilities for adult life. Research (Hasazi et al., 1989; Morningstar, Turnbull, & Turnbull, 1996) suggests that the family unit may be the single most powerful force in preparing the adolescent with disabilities for the adult years.

In this chapter, we examine families and the transition years for individuals with disabilities from three perspectives: (1) understanding valued postschool outcomes; (2) defining transition; and (3) developing a student- and family-centered transition planning process.

## VALUED POSTSCHOOL OUTCOMES FOR PEOPLE WITH DISABILITIES

 For most of the twentieth century, social policy in the United States viewed the provision of services for people with disabilities as a privilege and not a right.  When services were made available, they were primarily oriented toward protecting and caring for the individual in isolation from the family and society. The prevailing view was that people with disabilities were "sick" and needed to be "quarantined" (institutionalized) in order to protect them from society. In turn, isolating people with disabilities would protect society as well.

Within the past thirty years, dramatic changes have occurred in U.S. social policy regarding programs and services for people with disabilities. The policy of social exclusion, which dominated human services for most of the twentieth century, has been replaced with one of inclusion for people with disabilities. This transformation has been described "as one of the great social reform movements of our time" (President's Committee, 1995, p. 8), and has resulted in a changing emphasis away from social isolation to (a) employment, useful work, and valued activity; (b) access to further education when desired and appropriate; (c) personal autonomy, independence, and adult status; (d) social interaction and community participation; and (e) participation within the life of the family.

Within the framework of social inclusion, the expectations for people with disabilities during the adult years are no different from those who are not disabled. However, the content of the preparation in school may differ depending on the needs and abilities of the individual (such as an academic vs. a functional life orientation). The outcomes remain the same. A common set of quality indicators during adult life may be applied to both disabled and nondisabled individuals. These indicators include being able to make choices, feeling valued, and participating in all aspects of community life.

---

### ⊕ FOCUS 1

*Identify three quality of life indicators that are common to most adults.*

---

### Quality of Life during the Adult Years

What constitutes a quality life during the adult years is personally driven. However, as suggested by Hardman, Rouse, and McDonnell (1994), there are some indicators that appear to be common for most adults.

*Everyone should be able to make their own choices about adult living, including selecting friends, where they will live, and what jobs they will hold.* Issues regarding choice may be characterized by three factors: controlling the environment, involvement in community life, and social relationships. The determination of quality can be addressed through questions like these:

- "Do you have a key to the house in which you live?" (controlling the environment)
- "Do you earn enough money to pay for your basic needs, including housing and food?" (involvement in the community)

- "Do you have the opportunity of interacting with family, friends and neighbors?" (social relationships)

*Each person is valued as an individual capable of personal growth and development. As such, everyone has the opportunity to participate in all aspects of community life.* Participation in community life includes (a) access to adequate housing, (b) opportunities to exercise citizenship (e.g., voting), (c) access to recreation and personal services (parks, theaters, grocery stores, restaurants, public transportation, etc.), and (d) access to medical and social services as needed.

*Each person has the opportunity to participate in the economic life of the community.* Work is important for reasons beyond monetary rewards, such as social interactions, personal identity, and economic contributions to the community. Work removes the individual from being viewed solely as a consumer of service. Hackman and Suttle (1977) suggest that the indicators of a quality work life include adequate and fair compensation, safe and healthy environments, development of human capacities, growth and security, social integration, constitutionalism (the rights of the worker and how these rights can be protected), the total life space (the balanced role of work in one's life), and social relevance (when organizations act in socially irresponsible ways, employees depreciate the value of their work and careers).

## TRANSITION PLANNING AND THE FAMILY

Transition planning is a complex and dynamic process involving students with disabilities, parents, school personnel, and other appropriate human service agencies in making choices about which experiences will best enhance the opportunity for the individual to achieve valued postschool outcomes. As described by Will (1984), transition planning is the bridge between school and adult life. Effective transition planning requires "a sound preparation program during high school, support for individuals as they finish school, and opportunities to access services when needed during the adult years" (Hardman, Drew, & Egan, 1996, p. 146).

### Public Policy Frameworks for Transition Services

⊞   **FOCUS 2**

*How does the Individuals with Disabilities Education Act (IDEA) define transition services?*

The legal requirement that students with disabilities are to receive transition services was initially enacted into federal law through the Individuals with Disabilities Education Act (IDEA). IDEA requires that every student with a disability receive transition services beginning no later than age 16, or younger when appropriate. The law defines these services as follows:

> a coordinated set of activities for a student, designed within an outcome-oriented process, which promotes movement from school to post-school activities, including post secondary education, vocational training, integrated employment (including supported employment), continuing and adult education, adult services, independent living, or community participation. The coordinated set of activities shall be based upon the individual student's needs, taking into account the student's preferences and interests, and shall include instruction, community experiences, the development of employment and other post-school adult living objectives, and, when appropriate, acquisition of daily living skills and functional vocational evaluation. (PL 101-476, 602[a][19])

The legislation's intent is to facilitate a successful transition to adult life for the student with disabilities and to continue providing formal support as appropriate during the adult years. To better facilitate a successful transition from school to the adult services system, federal regulations require representatives from public agencies to participate in meetings to develop, review, or revise the coordinated set of activities for transition within the IEP. Participants must include the student, parents, school personnel, and representatives of any other agencies that are likely to be responsible for providing or paying for transition services (34 C.F.R. § 300.344).

Vocational rehabilitation often plays an important role in facilitating transition from school to adult life. It provides services through counselors in several different areas (such as guidance and counseling, vocational evaluation, vocational training and job placement, transportation, family services, interpreter services, and telecommunication aids and devices). Strong linkages between educators and vocational rehabilitation counselors help facilitate access to postsecondary education and/or employment opportunities

Rehabilitation services are funded through the Rehabilitation Act of 1973, which was amended in 1992 to encourage stronger collaboration and outreach between the schools and rehabilitation counselors in transition planning. The Rehabilitation Act emphasizes that disability is a natural part of the human experience and in no way diminishes the right of individuals to (a) live independently; (b) enjoy self-determination; (c) make choices; (d) contribute to society; (e) pursue meaningful careers; and (f) enjoy full inclusion and integration in the economic, political, social, cultural, and educational mainstream of American society (Rehabilitation Act Amendments of 1992: Section 2: Findings, Purpose, Policy).

Another important piece of federal legislation that promotes social inclusion and plays a role in transition planning is the Americans with Disabilities Act of

1990 (ADA) (discussed in depth in Chapter 10). ADA prohibits discrimination against people with disabilities in public accommodations, transportation, tele-communication services, and employment. Employment is an area that is often directly targeted for training as a part of the student's transition plan. Under ADA, employment discrimination on the basis of an individual's current, prior, or perceived disability or an individual's known association or relationship to a person with a disability is prohibited. Further, the employer must provide "reasonable accommodations" to qualified employees to perform essential job functions as long as these accommodations don't impose "an undue hardship" on the employer.

## The Individualized Transition Plan (ITP)

### ⊞   FOCUS 3

*How does the individualized transition plan (ITP) relate to the individualized education program (IEP)? What is the purpose of the ITP?*

Under IDEA, transition services are delivered directly through the individual education program (IEP). The IEP must include the following:

> A statement of the needed transition services for students beginning no later than age 16 and annually thereafter (and, when determined appropriate for the individual, beginning at age 14 or younger), including when appropriate, a statement of the interagency responsibilities or linkages (or both) before the student leaves the school setting. (PL 101-476, 602[A], 20 U.S.C. 1401 [A])

The vehicle for identifying and delivering transition services for students with disabilities is the individualized transition plan (ITP). By definition, the ITP is a component of the IEP for students with disabilities during the secondary school years. Its purpose is to identify the needed transition services for the student based on projected postschool outcomes. For one student, the ITP may reflect services and supports necessary for access to postsecondary education; for another, the ITP may focus on employment, supported living, and recreation/leisure. The ITP for Lisa (see Window 9.1) focused on employment in outdoor recreation as the immediate goal following school. To accomplish this overriding goal, Lisa, her parents, and the school team decided on several objectives to be completed during the year in addition to the requirements for high school graduation. These objectives included the development of organizational and independent living skills, as well as work experience in an outdoor setting (see Figure 9.1, Lisa's ITP in the Area of Work Experience). As suggested by Smith and Luckasson (1995), "In most cases, the ITP supplements and complements the school-based IEP process. While the

**FIGURE 9.1**    *Lisa's ITP in the Area of Work Experience*

Student:  *Lisa O'Neil*                                 Meeting Date: 3/25/97

Place:  Eastridge High School                           Proposed Graduation Date: 6/99

Participants:
     Parents:                            *Sarah and Gene O'Neil*
     School Principal:                   *Sally Monroe*
     Special Education Teacher:   *Dennis Cochran*
     School Psychologist:              *George Rivera*

Planning Area:   Work Experience in Outdoor Recreation

*Transition Goal:*   Lisa will initiate a work experience program for a minimum of 10 hours per week through the local parks and recreation program, state fish and game department, and/or national forest service.

| Support Activities | Responsible Person | Time Line |
|---|---|---|
| Complete application to the appropriate agency for work experience program | Lisa O'Neil w/support from Dennis Cochran | 4/15/97 |
| Determine most appropriate work experience site along public transportation route | Team members | 5/15/97 |
| Contact vocational rehabilitation and local job service agency to identify personnel to be involved in transition plan | Dennis Cochran | 5/15/97 |
| Schedule work experience program into school schedule | Dennis Cochran George Rivera | 6/1/97 |
| Meet with director of selected agency to set up logistics for work experience program | Lisa O'Neil Mr. and Mrs. O'Neil Dennis Cochran | 9/15/97 |
| Handle logistics for public transportation to and from work experience site (e.g., insurance, backup, etc.); approve off-campus community-based program | Sally Monroe | 9/15/97 |
| Obtain public transit bus pass | Mr. and Mrs. O'Neil | 9/15/97 |
| Teach bus route to and from work experience site | Dennis Cochran | 10/1/97 |
| Develop objectives for Lisa based on work experience requirements on site | Team Members and identified agency supervisor | 10/1/97 |
| Begin work experience program | School: Dennis Cochran Training Site: Identified agency supervisor | 10/15/97 |
| Evaluate progress toward identified work experience objectives | Team members | ongoing |

IEP describes the educational goals and objectives that a student should achieve during a school year, the ITP addresses the skills and the supportive services required in the future" (p. 116).

In addition to the student with disabilities, parents, and school personnel, the ITP team may also involve professionals from adult services (such as vocational rehabilitation counselors, representatives from university/college centers for students with disabilities, the state developmental disability agency, etc.). The team may also include friends and extended family members who will become important elements of a student's natural support network following school.

Wehman (1996a) identifies seven basic steps in the formulation of a student's ITP: (1) Organize ITP teams for all transition-age students; (2) Organize a circle of support; (3) Identify key activities; (4) Hold initial ITP meetings as part of annual IEP meetings; (5) Implement the ITP through secondary school and adult service provision; (6) Update the ITP annually during the IEP meetings and implement quarterly follow-up procedure; and (7) Hold an exit meeting (see Table 9.1).

The ITP process facilitates a working relationship among the family, schools, and various agencies in the local community. Working together, the team identifies the services and supports that will facilitate the student moving toward valued postschool outcomes while still in school. It also establishes agreements among agencies to ensure services remain in place once the student exits school. Wehman (1996b) indicates that "formal interagency agreements at both the state and local levels are necessary in order for comprehensive planning and service implementation to occur" (p. 127). Furthermore, each agency must be knowledgeable about the purpose and capabilities of other participating agencies.

## STUDENT-CENTERED TRANSITION PLANNING

In order for schools and other human services agencies to prepare students with disabilities for active participation in the lives of their family and community, they must emphasize the skills that will facilitate access to these natural environments. However, research indicates that graduates exiting school have not been adequately prepared for postsecondary education or employment, and generally do not access resources and services that would enhance community participation (Bursuck & Rose, 1992; National Council on Disability, 1989; Peraino, 1992; Valdes, Williamson, & Wagner, 1990). In a survey of students with learning disabilities one year after exiting high school, Sitlington and Frank (1990) found that, although 50 percent of these students had enrolled in postsecondary programs, less than 7 percent were still in school. A Harris Poll (Harris & Associates, 1994) found that compared to students without disabilities, individuals with disabilities tend to experience less job satisfaction, social involvement, and gratification, as well as a tendency to live with family members rather than on their own. The poll also found that only 30 percent of adults with disabilities were working full or part time. Yet 79 percent of those not working, and of working age, indicated they would like to have a job.

Given that many of the valued postschool outcomes for students with disabilities are not being fully realized, parents and professionals are turning their attention to identifying which factors during the transition years have the greatest chance of enhancing postschool success. Although undoubtedly many com-

**TABLE 9.1**    *Basic Steps in the Formulation of an ITP*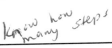

*Step One: Organize ITP teams for all transition-age students.*

- Identify all students who are transition age.
- Identify appropriate school service personnel.
- Identify adult services and agencies.

*Step Two: Organize a circle of support.*

- Meet with transition-age student and small circle of friends, family members, co-workers, neighbors, church members and staff to establish individual's needs and preferences for adult life.

*Step Three: Identify key activities.*

- Identify those items that are most important to the individual in the transition from school to adult years.

*Step Four: Hold initial ITP meetings as part of annual IEP meetings.*

- Schedule the ITP meeting.
- Conduct the ITP meeting.
- Develop the ITP.

*Step Five: Implement the ITP.*

- Operate according to guidelines defined in local interagency agreements.
- Use a transdisciplinary and cross-agency approach.

*Step Six: Update the ITP annually during the IEP meetings and implement follow-up procedures.*

- Phase out involvement of school personnel while increasing involvement of adult service personnel.
- Contact persons responsible for completion of ITP goals to monitor progress.

*Step Seven: Hold an exit meeting.*

- Ensure most appropriate employment outcome.
- Ensure most appropriate recreation outcome.
- Ensure most appropriate community living outcome.
- Ensure referrals to all appropriate adult agencies and support services.

*Source:* Adapted from *Life beyond the classroom: Transition strategies for young people with disabilities* by P. Wehman. Copyright © 1996 by Paul H. Brookes Publishing Co., P.O. Box 10624, Baltimore, MD 21285-0624.

plex elements contribute to an enhanced quality of life for people with disabilities, two specific factors appear to play a critical role: (1) the promotion of self-determination (personal choice) (McDonnell et al., 1991; Shulman, 1989; Wehmeyer, 1992a, 1992b), and (2) strong parent involvement in planning for the future (Morningstar, Turnbull, & Turnbull, 1996; Nisbet, Covert, & Schuh, 1992; Wehman, 1996a; Wehmeyer & Metzler, 1995).

## Promoting Self-Determination in Transition Planning

**⊕   FOCUS 4**

*What is self-determination?*

Professionals increasingly believe that teaching self-determination enables students with disabilities to become more efficient in knowledge acquisition and flexible in their ability to problem-solve (Ward, 1991). Yet self-determination, as a goal in transition planning, is a significant challenge for people with disabilities, their families, and professionals. Deci and Ryan (1985) define self-determination as

> the capacity to choose and to have those choices be the determinants of one's actions. However, it is more than a capacity . . . it is a need, an innate propensity to be self-determining that leads organisms to engage in interesting behaviors. When self-determined, one acts out of choice rather than obligation or coercion. . . . People who are self-determined operate from an autonomy-orientation in which they use information to make choices and to regulate themselves in pursuit of self-selected goals. (pp. 38–39)

Instruction in self-determination helps students achieve initial goals that maximize potential while making them aware of the specific barriers they will face. It is also the responsibility of the schools to provide the support necessary to overcome these barriers (Ward, 1991). Ultimately, the student comes away from school with a more well-developed sense of personal worth and social responsibility (Deci et al., 1991). Wehmeyer (1992a) suggests several ways that schools and parents can support the development of self-determination in students with disabilities:

1. Teach skills that promote self-regulation.
2. Emphasize psychosocial skills needed in the workplace.
3. Structure environments to ensure opportunities for students to make choices.
4. Organize instruction to promote self-determination.
5. Use teaching strategies that promote self-determination.

Building the capacity to support self-determination for students with disabilities will require schools to rethink their instructional approaches on two levels. First, students with disabilities must receive direct instruction on the skills necessary to be self-determined. Second, changes must be made in the current instructional paradigm away from professional-driven goals and objectives to an emphasis on personal choice and decision making.

### ⊕   FOCUS 5

*Identify factors critical to the development of self-determination.*

***Developing Skills for Personal Choice and Decision Making.***  As we move into the next century, creating opportunities for individual choice and decision making is a critical issue in the school to adult life transition of people with disabilities (Wehman, 1996a). Each individual must be able to consider options and make appropriate choices free from undue external influence or interference. The individual should act as the primary causal agent in his or her life (Deci & Ryan, 1985; Schloss, Alper, & Jayne, 1993; Wehmeyer, 1992a), which means less decision making from service providers and family members and more of a focus on teaching and promoting personal choice, self-determination, and self-advancement (Turnbull et al., 1989). This is not always so easy and straightforward, as evidenced by Christian's family from Window 9.2 (see pages 226–227). Christian's mother, although advocating strongly for his independence, often faced situations in which he made decisions that she did not agree with or saw as clearly dangerous. It took a great deal of inner strength for Christian's mother to come to a realization that although "not all his choices were safe, physically or emotionally," they were his choices.

Factors related to the development of self-determination include (a) optimal challenge, (b) autonomy, (c) competence, (d) involvement, (e) rationale, and (f) acknowledging feelings. Activities which optimally challenge students are those that are neither too easy nor too difficult (Deci & Chandler, 1986). Excessive repetition, overlearned tasks, or activities far beyond a student's achievement level decrease motivation. The issue of optimal challenge is particularly salient to the education of students with cognitive disabilities (such as mental retardation, autism, traumatic brain injury). These students often require repeated exposure to a task for skill acquisition. Providing optimal challenges to learners requires a degree of individualized instruction for all students, but is critical in the design of instruction for students with disabilities.

Home and school environments that allow for choice and encourage adolescent-initiated activities have a higher probability of promoting self-determination (Deci & Chandler, 1986). Development of opportunities to express preference, make choices, and experience the outcomes of these choices are characteristics of environments that support student autonomy. Unfortunately, many of the professional and parent-training programs in special education have not focused on developing

**✴ WINDOW 9.2**

## Standing Together: One Family's Lessons in Self-Determination

SELF-DETERMINATION IS NOT SYNONYMOUS WITH INDEPENDENCE. Rather, it is best facilitated by interdependence: connections and support from those around us. Our brain, our spirit, our emotions, our psyche, and our sexuality all function better in social interaction than in isolation. For my son, Christian, it has been this positive interaction that has allowed him to experience more choices and opportunities, leading to his determined spirit. These are some example that he would like shared with everyone:

- Christian stood up and lowered his eyes. He spoke clearly and was firm. "I will not take Speech and Language anymore. It's always the same thing and it's for babies. I will take a language class, but no more therapy!"

- It was the second week on a new job and Christian noticed that all the employees went to a meeting, but that he was not included. He said nothing, but brought home his anger. The next day he went to his supervisor and said, "I work here, too. Why can't I go to the meetings?"

- He woke at 5:30 every morning and caught the bus for school at 6:15, arriving home at 4:30. Of those 10 hours, half were spent on the bus. In addition to the frustrations of this demanding schedule, he had a new job "experience" across town starting at 1:00. The criteria for success established by his school was that his work had to approach 95% of the quantity and quality of a person without mental retardation. He failed . . . week after week. On the fifth week he announced, "I keep telling you, this is the best that I can do. If it isn't good enough, I'm not coming anymore."

I am always in awe of Christian's tenacity. I remember all the days and nights in hospitals, feeling helpless to free him from painful, restrictive treatments and procedures. I remember being unable to speak up when he was treated as if he were invisible by doctors and teachers, simply because he was a child . . . and "retarded." I remember the past 18 years of special education and IEPs and feeling incompetent and alone at the table at which professionals typically used acronyms and languages I didn't understand or agree with. The words "severe," "profound," "can't," "flat scale," and "inappropriate" will always send shivers up my spine. I remember when the neighbor kids started the name calling: "fag," "retard," and "cripple."

It was difficult for me to move past the pity and protection. However, my basic values dictated that I raise all of my four children in a home that valued their voices and encouraged discussions about their thoughts and feelings. Also, before I ever had children, I knew that the first priority to teach them was compassion. I didn't know anything about self-determination, but Christian was able to risk saying the wrong thing or making a mistake because he knew no matter what happened, home was a place where he was valued, accepted, and loved.

By the time Christian was seven, he was frustrated and angry about his disability. My first reaction was to protect him from experiences that would cause pain or frustration. I felt that was part of my job description as a parent. By the time he was 10, I knew I was not doing him a favor. I began to question if I was responding out of pity or love. I quit feeling sorry for Christian. We regularly discussed how he had to live with himself and

*continued*

★ **WINDOW 9.2** *(continued)*

learn to understand what seizures were and what mental retardation meant for him. At the same time the family, including his brother and sisters, supported and went to bat for him when attitudes and programs he experienced demeaned and devalued him.

Self-advocacy and self-determination begin with advocacy. Christian observed his dad, myself, and his siblings all standing up for his rights. Not only did that allow him to learn behaviors, but he knew he was worth the fight. For example, it was wrong for a teacher to set up a classroom reward system with criteria that never allowed success for Christian. When he displayed anger, he was called psychotic; we went through due process. It was also wrong for hospital staff to continue to insist on further sedative when they had already administered a high enough dose to put a 200-pound man out cold: we left AMA (Against Medical Advice).

As an advocate I could be in charge and direct the course of action and be the decision maker. The real challenge for me was when adolescence arrived. All the skills I'd hoped Christian would have, appeared. I was disjointed, fearful, confused, and struggled with his "noncompliant, inappropriate and aggressive" behaviors. Oops! The change meant I had to look at my values again in order to step back and support Christian in decisions I didn't always agree with and often thought were dangerous. I needed to believe that he would make decisions that would keep him safe physically and emotionally. In the beginning I also needed to believe that "the world" would view his contributions as important. I struggled with my perceptions of mental retardation being at the bottom of the disability list and the possibility that he would have no caring person in his adult life. Not all the choices that Christian has made have been safe, physically or emotionally, but they have been his choices.

For instance, Christian's first major purchase with his SSI money was a chain saw. In another instance, Christian, who cannot drive a car, bused around the city, found a 19-foot boat to purchase, and now is looking for a "friend" (paid or unpaid) to get the boat to water. Two days ago he was at the corner waving cars down and offering to pay $100 for a drive to a lake. He recently announced that there must not be any available women who could possibly like him so he was going to pay for that service also. I have learned to spend a great deal of time taking hot baths or putting invisible masking tape over my mouth.

Self-determination requires that a person have rich and abundant experiences. In order for growth in confidence and the ability to make choices, a person must have successful and unsuccessful experiences. Christian has used that chain saw and other power tools to help clear a wooded area and build a deck. He is currently enrolled in a technical college in the chef program, using meat cleavers and very sharp knives; a few supportive people in the decision-making role decided not to be afraid that he would have a seizure and get hurt. When he goes to the lake with the family, Christian drives that 19-foot boat and skillfully docks it because his dad and I decided that to risk paying for a dent in another boat was worth building Christian's confidence. Christian can say no to drugs, alcohol, and abuse because his siblings have included him in their typical teen parties and he's had the opportunity to say no.

Christian may still be vulnerable, and may still get frustrated by his mistakes and angry about attitudes that isolate him. But, he has a strong determination to know, understand, and like himself . . . and he knows that he is worth it.

*Source:* Reprinted with permission from "Standing Together: One Family's Lessons in Self-Determination," by Kris Schoeller. Published in *Impact: Feature Issue on Self-Determination*, Vol. 6(4), Winter 1993–1994, Institute on Community Integration, University of Minnesota, Minneapolis.

these opportunities (Wehmeyer, 1992b). For the most part, training has encouraged highly structured, tightly controlled classrooms and instruction. However, promoting self-determination should not be equated with removing all structure from a classroom environment. Parents and professionals must work together to promote self-determination without placing students in life-threatening situations.

Competence and involvement are considered basic human needs (Deci & Ryan, 1985, 1987, 1991). Competence involves understanding how to attain various outcomes and being efficacious in performing the required actions to achieve these outcomes. This notion is also referred to as self-efficacy—an individual having confidence in being able to perform a particular task (Bandura, 1977; Gillespie & Hillman, 1993). Involvement depends on an individual developing secure and satisfying connections with others in one's social environment (Deci et al., 1991). The most desirable outcomes for individuals are achieved when involvement or "caring" occurs in conjunction with support for autonomy and competence (Deci & Chandler, 1986).

Self-determination may be also enhanced by providing a rationale for specific task completion and acknowledging the individual's feelings. Although everyone has to engage in tasks they feel are uninteresting, self-determination is strengthened when a reason for participation is provided and the individual's questions or concerns are acknowledged (Deci & Chandler, 1986).

Although providing opportunities for students to make choices and decisions is paramount in developing self-determination, parents and professionals must also assist youths in (a) identifying options from a range of alternatives, (b) identifying the associated consequences, (c) selecting and implementing options, (d) evaluating results, and (e) adjusting future directions. Self-evaluation, self-monitoring, self-management, and self-instruction techniques are skills supportive of autonomy. The development of these skills is a complex and long-term process. Instructional programs that promote self-determination must begin laying the groundwork early on in the child's life. As suggested by Abery (1994), "striving to attain self-determination doesn't begin (or end) during adolescence or early adulthood. Rather it is initiated shortly after birth and continues until we have breathed our last breath" (p. 2).

### ⊞  FOCUS 6

*Describe three ways to provide meaningful opportunities for students with disabilities to participate in transition planning.*

***Promoting Active Student Participation in Program Planning and Implementation.*** The development of self-determination in an adolescent with disabilities may be the single most important outcome for successful transition to adulthood (Halloran & Henderson, 1990; Wehman, 1996a; Wehmeyer, 1992a; Wehmeyer & Metzler, 1995). As we already discussed, having meaningful opportunities to assume control in one's life by expressing preferences and making choices and decisions are important aspects of this concept. The development of the individualized education program (IEP) is an excellent vehicle for providing necessary opportunities for self-determination. Unfortunately, very few adolescents with disabilities attend their program planning meetings and fewer yet *actively* participate (Wehman, 1996a). However, as Morningstar, Turnbull, and Turnbull (1996) point out, the lack of student attendance may be just a small part of the problem. In a recent study by these authors, the majority of students with disabilities reported their perception of the IEP process as irrelevant.

Active participation in the IEP process begins with encouraging students to communicate their needs and preferences. To do so requires strong support from both families and professionals. This was certainly true for Lisa in Window 9.1. It took some careful prompting from her parents and school personnel for Lisa to share some of her feelings about the future. When she did so, Lisa was clear about her desire to work in the outdoors, and perhaps eventually become a fish and game warden. The development of Lisa's ITP is indicative of the partnership of students, parents, extended family members, and professionals who must work together to assist the individual in developing preferred goals and objectives. Several models are currently available to support this process (see Point of Interest 9.1).

---

**♦ POINT OF INTEREST 9.1**

## *Person-Centered Planning Models*

### *McGill Action Planning System*

IQ scores and disability labels can sentence certain children to lifelong failure. MAPS (Making Action Plans) is a collaborative process that brings the key actors in a child's life together to create an action plan to be implemented in a regular classroom setting. MAP is an eight-step planning process (Forest & Pearpoint, 1992).

### *Personal Futures Planning*

Personal futures planning is a tool for fostering new ways of thinking about people with developmental disabilities. Futures planning helps groups of people focus on opportunities for people with disabilities to develop personal relationships, have positive roles in community life, increase their control of their own lives, and develop the skills and abilities to achieve these goals (Mount & Zwernik, 1989).

### *Group Action Planning*

Group Action Planning supports infants and toddlers with disabilities and their families in inclusive environments. Practical suggestions for implementing Group Action Planning are offered, as is a longitudinal vignette of its application with one individual with Down syndrome (Turnbull, Turnbull, & Blue-Banning, 1994).

Students must also be taught the skills necessary for their active participation. Options available to professionals include videotaped presentations of real or staged IEP meetings as a way to prepare students for their own conferences. Similarly, students may be coached via role playing and rehearsal as part of social skills or other communication skills development. Goals and objectives in these communication areas are typical in secondary-age student IEPs. It is with relative ease that professionals have included training and practice specifically targeted to a student's participation in their own IEP meetings (Peters, 1990; Van Reusen & Bos, 1990, 1994) (see Point of Interest 9.2).

---

◆ **POINT OF INTEREST 9.2**

*Guidelines for Successful Student Participation*

*Facilitating Communication*

- Give the student ample time to respond.
- Use good eye communication with the student.
- Ask the student to share information relevant to planning.
- Take notes and integrate the student's input.
- Ask for the student's opinion.

*Source:* Van Reusen & Bos (1990).

*Questions to Ask Students*

1. (Student's name), what do you think are your strongest learning skills?
2. What skills do you want to learn or improve?
3. What goals do you want to work on next year to help you do better in school?
4. What goals do you want to work on next year to help you get along better with other people?
5. What vocational goals do you want to work on next year?
6. Are there any after school activities in which you want to become involved, such as sports, jobs, clubs, etc.?
7. Many students your age have begun to think about careers or jobs they might like after they finish school. What kind of job or career training do you think you would like to start after you finish school?
8. Are there any materials that have been particularly helpful in learning information or skills?
9. What kinds of activities help you learn best?
10. What size learning or study group works best for you?

*continued*

---

◆ **POINT OF INTEREST 9.2** *(continued)*

11. I'm sure you've taken a lot of tests during your years in school. Can you name or describe the type of test questions on which you do best?

12. Is there anything we've overlooked or something you'd like to say about school or any other area you are concerned about?

*Source:* Van Reusen, Bos, Schumaker, & Deshler (1987).

*Guidelines for Successful Student Participation in the IEP Conference*

1. Inform parents, administrators, and other team members prior to the conference that the student will be attending.

2. Make provisions in advance for allowing an adequate amount of time for the conference.

3. Prepare the student before the conference.

4. Outline the agenda/objectives for the meeting for all team members at the start.

5. Remind all team members to address the student directly, maintaining eye contact.

6. Use nontechnical language to convey information.

7. Highlight the student's strengths, keep remarks positive, and make specific suggestions regarding weaknesses.

8. Allow the student opportunities to ask questions and request clarity.

9. Provide opportunities for student contributions and reactions to recommendations.

10. Offer a statement summarizing decisions, goals, and suggestions, and invite final questions and comments.

*Source:* Adapted from Peters (1990).

---

## ENHANCING FAMILY INVOLVEMENT DURING THE TRANSITION YEARS

In addition to a student-centered orientation, a quality transition program is characterized by active parent involvement (Bates, 1990; Wehman, 1996a). Families are a major force behind a successful transition from school to adult life (Nisbet, Covert, & Schuh, 1992). Yet evidence suggests that parents and other family members have not been active participants in identifying transition goals and program options for their adolescent children (Gerry & McWhorter, 1991; Lichtenstein & Nisbet, 1992; Mallory, 1996). Cindy Sirois of Boston, a parent of a child with disabilities, puts it this way:

Unfortunately [during] his first eight years of schooling, I didn't know as a parent that I had any rights or any power or responsibilities. At that time I was undereducated myself. I have a ninth grade education and I sat . . . with people who I perceived to have the knowledge to teach my child and felt that, even though my gut told me it wasn't right, they must know. (National Council on Disability, 1995, p. 107)

This lack of parent participation can have a direct detrimental effect on post-school outcomes for the student with disabilities. Peraino (1992) suggests that one reason people with disabilities are not accessing valued outcomes when they enter adult life is because there is a lack of information and training regarding available resources following school. To facilitate parent participation in transition planning, schools can use two broad strategies: (1) provide information and training on transition issues; and (2) create opportunities to be active participants in the IEP/ITP process.

### Parent Information and Training

**⊞   FOCUS 7**

*Identify six possible topics for parent information and training during the transition from school to adult life.*

In order for parents to be integrally involved in assisting their son or daughter in making choices about life after school, they need information and training across several areas related to transition planning. Parents need information in such areas as (a) the components of effective secondary and transition programs; (b) the characteristics of adult service programs; (c) criteria for evaluating postschool services and supports; (d) possible service alternatives; (e) the current status of services in their local community, and (f) the identification of innovative programs (Hardman & McDonnell, 1987; McDonnell et al., 1991).

Professionals need to create opportunities for families to engage in person-centered futures planning. Information and training for parents may be provided in a variety of written formats, such as pamphlets, guides, or Internet web pages (see Point of Interest 9.3). One written format specific to the area of transition services is a step-by-step planning guide for parents. This guide could include a checklist of transition planning activities to be completed prior to the student leaving school, along with time lines and contact persons (see Figure 9.2 on page 235). Information could also be made available through videotaped presentation or via live in-service training programs, such as those offered through Parent Information and Training Centers (PTICs) (see Point of Interest 8.3).

♦ **POINT OF INTEREST 9.3**

*The Family Village*

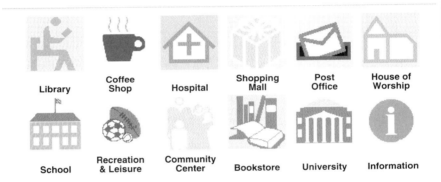

T HE FAMILY VILLAGE, A COOPERATIVE VENTURE of the Waisman Center at the University of Wisconsin-Madison, the Joseph P. Kennedy, Jr., Foundation, and the Mitsubishi Electric America Foundation, went on-line as an Internet home page in April 1996. The Village is an information resource for families with children and adults who are disabled as well as professionals around the world. Using the Internet (http://www.familyvillage.wisc.edu), families and professionals can stop in, stroll around, and visit these Family Village attractions:

- A Family Village school with information on various government agencies concerned with needs of persons with disabilities, inclusive education resources, early intervention resources, individual education plan resources, parent training and information centers, assistive technology, and university special education training programs.

- A library containing general information on people with disabilities as well as a section on diagnoses of specific conditions.

- A coffee shop where families can make direct connections with other families and professionals via the Internet. The coffee shop also includes specific information on national parent-to-parent and sibling-to-sibling programs.

*continued*

◆ **POINT OF INTEREST 9.3** *(continued)*

- A community health center with information for families on emergency services, hospitals, pharmacies, dentists, and so on, in their local community.

- A shopping mall containing information about groups and vendors that supply assistive technology to children with disabilities, including toys, computers, adaptive devices, shoes, and clothing.

- A post office with a parent-to-parent web board for posting messages.

- A listing of worship resources for individuals with disabilities and their families.

- A family resource center with information on day-care resources, new parents/baby care information, positive parenting resources, parenting a teenager, as well as resources related to ethnic diversity, single parents, adoptive families, foster families, military families, and extended family members.

- A sports and recreation center with a listing of Special Olympics chapters from around the country, information on Paralympic Games, and special camps for children with disabilities.

- A Family Village university containing information on web sites of major national disability organizations, and universities around the countries with programs in the area of disability.

- A book store with a listing of books, magazines, journals, and newsletters with a focus on disability.

Providing parents a range of options for acquiring information and building on their strengths will enhance their involvement during school. It will also facilitate the improvement of outcomes for students with disabilities as they enter adult life. Parents face many difficult decisions as they plan with their son or daughter the transition out of school: Should employment or further education be a priority immediately following school? What are the government-sponsored services and supports available within our local community that are consistent with the needs, preferences, and functioning level of our son or daughter? What are the eligibility requirements? What if there are no appropriate programs or services available? Where do we get the assistance to help us obtain the appropriate services if they are not available? How do we know what is taught in school will help our son or daughter access valued postschool outcomes?

Parents may need help understanding the status of current programs and supports in the local community and advocating for services not presently available. The evaluation of current programs should address such issues as accommodations/supports available in postsecondary institutions (such as universities/colleges or vocational training programs), average wages in various jobs, contact with nondisabled peers, independent and supported living, the size of waiting lists

**FIGURE 9.2**    *Transition Planning Checklist for Parents*

| Date Completed | Activity | Time Line | Contact Person |
|---|---|---|---|
| _____ | 1. Attend transition meeting | Year 1 | Classroom Teacher |
| _____ | 2. Attend parent workshop on entitlement programs | Year 1 | Classroom Teacher |
| _____ | 3. Attend parent workshop on eligibility programs | Year 1 | Classroom Teacher |
| _____ | 4. Apply for supplemental Social Security income | Year 2 | Mr. Larry W. Social Security Office |
| _____ | 5. Visit vocational programs | Year 2 | Ms. Susan L. Developmental Disability Agency Field Office |
| _____ | 6. Visit residential programs | Year 2 | Ms. Susan L. Developmental Disability Agency Field Office |
| _____ | 7. Target potential postschool services | Year 3 | Classroom Teacher Ms. Susan L. Developmental Disability Agency Case Manager |
| _____ | 8. Develop formal transition plan | Year 4 | Classroom Teacher Ms. Susan L. Developmental Disability Agency Case Manager |
| _____ | 9. Make applications to targeted service programs | Year 4 | Ms. Susan L. Developmental Disability Agency Field Office |
| _____ | 10. Update formal transition plan plan prior to graduation | Year 5 | Classroom Teacher |

*Source:* From *Secondary programs for students with developmental disabilities* by John McDonnell et al. Copyright © 1991 Allyn and Bacon. Reprinted with permission.

for various services, long-term security, and procedures for accessing programs. Helping parents understand and identify innovative programs not readily available for their son or daughter gives them a base from which they are able to better support their son or daughter's access to an appropriate community service system. Without assistance from professionals, it is difficult for students with disabilities and their parents to make appropriate choices prior to leaving school.

## Parents as Active Participants in the IEP/ITP Process

⊕　　**FOCUS 8**

*Identify the four steps of "The Big Picture Transition Planning Analysis."*

Although parent involvement in the IEP/ITP process is mandated under the provisions of IDEA, in actual practice the role of parents in transition planning varies greatly. Harris and Associates (1989) found that only 79 percent of the parents surveyed had attended their child's IEP meeting in the past year; 73 percent indicated that they had made some contribution to the development of their son or daughter's IEP objectives. Twain (1986) found that parent nominations of IEP goals were usually ranked as lower priorities than teacher-nominated goals. Additionally, few parents were receiving ongoing information relevant to transition planning. In a survey of parents of adolescent with disabilities, Pratt, Panzer, and Wilcox (1989) reported that 55 percent had never even heard of a formal transition plan. These authors also indicated that whereas teachers rate parent participation in transition planning as high, only 25 percent of the parents surveyed indicated that they had any choice in the kind of community training their son or daughter received.

Given the variability of parent involvement as described here, it becomes critical for schools to make a concerted effort to develop strategies that promote and support active participation in transition planning. McDonnell and McDonnell (1992) offer many strategies that schools can employ to facilitate parent involvement. They suggest a procedure referred to as "The Big Picture Transition Planning Analysis" (see Table 9.2).

Although the big picture analysis may be helpful, there is still the concern that even when parents are involved in planning they still need support in setting challenging and realistic future goals. Low expectations and inappropriate goal selection by students and/or families are sometimes cited by professionals as barriers to successful transition (McNair & Rusch, 1991). For example, McNair and Rusch found that parent attitudes toward competitive employment in the community, although improving, were still somewhat negative. One way to change parent attitudes about community living and employment is to demonstrate that adolescents with disabilities can participate in community activities and work competitively while still in school. It is also important for parents to see that their son or daughter can be reemployed if jobs are lost. Employment information along with residential living options and social activities have been identified by parents as their most important needs (Botherson et al., 1988). Included within these broad categories is information about SSI benefits, transportation, co-worker attitudes, health-care benefits, and supervision and safety.

**TABLE 9.2**    *The Big Picture Transition Planning Analysis*

*Step 1: Present Picture*

A. History—Ask parents to list important events which have occurred in the life of the individual, then list the individual's strengths and challenges (particularly those which may require accommodation in the realization of preferences/needs).

B. Preferences—Ask parents to list their son or daughter's favorite things! (may include: activities, foods, TV programs, etc.)

C. Friends and Relationships—Ask parents to list the social and emotional connections their son or daughter has established. It may also be helpful to identify the type of relationship (e.g., Bobby—friend; Kate—babysitter)

D. Community Access—Ask parents to identify the places, events and activities the individual participates in within the community. It may be helpful to indicate who he or she participates with (e.g., church, family; youth group; convenience store, sister, mom, school).

E. Living Arrangements—Identify where the individual presently lives, also identify significant people in these settings such as family members, staff, roommates, etc.

F. School or Work—Identify present school or work arrangements, and any specific situational information (e.g., self-contained or home-school, workshop, or community employment).

G. Resource Management—Identify current resources (e.g., monetary, personal belongings, and services), who manages them, and how they are managed.

H. Transportation—List the ways in which the individual gets around the community.

*Step 2: Future Picture*

A. Living Arrangements—Where would the individual like to live?

B. Resource Management—Would the individual like to change how his or her personal resources are managed, or who manages them?

C. School or Work—What would the individual like to have happen in regard to current school program and future work opportunities? What changes would he or she like to see?

D. Transportation—Would the individual like to add or change the means of transportation presently available? If so, how?

E. Community Access—Are there community events, activities, and/or locations that the individual would like to participate in or access?

F. Friends and Relationships—Would the individual like to change the status of his or her relationships? If so, how?

G. Needs—What are the individual's needs which should be considered to allow fulfillment of the "Big Picture"?

H. Self-advocacy—In what areas would the individual like to have more control and choices?

**TABLE 9.2**    *(continued)*

*Step 3: Big Picture Planning*

A. Priorities—Identify those areas which have a high priority for the individual.

B. Solutions—As a team, brainstorm solutions which might lead to the realization of this priority. List them.

C. Resources—Brainstorm the possible resources available to accomplish the solutions. Consider the following resources: physical (e.g., belongings, materials, devices, adaptive equipment); people (e.g., family, friends, persons from the community, paid support); community (e.g., establishments, activities, events); social/educational (e.g., SSI, Voc Rehab, JTPA, public school, tech schools, etc.); and financial (e.g., trusts, SSI, insurance, charitable contributions, grants).

D. Most Promising Solutions—Identify the most promising solutions and number those in order of likely success (1 being most likely). Identify the necessary resources required to accomplish the solution. Continue with the next highest priority. The team should determine how many priorities to address depending on the complexity of the solutions selected and the timelines to accomplish them.

*Step 4: Big Picture Action Plan*

A. List the prioritized solutions in sequential order (1's first, etc.) from the "Big Picture" planning meeting.

B. Specify the targeted resources for the first priority. Include who is responsible, and what he or she will do. Determine timelines to accomplish the goal.

C. Complete action plan on remaining priorities as listed.

D. At least annually, the team should make notes in the follow-up section regarding the status and effectiveness of the action for each solution.

*Source:* From *The School and Community Integration Program curriculum and IEP process* by John McDonnell. Copyrighted © 1992 University of Utah. Reprinted with permission.

## REVIEW

*FOCUS 1:  Identify three quality of life indicators that are common to most adults.*

• Everyone should be able to make their own choices about adult living, including selecting friends, where they will live, and what jobs they will hold.

• Each person is valued as an individual capable of personal growth and development. As such, everyone has the opportunity to participate in all aspects of community life.

• Each person has the opportunity to participate in the economic life of the community.

*FOCUS 2: How does the Individuals with Disabilities Education Act (IDEA) define transition services?*

- Every student with a disability must receive transition services beginning no later than age 16, or younger if appropriate.
- Transition services include a coordinated set of activities, designed within an outcome-oriented process, that promote movement from school to post-school activities, including postsecondary education, vocational training, integrated employment (including supported employment), continuing and adult education, adult services, independent living, or community participation.

*FOCUS 3: How does the individualized transition plan (ITP) relate to the individualized education program (IEP)? What is the purpose of the ITP?*

- The ITP is a component of the IEP for students with disabilities during the secondary school years. Whereas the IEP describes the goals that a student should achieve during the school year, the ITP addresses the skills and the supportive services required in the future.
- The purpose of the ITP is to identify the transition services that need to be in place for the student based on projected postschool outcomes.

*FOCUS 4: What is self-determination?*

- Self-determined people use information to make choices in pursuit of self-selected goals.
- Self-determination is an important element for preparing youth to contribute to a living democracy.
- The school plays a significant role in developing this ability, but doing so will require restructuring of both the content and delivery of instruction.
- Self-determined youth develop a greater sense of personal worth and social responsibility.

*FOCUS 5: Identify factors critical to the development of self-determination.*

- Choice and decision making.
- Optimal challenge.
- Autonomy.
- Competence.
- Involvement.
- Providing a rationale.
- Acknowledging feelings.

*FOCUS 6: Describe three ways to provide meaningful opportunities for students with disabilities to participate in transition planning.*

- Encourage students to express preferences and make choices in selecting activities, schedules, areas of study, and work experiences.
- Encourage students to attend and actively participate in their IEP meetings.
- Provide instruction in the areas of communication, decision making, and other skills that support active participation.

*FOCUS 7: Identify six possible topics for parent information and training during the transition from school to adult life.*

- Components of effective secondary and transition programs.
- Characteristics of adult service programs.
- Criteria for evaluating postschool services.
- Service alternatives.
- Current status of services in their local community.
- Identification of innovative programs.

*FOCUS 8: Identify the four steps of "The Big Picture Transition Planning Analysis"*

- Present picture: Includes history, current preferences, friends and relationships, community access, living arrangements, school or work, resource management, and transportation.
- Future picture: Includes preferred and/or projected living arrangements, resource management, school or work, transportation, community access, friends and relationships, needs, and self-advocacy.
- Big picture planning: Includes identification of priorities, solutions, needed resources, and most promising solutions.
- Big picture action plan: Includes listing of prioritized solutions, specification of targeted resources for first priority, completion of action plan with remaining priorities, and annual evaluation regarding status and effectiveness of action taken.

# REFERENCES

Abery, B. (1994). Self-determination: It's not just for adults. *Impact,* 6(4), 2. (ERIC Document Reproduction Service No. ED 368 109)

Americans with Disabilities Act of 1990, 42 U. S.C. §§ 101–108 (1991).

Bandura, A. (1977). *Social learning theory.* Englewood Cliffs, NJ: Prentice-Hall.

Bates, P. (1990). *Best practices in transition planning: Quality indicators.* Carbondale: Illinois Transition Project.

Bursuck, W. D., & Rose, E. (1992). Community college options for students with mild disabilities. In F. R. Rusch, L. Destefano, J. Chadsey-Rusch, L. A. Phelps, & E. Syzmanski (Eds.), *Transition from school to adult life* (pp. 71–91). Sycamore, IL: Sycamore.

Deci, E. L., & Chandler, C. L. (1986). The importance of motivation for the future of the LD field. *Journal of Learning Disabilities, 19*, 587–594.

Deci, E. L., & Ryan, R. M. (1985). *Intrinsic motivation and self-determination in human behavior.* New York: Plenum.

Deci, E. L., & Ryan, R. M. (1987). The support of autonomy and the control of behavior. *Journal of Personality and Social Psychology, 53*, 1024–1037.

Deci, E. L. & Ryan, R. M. (1991). A motivational approach to self: Integration in personality. In R. Dienstbier (Ed.), *Nebraska Symposium on Motivation: Vol. 38. Perspectives on motivation* (pp. 237–288). Lincoln: University of Nebraska Press.

Deci, E. L., Vallerand, R. J., Pelletier, L. G., & Ryan, R. M. (1991). Motivation and education: The self-determination perspective. *Educational Psychologist, 26*, 325–346.

Forest, M., & Pearpoint, J. C. (1992). Putting all kinds on the MAP. *Educational Leadership, 50*, 26–61.

Gerry, M. H., & McWhorter, C. M. (1991). A comprehensive analysis of federal statutes and programs for persons with severe disabilities. In L. H. Meyer, C. A. Peck, & L. Brown (Eds.), *Critical issues in the lives of people with severe disabilities* (pp. 495–526). Baltimore: Brookes.

Gillespie, D., & Hillman, S. B. (1993, August). *Impact of self-efficacy expectations on adolescent career choice.* Paper presented at the meeting of the American Psychological Association, Toronto, Ontario, Canada.

Hackman, J. R., & Suttle, J. L. (1977). *Improving life at work: Behavioral science approaches to organizational change.* Santa Monica, CA: Goodyear.

Halloran, W., & Henderson, D. R. (1990). Transition issues for the 1990s. *Impact, 3*, 2–3.

Hardman, M. L., Drew, C. J., & Egan, M. W. (1996). *Human exceptionality* (5th ed.). Boston: Allyn & Bacon.

Hardman, M. L., & McDonnell, J. (1987). Implementing transition initiatives for youths with severe handicaps: The Utah Community-based Transition Project. *Exceptional Children, 53*(6), 493–498.

Hardman, M. L., Rouse, M., & McDonnell, J. (1994). Transition to adult and working life. In T. Husen & T. N. Postlethwaite (Eds.), *The International Encyclopedia of Education* (2nd ed.). Oxford, England: Pergamon.

Harris, L., and Associates (1989). *The ICD survey III: A report card on special education.* New York: Author.

Harris, L., and Associates (1994). *National Organization on Disability/Harris Survey of Americans with Disabilities.* New York: Author.

Hasazi, S. B., Johnson, R. E., Hasazi, J., Gordon, L. R., & Hull, M. (1989). A statewide follow-up survey of high school exiters: A comparison of former students with and without handicaps. *Journal of Special Education, 23*, 243–255.

Hendry, L. B., Glendinning, A., Shucksmith, J., Love, J., & Scott, J. (1993). The developmental context of adolescent life-styles. In R. K. Silbereisen & E. Todt (Eds.), *Adolescence in context: The interplay of family, school, peers, and work in adjustment* (pp. 66–81). New York: Springer.

Individuals with Disabilities Education Act (IDEA), 33 U. S. C. §§ 1400–1485 (1990).

Individuals with Disabilities Education Act Part B Regulations, 34 C. F. R. § 300–500 (1992).

Lichtenstein, S., & Nisbet, J. (1992). *From school to adult life: Young adults in transition, a national and state overview* (Vol. 1). Durham: University of New Hampshire, Institute on Disability/UAP.

Mallory, B. L. (1996). The role of social policy in life-cycle transitions. *Exceptional Children, 62,* 213–223.

McDonnell, J., & McDonnell, A. (1992). *The School and Community Integration Program curriculum and IEP process.* Salt Lake City: University of Utah, Department of Special Education.

McDonnell, J., Wilcox, B., & Hardman, M. L. (1991). *Secondary programs for students with developmental disabilities.* Boston: Allyn & Bacon.

McNair, J., & Rusch, F. R. (1991). Parent involvement in transition programs. *Mental Retardation, 29,* 93–101.

Morningstar, M. E., Turnbull, A. P., & Turnbull, H. R. (1996). What do students with disabilities tell us about the importance of family involvement in the transition from school to adult life? *Exceptional Children, 62,* 249–260.

Mount, B., & Zwernik, K. (1989, Oct.). It's never too early, it's too late. St. Paul, MN: Metropolitan Council of the Twin Cities Area. (ERIC Document Reproduction Service No. ED 327 997).

National Council on Disability. (1989). *The education of students with disabilities: Where do we stand?* Washington, DC: Author.

National Council on Disability. (1995). *Improving the implementation of the Individuals with Disabilities Education Act: Making schools work for all of America's children.* Washington, DC: Author.

Nisbet, J., Covert, S., & Schuh, M. (1992). Family involvement in the transition from school to adult life. In F. R. Rusch, L. Destefano, J. Chadsey-Rusch, L. A. Phelps, & E. Szymanski (Eds.), *Transition from school to adult life: Models, linkages, and policy* (pp. 407–424). Pacific Grove, CA: Sycamore.

Peraino, J. M. (1992). Post-21 follow-up studies: How do special education graduates fare? In P. Wehman (Ed.), *Life beyond the classroom: Transition strategies for young people with disabilities* (pp. 21–70). Baltimore: Brookes.

Peters, M. T. (1990). Someone's missing: The student as an overlooked participant in the IEP process. *Preventing School Failure, 34,* 32–36.

Pratt, C., Panzer, J., & Wilcox, B. (1989, December). *Parent involvement in transition planning: What goes on? What should?* Paper presented at the Annual Conference of the Association for Persons with Severe Handicaps, San Francisco.

President's Committee on Mental Retardation. (1995). *The journey to inclusion: A resource guide for state policy makers.* Washington: DC: Author.

Rehabilitation Act of 1973, as Amended, 29 U.S.C. §§ 720 et. seq., 1992.

Schloss, P. J., Alper, S., & Jayne, D. (1993). Self-determination for persons with disability: Choice, risk and dignity. *Exceptional Children, 60,* 215–225.

Schoeller, K. (1994). One family's lesson in self-determination. *Impact, 6*(4), 1, 19.

Shulman, L. S. (1989). Teaching alone, learning together: Needed agendas for the new reforms. In T. J. Sergiovanni & J. H. Moore (Eds.), *Schooling for tomorrow: Directing reforms to issues that count* (pp. 166–186). Boston: Allyn & Bacon.

Sitlington, P., & Frank, A. (1990). Are adolescents with learning disabilities successfully crossing the bridge to adult life? *Learning Disability Quarterly, 13,* 97–111.

Smith, D. D., & Luckasson, R. (1995). *Introduction to special education: Teaching in an age of challenge.* Boston: Allyn & Bacon.

Szymanski, E. (1994). Transitions: Life-span and life-space considerations for empowerment. *Exceptional Children, 60*, 402–410.

Turnbull, A. P., Turnbull, H. R., & Blue-Banning, M. (1994). Enhancing inclusion of infants and toddlers with disabilities and their families: A theoretical and programmatic analysis. *Infants and Young Children, 7*(2), 1–14.

Turnbull, A. P., Turnbull, H. R., Bronicki, G. J., Summers, J. A., & Roeder-Gordon, C. (1989). *Disability and the family: A guide to decisions for adulthood.* Baltimore: Brookes.

Twain, K. (1986). *Parental participation in IEP conferences.* Unpublished master's thesis, University of Oregon, Eugene.

Valdes, K. A., Williamson, C. L., & Wagner, M. M. (1990). *The National Longitudinal Transition Study of Special Education Students, Statistical Almanac: Vol. 5. Youth Categorized as Mentally Retarded.* Menlo Park, CA: SRI International.

Van Reusen, A. K., & Bos, C. (1994). Facilitating student participation in individualized education programs through motivation strategy instruction. *Exceptional Children, 60*, 466–475.

Van Reusen, A. K., & Bos, C. S. (1990). IPLAN: Helping students communicate in planning conferences. *Teaching Exceptional Children, 22*(4), 30–32.

Ward, M. J. (1991). Self-determination revisited: Going beyond expectations. In C. Valdisision (Director), Transition Summary, Number 7: *Options after high school for youth with disabilities.* Washington, DC: NICHCY. (ERIC Document Reproduction Service No. ED 340 170)

Wehman, P. (1996a). Individualized transition planning. In P. Wehman (Ed.), *Life beyond the classroom: Transition strategies for young people with disabilities* (2nd edition) (p. 77–103). Baltimore: Brookes.

Wehman, P. (1996b). Interagency cooperation. In P. Wehman (Ed.), *Life beyond the classroom: Transition strategies for young people with disabilities* (2nd edition) (pp. 107–136). Baltimore: Brookes.

Wehmeyer, M. (1992a). Self-determination: Critical skills for outcome-oriented transition services. Steps in transition that lead to self-determination. *Journal for Vocational Special Needs Education, 16*(1), 3–7.

Wehmeyer, M. (1992b). Self-determination and the education of students with mental retardation. *Education and Training in Mental Retardation, 27*, 302–314.

Wehmeyer, M. L., & Metzler, C. A. (1995). How self-determined are people with mental retardation? The national consumer survey. *Mental Retardation, 33*, 111–119.

Will, M. (1984). *OSERS programming for the transition of youth with disabilities: Bridges from school to work life.* Washington, DC: Office of Special Education and Rehabilitative Services.

# CHAPTER TEN

# Families and the Adult Years

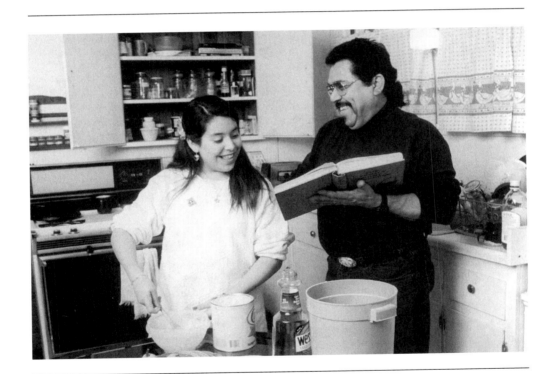

★ **WINDOW 10.1**

*Steve*

OVER THE PAST SEVERAL YEARS, many changes have occurred in Steve's life. After spending most of his adolescence in a large institution, Steve moved into a group home with seven other adults with disabilities during his early thirties. Now in his mid-forties, Steve lives in an apartment with two other individuals with disabilities, receiving on-going training and assistance from a local supported living program. His parents and three older brothers all live within five miles from the apartment, maintaining regular contact via the phone, visits, or family functions. Steve used to go to his parents' house on weekends, but now prefers to spend the time in his apartment watching videos, or going out with his roommates or the supported living staff.

Steve has had many labels describing his disability over the years, including mental retardation, epilepsy, autism, physical disability, chronic health problems, and serious emotional disturbance. He is very much challenged both mentally and physically. His medical problems associated with epilepsy have resulted in the use of medications that affect his behavior (motivation, attitude, etc.), and his physical well-being. During his early twenties, Steve had a seizure while walking up a long flight of stairs which resulted in a fall that broke his neck. The impact from the fall was a paralyzed right hand, and the limited use of his left leg. He must visit a local neurologist on a frequent basis, and a nurse comes to his apartment almost daily to ensure proper use of medications.

A lifelong goal for Steve has been to be able to work in a real job, make money, and have choices about how he spends it. For most of his life the goal has been out of reach. His only jobs have been in sheltered workshops, where he worked for next to nothing doing piecemeal work such as sorting envelopes, putting together cardboard boxes, or folding laundry. While most of the focus in the past has been on what he "can't" do (can't read, can't get along with supervisors, can't handle the physical requirements of a job, etc.), his parents and siblings are looking more and more at his very strong desire to succeed in a job.

A job has opened up for a stock clerk at a local video store about three miles away from Steve's apartment. The store manager is willing to pay minimum wage for someone to work 4 to 6 hours a day stocking the shelves with videos, and handling some basic custodial tasks (such as cleaning floors, washing windows, and dusting furniture). Steve loves movies and is really interested in this job. With the support of family and a local supported employment service provider, he has applied for the position.

*Source:* Adapted from *Human Exceptionality* by Michael Hardman et al. Copyright © 1996 by Allyn and Bacon. Reprinted with permission.

ADULTHOOD IS MOST TYPICALLY CONSIDERED as the period of life when we advance from relative dependence on our family or caregivers to more independence and increasing individual responsibility. This life passage also involves a legal change of status: a transition from minor child to adult. Legally, adult status is based on the premise that when people reach a specific age (usually 18 years old; 21 in some states), they attain a level of *competence* and parents should no longer have the right to make decisions on their behalf. As such, at the designated age of majority, a person is deemed competent and immediately given the right to make his or her own choices. With this newfound set of rights also comes a person's responsibility to meet the societal expectations of being an adult. If for whatever reasons those expectations are *not* met, consequences are imposed.

Adult status is also associated with the time when we finally move away from home, gain employment, and become self-supporting. However, if independence from parents was the sole criteria for being an adult, some people who reach the age of majority would not meet the standard. The fact is that parents often continue providing support after the age of 18. The purpose of the support may be to further their son or daughter's education or to allow them to stay at home while they work and save money before moving out on their own.

For families with a person who is disabled, adult status is a paradox. On the one hand, parents struggle with their child's right to grow up. On the other hand, they must continue to deal with the realities of their son or daughter's mental or physical limitations. The issues surrounding what legally or practically constitutes adult status are extremely complex for these families. Just as there is a great deal of variability in the needs and functioning level of people with disabilities, there is also a corresponding variability in lifestyle during the adult years. Adults with mild disabilities may lead a life similar to those who are not disabled, primarily because their challenges while growing up were mostly related to academic performance in school. Some adults with mild disabilities become self-supporting, eventually working and living independent of their immediate family. As is true for nondisabled people, however, some of these adults may still need support, whether it be government sponsored (such as vocational rehabilitation) or natural—family members, friends, and neighbors. Drew, Hardman, and Logan (1996) summarized some of the issues surrounding adult life for people with mild disabilities:

> What does society expect of an adult? Adults work, earn money, and buy the necessities of life and as many of the pleasures they want or can afford. An adult socializes, often marries, has children, and tries to live as productively and happily as possible. The adult with [mild disabilities] may be unable to find or hold a job, particularly without formal supports in place. If jobs are available, wages may be so low that even the necessities of life may be out of reach. What if the [individual] has no one to socialize with, no one to love or be loved by? There are many such "what ifs" for adults with [more mild disabilities], who may just exchange the frustrations of earlier life for new and sometimes harsher ones. (p. 283)

For adults with more severe disabilities, continuous government and natural supports are critical in order to ensure access and participation in employment, residential living, and recreation in their local community. Parents and family members of people with severe disabilities often face the stark reality that their caregiving role may not diminish during the adult years and could well extend through a lifetime. This is true for Steve (see Window 10.1 on page 246). Even though he is now in his mid-forties, Steve still requires both government and family support. Whether at work or home, Steve needs assistance from many people. He receives life skills training from his supported living program, and his medical needs are taken care of through frequent visits to a local physician. A nurse comes to Steve's apartment on a regular basis to ensure that his medications are being administered safely. Finally, he stays close to his immediate family members who live only a short drive away from his apartment.

This chapter examines adults with disabilities and their families from three perspectives: (1) making choices: issues of competence, consent, and guardianship; (2) understanding and exploring adult services; and (3) building a support network.

## MAKING CHOICES: ISSUES OF COMPETENCE, CONSENT, AND GUARDIANSHIP

Quality of life during the adult years may be defined by (1) employment, useful work, and valued activity; (2) access to further education when desired and appropriate; (3) personal autonomy and independence; (4) social interaction and community participation; and (5) participation within the life of the family. As one reaches the age of majority, decisions have to made relative to each of these five areas. What kind of career or job do I want? Should I go on to further education to increase my career choices? Where will I live and whom will I live with? How will I spend my money? Who do I choose to spend time with? Who will be my friends? Most people face these choices as a natural part of growing into adult life, but the initial questions often facing families with an adult who is disabled may be quite different. For these families, the issues may revolve around the competence of their son or daughter. Is this adult child competent to make decisions that are in his or her best interests, regardless of the fact that the age of majority has been reached? Is it possible to be competent in some areas and not others? How will competence be determined? Who will be making decisions in those areas where the person is not competent? How will consent be given to make such decisions?

### Competence

⊕   **FOCUS 1**

*What are the basic issues in determining whether or not an adult is mentally competent?*

It is fundamental in law that when a person reaches the age of majority, he or she is deemed mentally competent until determined otherwise. Every adult is presumed to be able to make rational and reasoned personal choices (see Win-

---

★ **WINDOW 10.2**

---

## *Making Adult Choices: Varying Perspectives from People with Disabilities*

- I want to be my own boss, be free, free to stay out, shop more.
- I want to live where it is more quiet. The reason I want to move is to get away from my Mom and Dad; I'd like to be on my own. I want to move in with my sister, but moving somewhere by myself would be even better.
- I would like to move in with my best friend. I see that my parents are getting older; pretty soon they won't be able to take care of me anymore. I don't want to be alone.
- I'd like very much to move in with my sister. I'd have more privacy and time for myself.
- I want to move in with my girlfriend. I'm in love.
- I want to stay with Mom. I take care of her and she takes care of me.
- The hard thing is leaving here . . . memories.
- I like my home. My parents care about me.
- I want to stay home; I don't want to be in a nursing home unless I am very old.

*Source:* From *Older adults with development disabilities* by E. Sutton et al. Copyright © 1993 by Brookes Publishing Co. Reprinted with permission.

---

dow 10.2). The legal presumption of mental competence removes from parents the obligation and power to make decisions for their adult child, a power that until this point in life could not be usurped unless it was abused. For professionals, this means no longer dealing directly with parents on issues related to the person who has reached the age of majority, but respecting the rights of the individual as an adult. Respecting these rights involves the obligation to maintain confidentiality from parents and others if the person so desires.

Although the presumption in law is that everyone is competent at the age of majority, this supposition can be overturned or set aside by the courts in certain circumstances. An adult can be deemed incompetent through a process known as adjudication. In adjudication, those seeking to have the individual declared incompetent must provide a preponderance of evidence that the person does not have the capacity to make rational choices. The courts evaluate a person's competence by asking these three basic questions:

- Does the person have the capacity to make rational and reasoned decisions consistently that are in his or her best interests and those of others that the individual has direct contact with?

- Is the individual only *partially* incompetent, and thus has the capacity to make some rational decisions at varying levels of complexity?

- Is the individual *totally* incompetent, and thus unable to make any reasoned personal decisions?

Determining incompetence is a very sensitive and complex process. It is further complicated by a somewhat unclear judicial criteria as to what differentiates complete competence from partial or total incompetence. Competence is not an all-or-nothing proposition. Certainly, few people are completely competent in everything; correspondingly, few people are totally incompetent as well. Any decision to remove or reduce an individual's right to make choices must be weighed very heavily because such rights are fundamental to adult status from a legal, moral, and practical standpoint.

One of the first challenges facing families when their son or daughter with a disability reaches the age of majority is weighing their adult child's right to self-determination against the mental competence to make reasoned choices. While other families with nondisabled adult children are in the process of letting go, families with a person who is disabled are trying to deal with whether they will continue as full or partial decision makers for their son or daughter. In making these decisions, parents may ask several questions:

- What is the capacity of my child to make reasoned choices?

- If there are clear limitations in capacity, are there some decisions that he or she can make on their own? What are these decisions?

- If the limitation is such that my child cannot make any reasoned decisions and requires someone to act continually on his or her behalf, what are my legal obligations and responsibilities?

- If I have to make some or all of the decisions for my child, do I have to get approval? If so, from whom?

To answer these questions, parents and professionals must first have an understanding of the basic elements and types of consent. Understanding the concept of consent gives parents the knowledge to deal with the issues relative to their child's ability to make decisions. From that point, parents can choose whether or not to pursue legal avenues, such as guardianship, as a means to gain full or partial control over their son or daughter's life.

## Elements of Consent

**FOCUS 2**

*Identify the three elements of consent.*

Consent may be defined as the act of giving or withholding approval to some action or procedure that affects the life of the individual (Turnbull et al., 1989). Giving or withholding approval is a routine aspect of adult life. On a formal basis, we may give or withhold our consent to creditors, such as banks or mortgage companies, to review our personal records. We may give or withhold consent to physicians to provide a needed drug or surgical procedure. On an informal level, we may give or withhold consent to a family member or friend who wants to borrow a car or use our computer. Regardless of why, how, or when we give or withhold consent, three factors must be taken into consideration to meet the legal definition of the term: capacity, information, and voluntariness (Turnbull, 1977).

**Capacity.** Capacity is the ability to acquire and retain knowledge, evaluate the information received, and make a choice based on the evaluation. In the judicial system, a person is deemed competent or incompetent based on the concept of *capacity.* The term also takes into account the person's ability to give consent. "Does the individual understand the nature and consequences of giving consent?" This issue is very relevant to persons with disabilities. It cannot be assumed that because individuals of adult age have identified disabilities they are not competent to make decisions about their lives.

**Information.** To meet the legal requirement of consent, information must be communicated effectively in both substance and manner. "In other words, what information was given, and how was it presented?" (Drew, Hardman, & Hart, 1996). It is not good enough that the communicator intends for the information to be understood; it must be comprehended by the receiver. As such, there is a clear obligation on the part of the person communicating to ensure that it was understood.

**Voluntariness.** Voluntariness refers to a person's ability to exercise free power of choice without the intervention of force, fraud, deceit, or duress. There must not be any constraint or coercion either explicit or *implicit* on the part of the part of the person seeking consent.

*Types of Consent*

**⊕    FOCUS 3**

*Describe the three types of consent.*

In addition to the three elements of consent, there are also three types of consent: direct, substitute, and concurrent. *Direct consent* is obtained directly from the person who is involved or affected by an action. As such, it is assumed that the person is completely competent to give or withhold approval. *Substitute consent* (sometimes referred to as third party consent) is given by someone other than the person who is involved or directly affected by an action. Substitute consent is appropriate only when it is determined that a person does not have the capacity to make the decision or is dependent on others for his or her welfare. *Concurrent consent* is a combination of both direct and substitute consent (Turnbull et al., 1989). Concurrent consent is appropriate when the person seeking consent is unclear whether or not the person is fully competent. To protect from liability, the person seeking consent involves another person in the decision making. Consent then becomes a joint process that involves the person who is affected by the action and at least one other individual who is knowledgeable about the other person and the situation. For example, a doctor is seeking consent from Lyle (an adult with a disability who has not been adjudicated as incompetent by the courts) to conduct a procedure using a laser that would improve vision. Although recognizing Lyle's right to give or withhold consent to the operation, the doctor is also concerned about whether he understands the substance of the information provided regarding the operation. As a protection, the doctor not only obtains consent from Lyle but from his father as well.

As parents gain more understanding of the issues surrounding consent, they eventually come to this question: "How much power or control over my adult child's life is necessary to protect him or her from harm and enhance opportunities for a successful adult life?" If the decision is that their son or daughter is either partially or totally incapable of making rational choices, then the exploration into guardianship may be an appropriate alternative.

*Guardianship*

**⊕    FOCUS 4**

*What is guardianship? Distinguish between full, limited, and temporary guardianship.*

Guardianship, a legal term, gives power to one individual to direct or control the life of another person. This power comes through the courts when it is determined that an individual is not capable of handling his or her personal life, including not being able to give consent. The term is most often applied after an individual reaches the age of majority. It is usually not necessary to establish guardianship for minor children whose parents are considered the legal and natural guardians. In some cases, however, guardians for children may be foster parents, adoptive parents, or the state social services agency.

There are many reasons why an adult with disabilities may need a guardian:

- The person has assets he or she cannot adequately manage. Someone is needed to be sure the assets are secure and used for the intended purpose.

- A person . . . needs medical care or other services that will not be provided unless there is a clear understanding about the person's legal capacity to consent to treatment or services. (Note: Health and [other] service providers are becoming more concerned about liabilities when providing service to someone who may not have the capacity to make an informed consent to treatment or services.)

- Parents or siblings cannot get access to important records or provide other help without guardianship. As a legal adult, a person [with disabilities] must often give consent for the release of health and other records to parents or others. Health and [other] service providers, unsure of the person's ability to give consent, may require documentation of the person's legal capacity before allowing access to records without the person's consent. (Davis & Berkobien, 1994, p. 44)

Guardianship may be full, limited, or temporary in its application. *Full guardianship* involves one person's full control over the decisions made in another person's life. Because full guardianship is very restrictive, it is applied only in those cases in which the person is not capable of making any rational choices. *Limited guardianship* allows an individual to keep some control over life decisions while giving another person authority in some areas consistent with the needs of the individual. Limited guardianship may be applied to a person and/or a person's property. The guardian of a person has authority over personal issues, such as consent for medical procedures, choosing where the person lives, arranging for transportation, and ensuring proper nutrition. The guardian of property is expected to protect a person's personal assets by investing them appropriately, and using them for care, education, and general welfare. *Temporary guardianship* is applicable under special circumstances and within a limited time frame. An example of a special circumstance may be a reaction to drugs that renders an individual mentally and physically incapacitated. In this case, family members can seek temporary guardianship to deal effectively with this emergency situation. Once the emergency is over, the guardianship is no longer applicable.

To assist parents in making decisions regarding whether or not to pursue guardianship over their adult child with disabilities, Turnbull et al. (1989) identified several questions for parents to ponder. These questions are concerned with issues of individual need, possible alternatives to guardianship, as well as service, family, and ideological considerations (see Table 10.1).

## UNDERSTANDING AND EXPLORING ADULT SERVICES

During the adult years, families must come to terms not only with the complex *process* of choice making relative to future planning for the family member with disabilities, but they must deal with the maze of options in adult services. Over the past thirty years, adult services have gone through major reform. The system has evolved from a sole focus on protecting, managing, and caring for persons with disabilities in segregated programs to one of providing the supports necessary for the individual to participate in family and community life. Gerry and Mirsky (1992) suggest five principles to guide adult services as we move toward the twenty-first century:

1. Services for people with disabilities should be based on the needs and wishes of the individuals themselves and, as appropriate, for their families.

2. Services for people with disabilities must empower consumers and be flexible enough to reflect the differing and changing needs of people with disabilities.

3. Every person with a disability must have a real opportunity to engage in productive employment.

4. Public and private collaborations must be fostered to ensure that people with disabilities have the opportunities and choices that are available to all Americans.

5. Social inclusion of people with disabilities in their neighborhood and communities must be a major focus of the overall effort (p. 341).

We begin this section on government-funded supports for adults with disabilities with an overview of the Americans with Disabilities Act (ADA). ADA is the most important civil rights legislation in the United States since the Civil Rights Act of 1964. From ADA, we move on to a discussion of what families need to know about government-funded programs, including the differences between entitlement and eligibility programs, financial security and health care, and institutional versus community-based services.

**TABLE 10.1**  *In Pursuit of Guardianship*

A. *Individual Needs*

1. For what kinds of decisions does your son or daughter need substitute consent?
2. For what steps of the decision-making process does your son or daughter need substitute consent?
3. For decisions at what level of complexity does your son or daughter need substitute consent?
4. Does your son's or daughter's decision-making capability tend to be stable or are there episodes when he or she needs more help than at other times?
5. What are your son's or daughter's preferences for how substitute consent is obtained?

B. *Alternatives to Guardianship*

1. Would protective services be sufficient to provide substitute consent in life-style decisions for your son or daughter?
2. Would implied onset be sufficient to obtain emergency services for your son or daughter?
3. Would establishing a representative payee be sufficient to provide substitute consent in financial management for your son or daughter?
4. Would establishing a Trust be sufficient to provide substitute consent in financial management for your son or daughter?

C. *Service Considerations*

1. Can your son or daughter get access to necessary services without guardianship?
2. Under what circumstances will guardianship be required for your son or daughter to obtain necessary services?
3. Under what circumstances might service providers seek unwarranted control over your son or daughter if he or she does not have a guardian?

D. *Family Considerations*

1. How available, willing, and able are family and friends to provide concurrent or substitute consent in an informal capacity and as a guardian?
2. What is the life expectancy and health of family and friends who might provide concurrent or substitute consent in an informal capacity and as a guardian?
3. What are the financial resources of your son or daughter that require concurrent or substitute consent for money management purposes?

E. *Ideological Considerations*

1. What is the ideology of parent and professional organizations concerning guardianship?
2. What is the ideology of the local courts concerning guardianship?

F. *Other Considerations*

1. Are there other considerations unique to your family circumstances that are important for you to consider?
2. Are there other people whom you need to consult?

G. *Decision*

1. Should you pursue guardianship for your son or daughter?

*Source:* From *Disability and the family: A guide to decisions for adulthood* by H. R. Turnbull, III, et al. Copyright © 1989 by Brookes Publishing Co. Reprinted with permission.

## The Americans with Disabilities Act (ADA)

**FOCUS 5**

*What is the purpose of the Americans with Disabilities Act (ADA)? Identify its basic provisions.*

ADA (Public Law 101–336) was signed into law on July 26, 1990, with the expressed purpose of protecting people with disabilities from discrimination. Unlike the Individuals with Disabilities Education Act (IDEA), ADA does not entitle people with disabilities to specific adult services (such as employment or housing). The law is intended to ensure that people with disabilities receive fair treatment—"a level playing field"—as they seek employment, access to public services, public accommodations, transportation, and telecommunications. Under ADA, businesses that serve the public are required to remove architectural barriers, such as curbs on sidewalks, narrow doorways, or shelving and desks that prevent access by a person with a disability. "Reasonable accommodations" must be made available to people with disabilities in hiring or promotion practices, restructuring jobs, and modifying equipment. All new public transit facilities (such as buses or train stations) must be accessible, and transportation services must be available to people with disabilities who can't use fixed bus routes. ADA also requires that public accommodations (restaurants, hotels, retail stores) and state and local government agencies be accessible to people with disabilities. Amtrak train stations must also be accessible by the year 2010. All companies who offer telephone service to the general public must provide telecommunication devices for people who are deaf (see Point of Interest 10.1).

## Distinguishing between Entitlement and Eligibility in Adult Services

**FOCUS 6**

*Distinguish between entitlement and eligibility programs for adults with disabilities.*

As families explore options for the adult family member with disabilities, they immediately discover a basic difference between education and adult services. Education is an entitlement program; many adult services are eligibility programs. Under an entitlement, all individuals who meet the eligibility requirements *must* be provided the service. For example, every student who is identified as "disabled" under the provisions of IDEA is entitled to special education services. These services must be provided by school districts regardless of the availability of funds. In an eligibility program, an individual may meet the eligibility requirements for a service, but he or she may not be able to receive it because there aren't enough funds to serve all eligible people. When funds are not available to purchase a needed service, the individual may be placed on a waiting list. Unfor-

## What Families with an Adult Who Is Disabled Want to Know about the Americans with Disabilities Act

### What Is the Americans with Disabilities Act?

ADA is a new law. It can protect your son or daughter against many kinds of discrimination. Discrimination keeps your son or daughter from getting a job just because someone says he or she has a disability. One part of ADA protects them against discrimination at work.

ADA can make it easier for your son or daughter to apply for a job. The law can help them get a job, learn to do the job, and keep the job.

ADA can "open doors" for your son or daughter. They can apply for more kinds of jobs. Their employer will help them work faster and learn the job more easily.

### Which Jobs Can My Son or Daughter Apply For?

They can apply for any job where they can do the important parts of the work, with or without help. ADA refers to the most important parts of a job as the "essential functions." They are the parts that must be done.

Here are some examples. If your son or daughter was a mailroom clerk, they might have three "essential functions." They would have to get mail from a bag, sort mail, and take mail to each person.

If the job was putting machine parts together, they might have four "essential functions." They would have to get supplies from a room, choose the parts needed, put the parts together, and pack shipping boxes.

These are only examples. Every job has its own "essential functions." Your son or daughter is qualified for a job if he or she can do the "essential functions," with or without help.

### What Are "Reasonable Accommodations"?

A "reasonable accommodation" is any change or help that makes it easier for your son or daughter to find a job and do the work. Some of the help may come from co-workers. Some may come from job coaches.

There are many kinds of "reasonable accommodations." Here are some examples. If help is needed getting a job:

- Your son or daughter can bring a friend or relative to apply for a job.
- Ask the employer to read the application to them.
- Ask the employer to write information on the application.
- Ask the employer to let your son or daughter show how they would do the job.

Remember: ADA protects your son or daughter against discrimination. Employers can not ask them if they have a disability. They can not ask if they take medicine or if they have been in an institution. They can ask them to have a medical exam, but only after they offer a job.

*continued*

♦ **POINT OF INTEREST 10.1** (*continued*)

If your son or daughter can't do some "non-essential" parts of a job, ask the manager for "job restructuring." This means someone else will do the less important parts of the job. Your son or daughter will still have to do the most important parts, or "essential functions."

### How Can My Son or Daughter Get "Reasonable Accommodations"?

Your son or daughter (with assistance as necessary) can talk to the employer. Together they can decide what "reasonable accommodations" will help at work. There are many "reasonable accommodations." They depend on the job and the individual's needs.

### What Kind of Help Can My Son or Daughter Ask For?

They can ask for help applying for a job. They can ask for a "reasonable accommodation" learning or doing the job.

They can also ask for help learning the rules at work. If they have trouble getting to work on time, they can ask to change the starting time.

### When Can My Son or Daughter Ask for the Help Needed?

They can ask for "reasonable accommodations" any time. They can ask when they apply for a job. They can ask when they start a job. They can ask after beginning work.

When they start a job, it's important to talk to the employer about the help they might need.

They may find that they need more help once they are working. They can ask the employer about a new "reasonable accommodation" anytime.

### Does the Employer Have to Give a "Reasonable Accommodation"?

Not always. Giving help may cause the employer "undue hardship." The employer doesn't have to give a "reasonable accommodation" if it costs too much. The employer doesn't have to give a "reasonable accommodation" if the work won't get done, even with help.

### Can Someone Come to Work with My Son or Daughter to Help?

Yes. A job coach or counselor can help your son or daughter learn a job. An agency may pay for a job coach or a counselor to help learn the job. Or the employer might let a friend or someone in your family help. The employer does not have to pay for these helpers.

### Can ADA Help My Son or Daughter Get Benefits?

ADA will help your son or daughter get the same benefits as co-workers who have the same hours and job. They might get job benefits like insurance or vacation time. The employer will tell them what benefits they get. He or she will show you how to sign up for them.

If you make too much money at work you may get less money from SSI or SSDI. You may also lose some Medicaid or Medicare benefits. Ask the job coach or counselor how your son's or daughter's benefits may change. Talk about this before they start work.

*Source:* Adapted from The Joseph P. Kennedy Jr. Foundation.

tunately, many adults services are eligibility programs. The result has been that in some states, adults with disabilities may wait months, even years, before they receive necessary employment assistance or housing.

## Financial Security and Health Care

### FOCUS 7

*What are the components of federal income support and health-care programs for adults with disabilities?*

A critical issue for many families centers around financial security and health care for the adult member with a disability. For a family with modest or very limited means, numerous questions surround how their family member will be supported. Will he or she be able to work? Will the income from employment be enough for the individual to be financially independent of the primary family? What is the role of government in ensuring financial support and providing medical benefits? How can we take advantage of the government assistance that is available?

***Income Support.*** Income support to people with disabilities is provided through federal legislation enacted under the Social Security Act. In 1972, amendments to the original Social Security Act of 1935 added a program entitled Supplemental Security Income (SSI). SSI provides direct cash payments to eligible disabled children and adults as well as to low-income elderly people. Recipients of these payments must meet the definitional criteria of disability and elderly and have income resources below a specified level. In order for a person to qualify, he or she must have a mental or physical disability that is expected to last for twelve months or longer, and be unable to engage in substantial gainful activity.

Beginning at age 18, SSI payments of approximately $400 per month are made to eligible people with disabilities. However, a variety of provisions in this act may reduce SSI cash payments. For example, individuals who live in a Medicaid-funded facility receive reduced payments, as do individuals who are employed and earning more than minimum wage.

Braddock and Fujiura (1988) describe the original SSI program as a strong disincentive to work: "Income maintenance benefits, under some circumstances, made it economically advantageous for the individual with a disability to remain unemployed" (p. 265). Under current law (the Employment Opportunities for Disabled Americans Act, Section 1619), the disincentive to work was reduced by continuing to maintain SSI payments for individuals who were above the 50 percent cutoff level. Under current regulations, SSI payments are reduced, not terminated, by $1 for every $2 earned above a monthly income of $85. The person seeking SSI payments must not have more than $2,000 in total assets.

In addition to SSI, people with disabilities may qualify for Social Security Disability Insurance (SSDI) for adult disabled children. This program, enacted in 1956, authorizes direct cash payments to disabled children 18 or older of retired, deceased, or disabled workers who are eligible for social security benefits. To be eligible for the SSDI program, parents or the adult child with a disability (described in law as "the workers") must have established a "work history" through paid premiums to the social security trust fund.

**Health Care.** Medicare and Medicaid are two federal-state programs providing health care for people with disabilities. Medicare, part of Title XVIII of the Social Security Act, is a national insurance program for individuals over the age of 65, as well as for eligible people with disabilities. To be eligible as a person with a disability, the individual must have been receiving social security benefits for at least two years. The two parts of Medicare are hospital insurance and supplementary medical insurance. The hospital insurance program pays for short-term hospitalization, related care in skilled nursing facilities, and, to a limited extent, home care. The supplementary medical insurance program covers physician services, outpatient services, ambulance services, some medical supplies, and medical equipment.

Medicaid was established in 1965 as a federal grant-in-aid program that pays for health-care services of people receiving SSI *cash payments* as well as those in low-income families unable to pay for medical needs. Eligibility criteria for Medicaid varies from state to state, but most often requires that the individual is currently receiving SSI. Medicaid is a federal-state partnership in which states choosing to participate must provide matching funds to the federal dollars based on state per capita income. The federal government currently contributes approximately 50 to 80 percent of the total cost for Medicaid services on a state-by-state basis. Medicaid is administered through the Health Care Financing Administration in the Department of Health and Human Services.

The Medicaid program pays for inpatient and outpatient hospital services, laboratory services, physician services, family planning, skilled nursing services, and early screening, diagnosis, treatment, and immunization for children. Because the states design their own plans for Medicaid within federal regulations, other services may also be provided depending on the individual state. For example, some states support dental work, eyeglasses, drugs, and allied services such as physical therapy and private nursing.

## Institutional Living

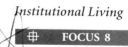

FOCUS 8

*What is an institution? Why are services for people with disabilities moving away from the institutional model?*

Throughout the twentieth century, adult services have been based on two predominant philosophies: People with disabilities should be isolated and protected from society versus people with disabilities should be included in the life of the family and community. One of the most predominant means of socially isolating people with disabilities is the large congregate care facility (institution). Institutions for people with disabilities are defined as large congregate living settings where (a) all aspects of life go on in the same place and under the same single authority; (b) activities are carried on in the immediate company of others, all of whom are treated alike and required to do the same thing together; (c) a system of explicit formal rulings and a body of officials govern tightly scheduled activities; (d) social mobility is grossly restricted; (e) work is defined as treatment, punishment, or rehabilitation; and (f) a system of rewards and punishments takes in the individual's total life situation (Goffman, 1975). Institutionalization of people with disabilities was widespread over the first half of the twentieth century, reaching peak levels in the 1970s. Scheerenberger (1976) reported a 74 percent increase in the number of institutions for persons with mental retardation over the ten-year period between 1964 and 1974. For most of the twentieth century, families with a disabled member have faced the dilemma of putting their son or daughter in an institution or keeping the individual at home with no medical, social, or educational services.

In the United States, the movement away from the institutional model came about for two reasons. First, many institutions had become dehumanizing warehouses with no adequate treatment programs and little effort to return people to their local communities (Balla, 1976; *Homeward Bound* v. *Hissom Memorial Center*, 1988; *Staff report*, 1985; *Wyatt* v. *Stickney*, 1972; Zigler, 1973). Professionals and parents alike questioned the basic assumptions that were driving institutional living. Evidence was emerging that people with disabilities could learn and apply skills such as employment and personal management if taught in less restrictive community and family environments (McDonnell et al., 1995). Second, a national mandate to educate children with disabilities in the public schools was passed in 1975. Public Law 94-142 (now IDEA) created a community-based alternative to institutionalization that focused on preparing the person with a disability to be a contributor rather than consumer of societal resources.

Today, institutions are widely viewed as a detriment to intellectual, psychological, and physical development. Menolascino, McGee, and Casey (1982) suggested that research data supports the following conclusions:

> (1) Prolonged institutionalization has destructive developmental consequences; (2) appropriate community-based residential settings are generally more beneficial than institutional placements . . . ; and (3) mentally retarded individuals with a wide spectrum of disabilities including the severely and profoundly retarded can be successfully served in community-based settings. (p. 65)

The number of people with disabilities living in institutional settings is declining significantly as we move toward the twenty-first century. Braddock et al. (1994) reported that since 1977, people living in state-operated institutions have been reduced by one-half, falling from 149,681 to 77,712. These authors further reported that 94 institutions are scheduled for, or have completed, closure in 20 states.

Although institutionalization is on the decline, the legal and moral debate continues regarding what is a good or bad institution or whether there is a need for any large residential facilities. Neither parents nor professionals have agreed on criteria for determining whether any institution is an appropriate living and learning environment for any person with a disability. What can be said, however, is that the accomplishments of institutions in the past ninety years add up to very little. Nisbet, Clark, and Covert (1991), summarizing the research on institutionalization, suggested that people who have lived in large institutional environments "do better in smaller ones when there is sufficient attention paid to their individual characteristics" (p. 115). Lakin and Bruininks (1985) indicated that "Once virtually the only model of extrafamilial care of [disabled] persons, [these facilities] are both aberrant social settings and have debilitating effects that increase the probability of segregated living" (p. 12).

Considerable debate surrounds the issue of how big a program has to be to be defined as an institution. Taylor, Biklen, and Knoll (1987) use the term *transinstitutionalization* to describe large congregate programs, such as nursing homes, which, although smaller than most public institutions, do not meet the criteria of a community-based supported living program (discussed later in this chapter). As suggested by Taylor et al., nursing homes can also be considered institutions, providing long-term medical support and personal care to individuals with more severe and profound disabilities.

Much of the funding for nursing homes and other large congregate programs comes through the Intermediate Care Facility/Mental Retardation (ICF/MR) program under Title XIX of the Social Security Act. Its purpose is to fund residential living and other services to people identified as mentally retarded and needing 24-hour care. In order to receive reimbursements under the program, the legislation requires states to provide "active treatment" that includes an individual written plan of care, interdisciplinary evaluations, and an annual review. The legislation also allows state-funded institutions for people with mental retardation to receive reimbursements as ICF/MRs. Thus the government has created a strong incentive within the states for continuation and expansion of institutional programs. Braddock and Fujiura (1988) reported that 87 percent of the funds budgeted under the ICF/MR program in 1986 were "associated with congregate care settings with capacities of 16 beds or larger. 75 percent of these funds supported care in large, state-operated institutions" (p. 262).

This strong incentive toward large congregate care living, including institutionalization, was contrary to the move toward more normalized, independent living for people with disabilities. Community service advocates argued that there was a need to move Title XIX funds to community alternatives. In response, the Congress authorized waivers in 1981, permitting the states to include community-based home care and related services in their Medicaid plans as long as they could demonstrate that such services were less expensive than institutional care. Despite the waiver program, the debate regarding expenditures of Title XIX funds for community service alternatives continues. Several pieces of legislation have been introduced over the past ten years targeting a "reform" of Medicaid and the ICF/MR provisions. These legislative proposals have centered around the expansion of the "menus" of services under Medicaid and the creation of incentives for the states to spend their federal Title XIX dollars on community service alternatives rather than large congregate care living arrangements.

## Community-Based Services

### ⊞  FOCUS 9

*Identify the basic components of community-based services in the areas of competitive employment, supported residential living, and recreation-leisure.*

The foundation of community-based services is *individualization*. Community services should be based on the needs and wishes of the person with disabilities, and when appropriate, their families (Gerry & Mirsky, 1992). Adults with disabilities receiving community-based adult services are entitled to an individualized program plan (IPP) (also referred to as individualized habilitation plans or individualized work rehabilitation plans). The IPP works essentially the same way as an individualized education plan (IEP) in the public schools. A multidisciplinary team that includes the adult with disabilities, parents and/or other family members (when appropriate), and professionals is established through the appropriate social services agency. The team meets to assess individual needs and preferences, set annual goals and objectives, determine the supports necessary to meet goals and objectives successfully, and evaluate the effectiveness of the program. Most often, the IPP concentrates on the areas of employment, residential living, and recreation-leisure.

**Employment.** Many adults with disabilities are unemployed or underemployed despite efforts to improve job preparation and accessibility for these individuals (Harris & Associates, 1994; Valdes, Williamson, & Wagner, 1990). Sustained employment is important for persons with disabilities for many reasons. A job provides monetary rewards, supports an adult identity, creates social contacts, promotes integration with nondisabled peers, and helps contribute to society.

High unemployment rates for people with disabilities may be attributable to traditional employment models that have been oriented to either no training for the individual after exiting school or short-term services. The expectation has been that the individual will not need ongoing support while on the job. Underemployment is also related to an emphasis on sheltered or protected work settings where the individual is placed for training but does not earn significant wages. We have reason to be optimistic about employment opportunities for persons with disabilities as we move into the twenty-first century. The concept of competitive employment for persons with disabilities has changed dramatically in recent years (McDonnell et al., 1995). Competitive employment can be described in terms of three service alternatives: (1) employment with no support services, (2) employment with time-limited support services, and (3) employment with ongoing support services.

*Employment with No Support Services*
Like most adults, people with disabilities may be able to locate and maintain a community job with no additional supports from public or private agencies. The person may locate employment either through contacts made during high school employment preparation programs or through such sources as employment agencies, want ads, and friends or family connections. For some people with a disability, community employment without support is possible if adequate vocational training and job experience are available during the school years.

*Employment with Time-Limited Training and Support Services*
An adult with a disability may be eligible for services through vocational rehabilitation. Under the Vocational Rehabilitation Act of 1973 (amended under P. L. 102–569 in 1992), federal funds are passed through to the states to provide services in counseling and job placement. To qualify for vocational rehabilitation, the individual must have an employment-related disability. The expectation is that the person will be independently employed following rehabilitation training. After the individual completes the training, rehabilitation services terminate, unless the individual fails on the job and has to be retrained.

Vocational rehabilitation has been historically viewed as a good investment, backed up by cost-benefit studies that indicate a positive ratio between the government costs and wages of former clients. However, more recently, the efficacy of rehabilitation services has been called into question (Government Accounting Office [GAO], 1993). The issues raised regarding services provided under the act are concerned with whether vocational rehabilitation "is able to serve all those who are eligible and desire services, whether the services provided are sufficient in scope and suitably targeted to meet the needs of a diverse client, and whether the program's effects persist over the long term" (GAO, 1993, p. 11). A relatively new government-funded program that responds directly to these concerns is called supported employment.

*Employment with Ongoing Supports: The Supported Employment Model*
Supported employment is defined as work in an integrated community setting for individuals with disabilities who require some type of ongoing support and for whom competitive employment has traditionally not been possible. Federally funded supported employment placements must meet the following criteria: (a) the job must provide between 20 and 40 hours of work weekly and be consistent with the individual's stamina; (b) the individual must earn a wage either at or above minimum wage, or a wage commensurate with production level and based on the prevailing wage rate for the job; (c) fringe benefits should be similar to those provided for nondisabled workers performing the same type of work; (d) employment must be community-based and provide the individual with regular opportunities for integration with nondisabled workers or with the public as a regular part of working; work should take place in settings where no more than eight persons with disabilities work together (the 1986 Amendments to the Vocational Rehabilitation Act; the Developmental Disabilities Act of 1984).

Over the past decade, the federal government has established programs funding states to initiate supported employment services through cooperative interagency services (education, vocational rehabilitation, developmental disabilities). Every state receives either matched federal funds or is provided stand-alone state dollars for supported employment services. In a relatively short time, supported employment has become a viable alternative for training and employment of individuals with disabilities.

Bellamy and Horner (1987) highlighted four critical features of supported employment. First, remuneration for the individual is a program goal. Wages are a primary index of employment success. Second, work should take place in socially integrated settings rather than segregated facilities. Job placement in an integrated setting allows the individual to learn appropriate social and vocational skills side by side with nondisabled peers and apply the skills in the environment. The nondisabled employer and co-workers also learn about the potential of the disabled individual as a reliable employee and friend. Third, support on the job is continuous, based on individual need, and is not time limited. Time-limited services like traditional vocational rehabilitation or vocational education have been restricted to individuals with disabilities who are supposed to need no support after reception of services. These time-limited services, then, terminate after the individual enters the work force. Unlike time-limited services, continuous services are made available as needed. Support does not end with placement in an employment setting or after a specified time for follow-up. Services are provided on the job and consist of whatever support is necessary to maintain employment. Continuous supports include job development, job placement, ongoing postemployment training, skill maintenance and generalization, and follow-up services. The amount and type of continuous support are related to individual need, job demand, and the organizational structure of the supported employment program (Rusch et al., 1992). Fourth, supported employment is for people with disabilities who have not usually been served in vocational programs. "There is . . . the clear possibility that supported employment may become the nation's first zero-reject employment program" (Bellamy & Horner, 1987, p. 498). Historically, adult services for people with more severe disabilities could only be described as prevocational or nonvocational with a focus on "getting people ready" or lifelong custodial care. As indicated by Bellamy et al. (1988), however, traditional models of preparing people for work in sheltered settings have not been effective.

*Supported Residential Living.* Today, most people with disabilities, along with their families and professionals, are advocating for the expansion of small supported living programs located in residential neighborhoods and staffed by highly trained personnel. In a supported living program, the adult with disabilities has access to existing services in the community for education, work, health care, and recreation. Other alternatives might also be appropriate, such as living with a local family, foster care, or adoption. Braddock et al. (1994) define supported living as "housing in which individuals with disabilities choose where and with whom they live, housing which is owned by someone other than the support provider (i.e., by the individual, the family, a landlord, or a housing cooperative), and housing in which the individual has a personalized support plan which changes as her or his needs and abilities change" (p. 26).

Several classifications of residential programs have been developed over the years (Baker, Seltzer, & Seltzer, 1977; Campbell & Bailey, 1984; McDonnell, Wilcox, & Hardman, 1991; Nisbet, Clark, & Covert, 1991; Schalock, 1986). We discuss three of the most widely used residential models: group homes, semi-independent homes and apartments, and foster family care.

### Group Homes

There are both large and small group home models. In a small group home, there are usually two to four persons living in a single dwelling. Large group homes may have as many as eight to fifteen or more residents. Both large and small homes emphasize programs that provide daily living experiences as similar as possible to those of nondisabled individuals. Group homes are funded through a combination of state and federal funding, supplemented by fees paid by the residents and/or their families.

### Semi-Independent Homes and Apartments

There are several variations on the semi-independent home or apartment:

1. *Apartment clusters.* Comprised of several apartments fairly close together. They function to some extent as a unit and are supervised by a resident staff member who lives in one of the apartment units.

2. *Single coresidence home or apartment.* Single home or apartment in which an adult staff member shares the dwelling with a roommate(s) who is disabled.

3. *Single home or apartment.* A home or apartment owned and/or occupied by an adult with disabilities whom a nonresident staff member(s) assists. This is the most independent kind of living arrangement in the model.

In a semi-independent setting, most residents are responsible for, or contribute to, apartment maintenance, meal preparation, and transportation to place of employment.

*Foster Family Care*

Foster family care provides a surrogate family for the adult with disabilities. It integrates the individual into the family setting as a means for the person with a disability to learn adaptive skills and be able to work in the local community. People who operate the foster homes generally receive a per capita fee from the state and accommodate from one to six adults.

**Recreation and Leisure.** Recreation and leisure-time opportunities for adults with disabilities vary substantially from community to community according to the person's age and the severity of the disability. Many adults with disabilities and their families find it difficult to access activities that would be considered a normal part of a nondisabled adult's life. Access may be limited in such activities as swimming, movies, hiking, and restaurants for several reasons. There may be physical barriers to participation, such as stairs that are difficult to access or doors that are too narrow to accommodate a wheelchair. Other barriers may be linked more to personal issues; no one is available or willing to go with the person to the activity. The individual has no friends. The result is that many adults may do little with their leisure time beyond watching television.

Too often people with disabilities lead inactive lives, although meaningful recreation and leisure experience should be an integral part of their community experience (Fain, 1986). Shannon (1985) found that many adults with retardation spend significant amounts of time alone at home. Typical activities include watching television, listening to music, and looking at books and magazines. A longitudinal study of adults with disabilities found that the time spent alone by these individuals may be decreasing. In a follow-up investigation of young adults with disabilities between the ages of 19 and 22, Valdes, Williamson, and Wagner (1990) found that about 75 percent of these individuals got together with friends at least once a week. Approximately 21 percent of the respondents were with friends more than five times a week.

Peck, Appoloni, and Cooke (1981) believe that successful training in leisure time could come about through the incorporation of systematic assessment, highly structured training procedures, and rigorous evaluation components.

Adults with disabilities are entitled to the pleasures of well-planned recreational activities that are consistent with their individual needs and preferences. Efforts in this direction by local community organizations, places of worship, schools, and family can help make life more meaningful for these adults. One example of an organized recreation program for adults with mental retardation is Special Olympics (a competitive sports program). Other community programs may include local skiing, hiking, or camping programs for adults with and without disabilities. These programs promote the participation of adults with disabilities by adapting to individual needs. Therapeutic recreation is a profession concerned specifically with this goal: using recreation to help people adapt their physical, emotional, or social characteristics to take advantage of leisure-time activities more independently in a community setting.

## BUILDING A FAMILY SUPPORT NETWORK DURING THE ADULT YEARS

Beyond formal government programs, an informal system of natural supports for adults with disabilities is provided by extended family members, friends, and neighbors. Through this network many families find a personal bonding with others who will listen, understand, and support them. Extended family members may be grandparents, aunts, uncles, or cousins who may or may not live in the same household but have ongoing contact with members of the nuclear family. In this section, we examine support networks in the context of perpetual parenthood and sibling roles during the adult years.

### Perpetual Parenthood and the Need for Both Formal and Natural Family Supports

⊞    **FOCUS 10**

*Identify the supports needed for parents who choose to keep their son or daughter with a disability at home during the adult years.*

Much of our discussion in this chapter has emphasized the need for formal government supports to help facilitate the adult with disabilities moving away from the primary family and becoming more independent. In some cases, adults with disabilities never move away from their primary family. Parents assume the major responsibilities of caregiving for a lifetime (see Point of Interest 10.2). In a study of forty-three adults with disabilities, Heller and Factor (1993) found that 63 percent of the persons interviewed indicated that they wanted to remain in the family home. Respondents suggested two reasons for not wanting to leave the primary family: fear of the alternatives and a desire to be near parents. In fact, 85 percent of adults with mental retardation live under the supervision of their parents for most of their lives (Seltzer & Krauss, 1994).

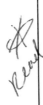

♦ **POINT OF INTEREST 10.2**

## *The Rain Man's Dad*

ACADEMY AWARD-WINNING SCREENWRITER Barry Morrow has christened him "Saint Francis—the unsung hero of a wonderful odyssey."

Murray, Utah resident Fran Peek, however, considers himself a regular guy who does what any father would do for his son.

Yeah, right. Maybe in the movies.

But in reality, how many fathers would devote their lives to caring for a 44-year-old son who can mesmerize audiences with his computerlike intellect, but who also requires the 24-hour-a-day nurturing of a mentally disabled child?

Friends say Fran Peek is one of a kind, quite possibly as unique as his son, Kim Peek—the savant who was an inspiration for the Academy Award-winning motion picture *Rain Man*.

Kim Peek was born in Salt Lake City on Nov. 11, 1951. From the beginning, his parents knew he was "different." A soft, baseball-size blister stretched across the back of his head, which was 30 percent larger than normal. At age 3, the blister retracted, destroying half of his cerebellum.

Doctors pronounced Kim mentally disabled and recommended that he be placed in an institution. The Peeks took him home and, over the years, watched their so-called retarded son display remarkable abilities.

Because of neurodevelopmental brain damage, Kim's motor skills are deficient. He has trouble doing such simple tasks as putting his shoes on the right feet. But his brain functions like a calculator/computer. He instantly absorbs and then retrieves virtually everything he reads.

On a recent afternoon in the front room of the condominium he shares with his father, Kim announced himself as "Rain Man" in a deep throaty groan. He went on to share "remember when" stories that exemplify his dad's compassion.

"[Dad] is a loving man," said Kim.

"I will give him a special love on Father's Day. He means a lot to me. He is a loving man," Kim repeated, before getting up to move to another chair in the room—to be alone, remove his specs and squint at the pages of the book he held close to his nose. Emitting a groan or low whistle now and then as he read, he listened to his father reminisce about their journey together—an exploration chronicled in *The Real Rain Man*, a book Fran recently wrote about his son and constant companion.

Fran, a former advertising executive and educator, became the day-to-day caregiver and "biggest fan" of his 200-pound son in 1979 when Fran and his wife separated, and ultimately divorced. Still a withdrawn, gentle child, Kim was sheltered, fiercely protected from outsiders. Even when traveling with Fran, "he opted to remain camouflaged in the background."

Then came *Rain Man* and Dustin Hoffman, who played the savant inspired in part by Kim in the movie. Kim and his father were thrust into the international spotlight. Their lives changed forever.

They became the "who's who" of the national speaking circuit. Everyone wanted to meet Kim—the living computer and perpetual calendar.

*continued*

◆ **POINT OF INTEREST 10.2** (*continued*)

From the beginning, Fran refused to take money for their appearances—only reimbursements for their travel expenses. Still, he has been accused by some, including members of his own family, of exploiting his son.

Fran calls it "sharing him."

"I couldn't put him back into an overprotective sheltered environment; he has too much to offer. I decided a long time ago that traveling would be our social life. But more than that, it has been a growing experience," he said. "We give hope to parents who have children born with brain problems and other kinds of disorders. Plus, it gives me a chance to talk one-on-one with them—and hopefully encourage them to give their children a chance to fail as well as succeed."

Fran's description of an average day:

- 5:15 A.M.—Father and son awaken. (Actually Kim goes into Fran's room and says, "Dad, aren't you up yet?") Fran goes downstairs to prepare the lunch Kim will take to work. Kim works on his "journal." Using telephone books, he matches the surnames of people with similar names who live in similar size cities and who have the same last four telephone digits. Fran doesn't know why he does it; Kim doesn't want to explain.

- 6:05–6:50 A.M.—They read the *Salt Lake Tribune*. Kim starts with the obituary section, "looking for names and addresses he has memorized," and goes on from there.

- 6:50 A.M.—Back upstairs. Fran helps Kim use the electric razor, shower and select the clothes he'll wear to work or wherever they are going that day. Kim relearns how to brush his teeth.

  Fran showers, dresses. Back downstairs. He fixes breakfast.

- 7:50 A.M.—They eat. Fran does the dishes. Back upstairs. He puts Kim's shoes in the proper position. Kim puts them on. Together they recomb Kim's hair and tuck in his shirt.

- 8:15 A.M.—Fran drives Kim to the Columbus Community Center, Salt Lake City. Fran returns home and corresponds with people who have invited them to speak and those to whom they have spoken.

- 3:00 P.M.—Fran picks up Kim at Columbus and takes him to the Salt Lake City Library. Kim studies more telephone and data books for his journal. Fran drives home to Murray.

- 5:45 P.M.—Fran picks up Kim. Both return home. Fran fixes dinner. Kim refreshes Dad's memory on tomorrow's schedule.

"As a father, my most important role is just being there when he has problems. When he is sad, I need to be there to comfort him," said Fran, whose vocabulary doesn't contain the word "sacrifice."

"He gave me a responsibility which is full time. I really had no choice," he continued. "I didn't weigh whether I was going to go out and get married again. I know I couldn't give a woman the attention she would deserve."

Fran Peek is too busy to wallow in self-pity. A sequel to *Rain Man* must be finished. If only he had a block of time. Alone. To write.

"Maybe from midnight to 3 A.M.," he pondered.

*Source:* The Salt Lake Tribune by JoAnn Jacobsen-Wells (1996).

Smith, Majeski, and McClenny (1996) characterize this situation as "perpetual parenthood" (p. 172). Perpetual parenthood is the result of an offspring's continuing dependency through the adult years either because there is a lack of formal resources for the family or the family simply chooses to keep the individual at home. This not to say that parents who choose to keep their adult offspring at home aren't in need of adult services. On the contrary, although they may choose not to access housing for their son or daughter, employment and recreation services will be needed as well as additional supports in the areas of respite care, in-home assistance, and counseling/training services. These services may be provided through formal and/or informal support networks.

***Respite Care and In-Home Assistance.*** Respite care and in-home assistance provide some additional relief and help for parents attempting to cope with the challenges of an adult with disabilities living in the home. In-home respite care may involve a paid companion spending some time with the adult who is disabled. Out-of-home respite care may be provided by families who are licensed to take adults with disabilities into their home for a limited period of time, or parent cooperatives, day-care centers, and community recreational services (Levy & Levy, 1986). Nisbet, Clark, and Covert (1991) suggest that respite care services may "enable family members to become more socially active and in turn reduce their feelings of social isolation" (p. 135). Examples of in-home assistance is help from a professional homemaker to reduce the family's time in dealing with household management tasks or a personal attendant to help with daily routines when the person has physical or cognitive limitations.

Extended family members are also sources of respite care and in-home assistance. These family members may periodically help prepare meals, clean the house, provide transportation, or just listen when everyone is overwhelmed. Hardman et al. (1996) suggest that grandparents and other extended family members are a critical resource for helping parents who choose to keep an adult family member at home. However, their effectiveness as a resource depends on their willingness to help, as well as how prepared and informed they are about how the family functions and the needs of the adult family member. These extended family members must be able to openly voice their questions, feelings, and concerns about the adult with disabilities living at home, including the emotional impact he or she is having on other family members. In turn, parents must be willing to share their own feelings to help extended family members learn as much as possible.

Many of the issues regarding whether or not extended family members are in a position to serve as a support network also apply to friends and neighbors. However, parents of an adult who is disabled may be less likely to reach out to friends and neighbors than to extended family members for several reasons. They may want to keep the family's personal business private or not burden a friend with their problems. They may fear rejection from friends or neighbors who don't understand their emotional needs and concerns. Nevertheless, it is possible for friends and neighbors to be part of a natural support network for the family. The nature and type of support is unique to the individuals involved and depends on a mutual level of comfort in both seeking and providing assistance. Clear communication regarding what friends or neighbors are willing to do and how that matches with what the family needs is essential if this support is to be meaningful.

*Counseling and Training.* In addition to respite care and in-home assistance, families may also receive counseling services and training to help them cope with the daily stress of caring for an adult member with disabilities. Counseling services and family training programs are most effective when they focus on the relationships and interactions between and among the members, and not just on the adult with disabilities. Such an approach, referred to as a "family systems perspective," is based on the premise that "all parts of the family are interrelated; furthermore, each family has unique properties, understood only through careful observation of the relationships and interactions among all members" (Turnbull & Morningstar, 1993, p. 22). (See Chapter 2 for an in-depth discussion on family systems.)

One relatively new and unique approach to counseling and training is psychoeducational support groups that are intended to assist parents whose adult child remains fully or partially dependent on the family for a lifetime (Smith, 1995). These groups provide an opportunity for older and aging parents to share their needs and concerns with others in similar circumstances regarding such issues as "making plans for when they can no longer care for their offspring due to their own disability or death" (Smith et al., 1996, p. 173). Psychoeducational support groups, facilitated by professionals knowledgeable in the areas of disability and the family, generally have five major goals: "(a) inform parents about the residential, financial, and legal aspects of [futures] planning, (b) promote acceptance of the relinquishment of care to others; (c) foster coping skills to deal with the impact of age-related changes on caregiving; (d) encourage knowledge and use of both formal and informal supports; and (e) instill solidarity among participants" (Smith et al., 1996, p. 173). Research on the effectiveness of this approach is extremely limited. However, in an initial case study on the impact of such groups on older parents of adults with disabilities, Smith et al. found that both the parents and the professionals involved saw the group as a worthwhile endeavor that was valuable for both future planning and the opportunity to be with other parents facing comparable challenges.

## Sibling Roles

**FOCUS 11**

*What roles do siblings play in the life of the adult family member with disabilities?*

Although some attention has been paid to the role of parents during the adult years, little has been written about siblings. What we do know suggests sibling concerns relative to their brother or sister with a disability change substantially from childhood to the adult years. During childhood, siblings focus on such questions as "Why did this happen to my family?" "What will I say to my friends?" "Is the disability inherited?" "Is it contagious?" "Can my friends catch it?" "Will my children get it too?" During adulthood, sibling concerns center more on "Who is going to take care of my brother or sister?" "When my parents die, who will be responsible?" "Am I going to have to take care of my brother or sister all of my life?"

A study by Griffith and Unger (1994) suggested that a majority of siblings believe that families should be responsible for the care of their disabled members. Most indicated that they were "willing to assume future caregiving responsibilities for their brothers/sisters" (p. 225). In a longitudinal study of 140 families who had adults with mental retardation still living at home, Krauss and colleagues (1996) found that many siblings remained very actively involved with their brother or sister well into the adult years. These siblings had frequent contact with their brother or sister and were knowledgeable about their lives. In addition, they played a major role in their parents' support network. Interestingly, about one in three of these siblings indicated that they planned to reside with their brother or sister at some point during adult life.

The reality is that sibling roles vary considerably depending on the attitudes and values of their parents, their own attitudes about responsibility, and proximity to their brother or sister (Hardman et al., 1996; McHale, Sloan, & Simeonsson, 1986). There are siblings who develop negative feelings very early in childhood and carry these feelings through to adult life. These siblings grew up resenting the time and attention parents gave to their disabled brother or sister, eventually becoming bitter and emotionally neglected adults. Such negative feelings often result in guilt that further isolates the individual from the primary family. Adult siblings, resentful of their brother or sister, may actively disengage themselves from parents and the disabled family member for long periods of time (Forbes, 1987; Seligman, 1991).

In contrast, some siblings play a crucial role during adult life, providing ongoing support to parents and spending time with their brother or sister who is disabled. In a seminal study of siblings of individuals with mental retardation, Grossman (1972) found that it was usually one sibling within the family who developed a strong bond with the family member. This sibling, often older than the disabled brother or sister, generally had a positive relationship during childhood that continued into the adult years. McHale et al. (1986) found that siblings who develop a positive relationship with a brother or sister who is disabled can play important roles in fostering learning and social development through the lifespan.

# REVIEW

*FOCUS 1: What are the basic issues in determining whether or not an adult is mentally competent?*

- Capacity to make rational and reasoned decisions consistently that are in his or her best interests and those of others that the individual has direct contact with (total competence).

- Capacity to make some rational decisions at varying levels of complexity (partial competence).

- Inability to make any reasoned decisions on their behalf (total incompetence).

*FOCUS 2: Identify the three elements of consent.*

- Capacity: The ability to acquire and retain knowledge, evaluate the information received, and make a choice based on the evaluation.

- Information: The ability to communicate effectively in both substance and manner. There is a clear obligation on the part of the person communicating to ensure that the information is understood.

- Voluntariness: A person's ability to exercise free power of choice without the intervention of force, fraud, deceit, or duress.

*FOCUS 3: Describe the three types of consent.*

- Direct consent is obtained directly from the person who is involved or affected by an action.

- Substitute consent (sometimes referred to as third party consent) is given by someone other than the person who is involved or directly affected by an action.

- Concurrent consent is a combination of both direct and substitute consent.

*FOCUS 4: What is guardianship? Distinguish between full, limited, and temporary guardianship.*

- Guardianship, a legal term, gives power to one individual to direct or control the life of another person. This power comes through the courts when it is determined that an individual is not capable of handling his or her personal life, including not being able to give consent.

- *Full guardianship* involves one person's full control over the decisions made in another person's life.
- *Limited guardianship* allows an individual to keep some control over life decisions while giving another person authority in some areas consistent with the needs of the individual.
- *Temporary guardianship* is applicable under special circumstances (such as physical incapacitation) and within a limited time frame.

*FOCUS 5: What is the purpose of the Americans with Disabilities Act (ADA)? Identify its basic provisions.*

- To protect people with disabilities from discrimination.
- To ensure that people with disabilities receive fair treatment as they seek employment, access to public services, public accommodations, transportation, and telecommunications.

*FOCUS 6: Distinguish between entitlement and eligibility programs for adults with disabilities.*

- Entitlement program: All individuals who meet the eligibility requirements *must* be provided the service.
- Eligibility program: An individual may meet the eligibility requirements for a service, but he or she may not be able to receive it because there aren't enough funds to serve all eligible people.

*FOCUS 7: What are the components of federal income support and health-care programs for adults with disabilities?*

- Income maintenance programs provide basic economic support for people with disabilities. SSI pays direct cash payments to eligible disabled children and adults as well as low-income elderly people.
- Federal health-care programs include Medicare and Medicaid. Medicare includes hospital insurance and supplementary medical insurance. The hospital insurance program pays for short-term hospitalization, related care in skilled nursing facilities, and home care to a limited extent. The supplementary medical insurance program covers physician services, outpatient services, ambulance services, some medical supplies, and medical equipment. Medicaid is a federal grant-in-aid program that pays for health-care services of people receiving SSI cash payments, as well as those in low-income families unable to pay for medical needs. Medicaid is a federal-state partnership program in which states choosing to participate must provide matching funds to the federal dollars based on state per capita income. It pays for inpatient and outpatient hospital services, laboratory services, physician ser-

vices, family planning, skilled nursing services, and early screening, diagnosis, treatment, and immunization for children.

FOCUS 8:  *What is an institution? Why are services for people with disabilities moving away from the institutional model?*

- An institution is a large congregate living setting in which (1) all aspects of life go on in the same place and under the same single authority; (2) activities are carried on in the immediate company of others, all of whom are treated alike and required to do the same thing together; (3) a system of explicit formal rulings and a body of officials govern tightly scheduled activities; (4) social mobility is grossly restricted; (5) work is defined as treatment, punishment, or rehabilitation; and (6) a system of rewards and punishments takes in the individual's total life situation.

- Many institutions had become dehumanizing warehouses with no adequate treatment programs and little effort to return people to their local communities. Evidence was emerging that people with disabilities could learn and apply skills such as employment and personal management if taught in less restrictive community and family environments.

- A national mandate to educate children with disabilities in the public schools was passed in 1975. Public Law 94–142 (now IDEA) created a community-based alternative to institutionalization that focused on preparing the person with a disability to be a contributor rather than consumer of societal resources.

FOCUS 9:  *Identify the basic components of community-based services in the areas of competitive employment, supported residential living, and recreation-leisure.*

- Competitive employment can be described in terms of three service alternatives: (1) employment with no support services, (2) employment with time-limited support services, and (3) employment with on-going support services. Time-limited services involves the expectation that the person will be independently employed following rehabilitation training. After the individual completes the training, the services terminate, unless the individual fails on the job and has to be retrained. Ongoing support services (supported employment) is defined as work in an integrated community setting for individuals with disabilities who require some type of continuous support, and for whom competitive employment has traditionally not been possible.

- Supported residential living programs include group homes, semi-independent homes and apartments, and foster care. There are both large and small group home models. In a small group home, usually two to four persons live in a single dwelling. Large group homes may have as many as eight to fifteen or more residents. There are three types of semi-independent homes and apartments: (1) apartment clusters (several apartments fairly close together supervised by a resident staff member), (2) single coresidence home or apartment (an adult staff member shares the dwelling with a roommate(s) who is disabled), and (3) single home or apartment (owned and/or occupied by an adult with disabilities whom a nonresident staff member(s) assists).

- Recreation and leisure programs, consistent with individual needs and preferences, include opportunities to participate in the same activities as nondisabled adults (such as going to restaurants and theaters, skiing, camping, hiking, etc.).

*FOCUS 10: Identify the supports needed for parents who choose to keep their son or daughter with a disability at home during the adult years.*

- Respite care and in-home assistance provide some additional relief and help for parents attempting to cope with the challenges of an adult with disabilities living in the home. In-home respite care may involve a paid companion and/or extended family members spending some time with the adult who is disabled. Out-of-home respite care may be provided by families who are licensed to take adults with disabilities into their home for a limited period of time, or parent cooperatives, day-care centers, and community recreational services. Examples of in-home assistance is help from a professional homemaker or extended family members to reduce the family's time in dealing with household management tasks, or a personal attendant to help with daily routines when the person has physical or cognitive limitations.

- Families may receive counseling services and training to help them cope with the daily stress of caring for an adult member with disabilities. Counseling services and family training programs are most effective when they focus on the relationships and interactions between and among the members, and not just on the adult with disabilities.

*FOCUS 11: What roles do siblings play in the life of the adult family member with disabilities?*

- During the adult years, sibling roles vary considerably depending on the attitudes and values of their parents, their own attitudes about responsibility, and proximity to their brother or sister.

- Some adult siblings, resentful of their brother or sister, may actively disengage themselves from parents and the disabled family member for long periods of time.

- Many siblings play a crucial role during adult life, providing ongoing support to parents, spending time with their brother or sister who is disabled, and becoming directly involved in future planning.

## REFERENCES

Baker, B. L., Seltzer, G. B., & Seltzer, M. M. (1977). *As close as possible: Community residences for retarded adults.* Boston: Little, Brown.

Balla, D. (1976). Relationship of institution size to quality of care: A review of the literature. *American Journal of Mental Deficiency, 81,* 117–124.

Bellamy, G. T., & Horner, R. H. (1987). Beyond high school: Residential and employment options after graduation. In M. E. Snell (Ed.), *Systematic instruction of persons with severe handicaps* (3rd ed.) (pp. 491–510). Columbus: Merrill.

Bellamy, G. T., Rhodes, L., Mank, D. & Albin, J. (1988). *Supported employment and community implementation guide.* Baltimore: Brookes.

Braddock, D., & Fujiura, G. (1988). Federal foundations for transitions to adulthood. In B. L. Ludlow, A. P. Turnbull, & R. Luckasson (Eds.), *Transitions to adult life for people with mental retardation—principles and practices* (pp. 257–274). Baltimore: Brookes.

Braddock, D., Hemp, R., Bachelder, L., & Fujiura, G. (1994). *The state of the states in developmental disabilities.* Chicago: University of Illinois Institute on Disability and Human Development.

Campbell, V. A., & Bailey, C. J. (1984). Comparison of methods for classifying community residential settings for mentally retarded individuals. *American Journal of Mental Deficiency, 89,* 44–49.

Davis, S., & Berkobien, R. (1994, August). *Meeting the needs and challenges of at-risk, two generation, elderly families.* Arlington, TX: The ARC—A National Organization on Mental Retardation.

Drew, C. J., Hardman, M. L., & Hart, A. (1996). *Designing and conducting research: Inquiry in education and social science.* Boston: Allyn & Bacon.

Drew, C. J., Hardman, M. L., & Logan, D. R. (1996). *Mental retardation: A life cycle approach.* Englewood Cliffs, NJ: Merrill.

Fain, G. S. (1986). Leisure: A moral imperative. *Mental Retardation, 24*(5), 261–283.

Forbes, E. (1987). My brother, Warren. *Exceptional Parent,* 50–52.

Gerry, M. H., & Mirsky, A. J. (1992). Guiding principles for public policy on natural supports. In J. Nisbet (Ed.), *Natural supports in school, at work, and in the community for people with severe disabilities* (pp. 341–346). Baltimore: Brookes.

Goffman, E. (1975). Characteristics of total institutions. In S. Dinitz, R. R. Dynes, & A. C. Clarke (Eds.), *Deviance: Studies in definition, management, and treatment* (p. 410). New York: Oxford University Press.

Government Accounting Office (GAO). (1993, August). *Vocational rehabilitation: Evidence of federal program's effectiveness is mixed.* Washington, DC: Author.

Griffiths, D. L., & Unger, D. G. (1994, April). Views about planning for the future among parents and siblings of adults with mental retardation. *Family Relations, 43,* 221–227.

Grossman, F. K. (1972). Brothers and sisters of retarded children. *Psychology Today,* 102–104.

Hardman, M. L., Drew, C. J., & Egan, M. W. (1996). *Human exceptionality* (5th ed.). Boston: Allyn & Bacon.

Harris, L., & Associates (1994). *National Organization on Disability/Harris Survey of Americans with Disabilities.* New York: Author.

Heller, T., & Factor, A. R. (1993). Support systems, well-being, and placement decision-making among older parents and their adult children with developmental disabilities. In E. Sutton, A. R. Factor, B. A. Hawkins, T. Heller, & G. B. Seltzer (Eds.), *Older adults with developmental disabilities* (pp. 107–122). Baltimore: Brookes

Jacobsen-Wells, J. (1996, June 16). Fatherhood at its peek. *Salt Lake Tribune*, pp. J-1, J-2.

Joseph P. Kennedy, Jr. Foundation (1993). *Opening doors for you.* Washington, DC: Author.

Krauss, M. W., Seltzer, M. M., Gordon, R., & Friedman, D. H. (1996, April). Binding ties: The roles of adult siblings of persons with mental retardation. *Mental Retardation, 34*(2), 83–93.

Lakin, K. C., & Bruininks, R. J. (1985). Contemporary services for handicapped children and youth. In R. H. Bruininks and K. C. Lakin (Eds.), *Living and learning in the least restrictive environment* (pp. 3–22). Baltimore: Brookes.

Levy, J. M., & Levy, P. H. (1986). Issues and models in the delivery of respite services. In C. L. Salisbury & J. Intagliata (Eds.), *Respite care: Support for persons with developmental disabilities and their families* (pp. 99–116). Baltimore: Brookes.

McDonnell, J. M., Hardman, M. L., McDonnell, A. P., & Kiefer-O'Donnell, R. (1995). *Introduction to people with severe disabilities: Educational and social issues.* Boston: Allyn & Bacon.

McDonnell, J., Wilcox, B., & Hardman, M. L. (1991). *Secondary programs for students with mental retardation.* Boston: Allyn & Bacon.

McHale, S. M., Sloan, J., & Simeonsson, R. J. (1986). Sibling relationships and adjustment of children with disabled brothers and sisters. *Journal of Children in Contemporary Society, 16,* 131–158.

Menolascino, F. J., McGee, J. J., & Casey, K. (1982). Affirmation of the rights of institutionalized retarded citizens (Implications of *Youngberg v. Romeo*). *TASH Journal, 8,* 63–71.

Nisbet, J., Clark, M., & Covert, S. (1991). Living it up! An analysis of research on community living. In L. H. Meyer, C. A. Peck, & L. Brown (Eds.), *Critical issues in the lives of people with severe disabilities* (pp. 115–144). Baltimore: Brookes.

Peck, C. A., Apolloni, T., & Cooke, T. P. (1981). Rehabilitation services for Americans with mental retardation: A summary of accomplishments in research and development. In E. L. Pan, T. E. Backer, & C. L. Vash (Eds.), *Annual Review of Rehabilitation* (Vol. 2). New York: Springer.

Rusch, F. R., Destefano, L., Chadsey-Rusch, J., Phelps, L. A., & Szymanski, E. (1992). *Transition from school to adult life: Models, linkages, and policy.* Sycamore, IL: Sycamore.

Schalock, R. (1986). *Transitions from school to work.* Washington, DC: National Association of Rehabilitation Facilities.

Scheerenberger, R. C. (1976). *Current trends and status of public residential services for the mentally retarded, 1974.* Madison, WI: National Association of Superintendents of Public Residential Facilities for the Mentally Retarded.

Seligman, M. (1991). Siblings of disabled brothers and sisters. In M. Seligman (Ed.), *The family with a handicapped child* (2nd ed.). Boston: Allyn & Bacon.

Seltzer, M. M., & Krauss, M. W. (1994). Aging parents with resident adult children: The impact of lifelong caregiving. In M. M. Seltzer, M. W. Krauss, & M. P. Janicki (Eds.), *Life course perspectives on adulthood and old age* (pp. 3–18). Washington, DC: The American Association on Mental Retardation.

Shannon, G. (1985). *Characteristics influencing current recreational patterns of persons with mental retardation.* Unpublished doctoral dissertation, Brandeis University, Waltham, MA.

Smith, G. C. (1995). Preventive approaches to building competencies. In G. C. Smith, S. S. Tobin, E. A. Robertson-Tchabo, & P. W. Power (Eds.), *Strengthening aging families: Diversity in practice and policy* (pp. 221–234). Newbury Park, CA: Sage.

Smith, G. C., Majeski, R. A., & McClenny, B. (1996). Psychoeducational support groups for aging parents: Development and preliminary outcomes. *Mental Retardation, 34*(3), 172–181.

*Staff report on the institutionalized mentally disabled.* (1985). Washington, DC: U.S. Senate Subcommittee on the Handicapped, Committee on Labor and Human Resources.

Taylor, S. J., Biklen, D., & Knoll, J. (1987). *Community integration for people with severe disabilities.* Baltimore: Brookes.

Turnbull, A. P., & Morningstar, M. E. (1993). Family and professional interaction. In M. E. Snell (Ed.), *Systematic instruction of persons with severe handicaps* (pp. 31–60). Columbus: Merrill.

Turnbull, H. R., III (Ed.). (1977). *Consent handbook.* Washington, DC: American Association on Mental Deficiency.

Turnbull, H. R., III, Turnbull, A. P., Bronicki, G. J., Summers, J. A., & Roeder-Gordon, C. (1989). *Disability and the family: A guide to decisions for adulthood.* Baltimore: Brookes.

Valdes, K. A., Williamson, C. L., & Wagner, M. M. (1990). *The National Longitudinal Transition Study of Special Education Students, Statistical Almanac: Vol. 5. Youth Categorized as Mentally Retarded.* Menlo Park, CA: SRI International.

Zigler, E. (1973). The retarded child as a whole person. In D. K. Routh (Ed.), *The experimental psychology of mental retardation.* Chicago: Aldine.

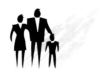

# Name Index

# Subject Index